The Side Effects Bible

The Side Effects Bible

THE DIETARY SOLUTION TO UNWANTED SIDE EFFECTS OF COMMON MEDICATIONS

FREDERIC VAGNINI, M.D.,

and

BARRY FOX, PH.D.

Broadway Books | New York

PRINTED IN THE UNITED STATES OF AMERICA

This book is not intended to take the place of medical advice from a trained medical professional. Readers are advised to consult a physician or other qualified health professional regarding treatment of their medical problems. Neither the publisher nor the author takes any responsibility for any possible consequences from any treatment, action, or application of medicine, herb, or preparation to any person reading or following the information in this book.

BROADWAY BOOKS and its logo, a letter B bisected on the diagonal, are trademarks of Random House, Inc.

Visit our Web site at www.broadwaybooks.com

First edition published 2005

Book design by Michael Collica

Library of Congress Cataloging-in-Publication Data

Vagnini, Frederic J.
The side effects bible : the dietary solution to unwanted side effects of common medications / Frederic Vagnini and Barry Fox.
p. cm.
Includes index.
1. Drugs—Side effects—Prevention. 2. Drugs—Side effects—Diet therapy. 3. Dietary supplements. I. Fox, Barry. II. Title.
RM302.5 V346 2005
615'.7042—dc22
2004054526

ISBN 0-7679-1883-5

1 3 5 7 9 10 8 6 4 2

CONTENTS

ACKNOWLEDGMENTS

I'd like to thank my wife Nadine, Greg Buie, and Ara DerMarderosian, Ph.D., Director of the Complementary and Alternative Medicine Institute at the University of the Sciences in Philadelphia, for their help in reviewing and correcting the manuscript.

B.F.

I would like to thank my coauthor, Barry Fox, who is the main person responsible for this important piece of work. I believe Barry is one of the foremost medical investigators and writers in the world and it has been a privilege to work with him. I would also like to thank my dedicated employees at the Heart, Diabetes, and Weight Loss Centers of New York, especially my nurses, Ms. Susan Hill and Ms. Carolyn Fredericks, who have established a world-class heart and blood vessel diagnostic center. My administrative staff, led by Ms. Mildred Napo and her associates, are also a mainstay to my busy centers. My nutrition and vitamin company has been directed by my very capable nephew Daniel Chaigis, and without him my nutritional center would not be possible. My special woman, Laurie, has stood by me during my many hours of long work on a number of different projects. I am especially thankful for my daughters, Grace Marie and Clare Ann, who are the most special people in my life and have enabled me to keep going and working and have been my inspiration.

F.V.

HOW TO USE THIS BOOK

Don't let the size of this book intimidate you; it's easy to use.

The first step is to get the generic name of your drug off the bottle/box/tube. Not the brand name, which is always capitalized and often sounds like it was invented by the pharmaceutical company's marketing department. Look for the generic name, which may be in lowercase and sounds like something a chemist would be comfortable saying.

Next, find that generic name in the index, which begins on page 552. (It's not a good idea to flip through the drug entries in Chapter 3 looking for the name of your drug. That might work, but many of the medications discussed are combined with others; it will be hard to find them because they'll be out of order in the otherwise alphabetical listing.)

Once you find your drug in the index, flip to the appropriate page, where you'll learn about the medication, some of its possible side effects, which nutrients it robs you of, additional ways it may upset your nutritional status, and what supplements and foods you can use to replenish your stores.

Then you can read about each of the nutrients robbed in Chapter 2. There, in individual listings for each nutrient, you'll learn what they do for you, the daily requirement, how safe the nutrient is, what side effects you may suffer if you get too much, and where to find it in foods. Each nutrient entry ends with a listing of drugs that rob you of that nutrient.

The final step is to discuss what you've learned with your physician. Remember, even though a drug may deplete you of a certain nutrient, you want your medical doctor to review the situation and make sure that taking that nutrient won't lessen the effect of the drug in question, won't interfere with other drugs you're taking, worsen a medical problem, and so on. Be sure to ask your physician what form of each nutrient is best for you.

By the way, you can also look through the index for your drug's brand name. We've listed many, but not all, of them for your convenience. If you're not sure which is the generic and which is the brand name, ask your doctor or show the medicine to your pharmacist—either one will know.

CHAPTER 1 | **Nutrient Robbery**

Sixty-five-year-old Hannah had been struggling with stiff and painful fingers for some time before she went to see her physician. The disturbing diagnosis was rheumatoid arthritis (RA), for which Hannah was given a drug named Naprosyn. This painkiller helped considerably, but after she had been taking it for a while, Hannah became concerned about the fact that she was bruising easily and often, and was constantly constipated.

Her doctor assured her that there was nothing to worry about, for these were common side effects of Naprosyn. "I'll give you another medicine, Dulcolax, for your bowels," he told her with a smile, "and we'll keep our eye on that bruising."

The Dulcolax worked well; Hannah's constipation quickly disappeared. But months later she started noticing that she felt weak all the time, and she could swear that her stomach was "funny."

When Hannah went back to see her doctor, he reassured her that these were "standard side effects, nothing to worry about." Reaching for his prescription pad, he began scribbling new prescriptions for drugs that would alleviate her weakness and stomach distress. He then warned her about the side effects she might experience from taking these new drugs.

Hannah's story is unfortunate, but very common. You may have experienced it yourself.

You have a problem, for which your physician prescribes a drug. That's Round One.

The medicine works, but it triggers a side effect—or maybe a few of them.

Diuretics help you expel fluid from your body. This is useful in treating elevated blood pressure—the idea is to reduce the blood volume by forcing "excess" fluid out of the body. As the volume of the blood drops, so does the blood pressure.

One family of diuretics, called the potassium-sparing diuretics, are specifically designed to prevent the loss of too much potassium. But while they're protecting the potassium, these drugs are encouraging the exodus of numerous other nutrients from the body, including:

- Calcium—possibly leading to osteoporosis, muscle cramps, heart palpitations, and, surprisingly enough, elevated blood pressure
- Folic acid—putting you at risk of headaches, fatigue, hair loss, appetite problems, and nausea
- Coenzyme Q_{10}—raising the odds of developing congestive heart failure, angina pain and stroke; plus, ironically, elevated blood pressure
- Magnesium—possibly triggering insomnia, loss of appetite, kidney stones, depression, and elevated blood pressure
- Vitamin B_6—placing you in jeopardy of suffering from PMS, anemia, and depression
- Zinc—raising the risk of joint pain, weakened immunity, and depression

Naturally, you return to your doctor, who gives you a new drug or two to eliminate the side effects of the first round of medicines. That's Round Two.

These new medicines take care of the side effects from Round One, but cause a few more of their own. So you go back to your doctor, who prescribes a new set of drugs. That's Round Three, and it may go on even further. Some people go through four, five, even ten rounds of drugs/side effects/new drugs, and end up taking a cornucopia of pills, most of which were given to cure the side effects caused by other drugs.

If this was absolutely necessary, you might just accept your fate, swallow your daily cocktail of chemicals, and suffer the consequences. But it's *not*. You don't have to swim in a sea of medications that can make you feel even worse just to keep yourself going.

It's Not the Drugs, It's the "Nutrient Robbery"

We think that the side effects of drugs are the inevitable by-products of mysterious biochemical processes that we can neither understand nor influence. Many side effects are, indeed, beyond our understanding and control. But others—10, 20, perhaps 30 percent of them—can be explained and cured. These millions of curable side effects are the direct result of drug-induced nutrient deficiencies. In other words, a drug "robs" you of one or more nutrients or other helpful substances, and the lack of the nutrient(s) causes unpleasant symptoms. In a sense, the drug acts as an "anti–vitamin pill," taking away the substances you need for good health.

The drugs aren't directly responsible for many of the side effects associated with them; it's really the nutrient robbery.

Remember the Naprosyn that Hannah took for her arthritis? This well-known painkiller, which has been prescribed to millions of people, depletes the body's stores of folic acid. A member of the B family of vitamins, folic acid helps the body produce red blood cells. A shortage of this vitamin means you'll have fewer red blood cells ferrying oxygen to your body tissues, which means that you'll soon start feeling very tired. A lack of folic acid can also set off gastrointestinal difficulties by triggering abnormal development of the cells lining the stomach and intestines.

MORE IS NOT NECESSARILY BETTER

We spend a lot of time talking about what happens when you run short of nutrients. But remember that too much of any nutrient can also be harmful. For example, having excessive amounts of vitamin A in your body can lead to loss of hair and appetite, dry skin, pain in the bones and joints, weakness, irritability, and other problems.

Some of the dangers of excess are listed in Chapter 2, in the "Safety and Side Effects" section that follows the introduction of each nutrient. And the fact that a drug may induce an excess of a nutrient is noted in the "Additional Ways This Drug May Upset Your Nutritional Balance" section in each of the drug entries in Chapter 3.

The obvious solution is to give everyone who takes Naprosyn a folic acid supplement—or to make sure that their diets contain plenty of the vitamin—to replace what the drug takes away. But very few physicians are aware of the Naprosyn–folic acid connection. Neither do they know that this drug-induced nutrient deficiency is the real cause of some of the drug's annoying side effects. Instead, when patients on Naprosyn complain of fatigue, diarrhea, nausea, or other problems, most doctors simply will prescribe another drug to fix these "unavoidable side effects."

The fix-it drug that Hannah was given, Dulcolax, depletes the body's potassium stores. Low potassium causes a variety of problems, including fatigue, dizziness, mental confusion, and continuous thirst, plus the weakness and irregular heartbeat that Hannah experienced. Instead of automatically heading for the prescription pad, Hannah's doctor should have recommended supplemental potassium or encouraged her to eat more bananas.

Hannah and millions of other Americans are suffering from an almost completely ignored epidemic of drug-induced nutrient depletion. They're tormented despite the publication of hundreds of scientific articles that prove numerous popular drugs rob the body of nutrients, and this nutrient robbery is the cause of many drug side effects.

A Major Problem

We don't know exactly how many millions of Americans are suffering from drug-induced nutrient depletion, but we do know that there are millions of instances of drug side effects every year. Even if only 20 percent of these side effects are, in fact, the result of "stolen nutrients," it means that hundreds of thousands of Americans suffer from this misunderstood and, therefore, undertreated problem. Despite the best intentions of doctors, all the fix-it drugs in the world won't get to the root of this problem.

A growing body of scientific evidence proves that many common drugs interfere with our ability to digest, absorb, transport, metabolize, synthesize, utilize, or excrete certain vitamins, minerals, and other vital substances. These drugs can also hamper the actions of these vital substances within the body.

Several drugs make it difficult to absorb nutrients. For example, Tagamet (cimetidine), a medicine used for ulcers, gastroesophageal reflux disease (heartburn), and other problems, can reduce the secretion of intestinal fluids needed to absorb vitamin B_{12}. When B_{12} levels fall, fatigue, allergies, and other problems may develop. The ability to absorb nutrients may also be hampered by drugs that damage the lining of the intestines, including Aldomet (methyldopa), which is used to treat elevated blood pressure, and colchicine, a medicine prescribed for gout. A chemotherapy agent named doxorubicin is close enough in structure to riboflavin to compete with it for binding sites on enzymes, thus "shutting out" the real vitamin and possibly triggering fatigue, a swollen and cracked tongue, bloodshot eyes, sensitivity to light, and painfully chapped lips. Questran (cholestyramine), a drug used to reduce elevated blood fats and cholesterol, can hamper the absorption of vitamins A, D, E, and K, causing a host of problems, including dry eyes, rough and scaly skin, increased vulnerability to colds and skin abscesses, muscle weakness, anemia, and easy bruising. "Bulk agents" such as psyllium gum, used to keep blood sugar under control and reduce weight, can diminish the absorption of riboflavin, vitamins A, C, and B_{12}, prompting increased susceptibility to infections, sore tongue, depression, anxiety, crusty skin, reproductive problems, and dry eyes. And that's just the beginning of the list of medications that can block the absorption of nutrients.

Unfortunately, even when nutrients are properly absorbed, they aren't necessarily "protected," because certain drugs increase their rate of excretion from the body. For example, the thiazide diuretics used to reduce blood pressure may speed up the rate at which magnesium, potassium, and sodium are flushed out of the body via the urine. A lack of magnesium can cause fatigue, muscle spasms, confusion, and irregular heartbeat, while a deficiency of potassium can trigger muscle weakness, nausea, vomiting, and diarrhea, among other things. And even the over-the-counter drugs found in almost everyone's medicine cabinet can be troublesome. Consuming large quantities of aspirin can increase the excretion of folic acid, which the body uses to synthesize DNA, regulate cell division and growth, and manufacture red blood cells. A deficiency of folic acid can trigger fatigue, shortness of breath, weakness, and irritability. Millions of people swallow large amounts of aspirin every day for headaches, joint pain, and other problems, and many of them wind up complaining of symptoms that are quite likely due to folic acid deficiency.

These are just a few examples of ways in which drugs can interfere with the digestion, absorption, transportation, metabolic activity, synthesis, utilization, or excretion of nutrients in the body—and the side effects that result. The only true solution to these problems is to replace the nutrients that have disappeared via supplements, wise dietary choices, or both.

DRUGS THAT ROB YOU OF MAGNESIUM

Magnesium is a vital mineral that helps the heart beat. It's also linked to migraine headaches: Up to 50 percent of those who suffer from these terrible headaches are deficient in magnesium.

You may develop a problem related to magnesium deficiency if you take any of these popular drugs, all of which rob the body of magnesium:

- Rhinocort (budesonide), used for hay fever and nasal inflammations
- Diprolene (betamethasone dipropionate), used for itchy rashes and inflammatory skin conditions
- Sandimmune or Neoral (cyclosporine), used for severe cases of psoriasis and rheumatoid arthritis
- Decadron (dexamethasone), used for asthma, rheumatoid arthritis, severe allergies, various anemias, severe psoriasis, lupus, ulcerative collitis, allergic conjunctivitis, and other ailments
- Lanoxin (digoxin), used for irregular heartbeats, congestive heart failure, and other heart ailments
- Doryx and Vibramycin (doxycycline), used for many bacterial infections, severe acne, and amoebic dysentery
- Lozol (indapamide), used for high blood pressure
- Deltasone and Orasone (prednisone), used for asthma, rheumatoid arthritis, severe allergies, and other ailments

And that's just the beginning of the list of magnesium-depleting drugs. All told, over 50 common drugs rob the body of magnesium.

BEWARE THE FOLIC ACID THIEVES

Aspirin, ibuprofen, Celebrex, hydrocortisone, birth control pills, the Tegretol used for seizures, the Tagamet given for ulcers, the Decadron prescribed for asthma and rheumatoid arthritis, the phenobarbital taken for seizures and insomnia, the Clinoril specified for ankylosing spondylitis, gout, and other forms of arthritis, and numerous other drugs can rob you of this member of the B family of vitamins.

A deficiency of folic acid can cause fatigue, shortness of breath, irritability, and weakness. A deficiency of folic acid during pregnancy can cause fetal abnormalities.

Even a Small Deficiency Can Be Dangerous

Most of us are well aware that a severe lack of vitamin C can cause scurvy and death, while a serious shortfall of calcium can cause osteoporosis. But what about the small to moderate nutrient deficiencies caused by the use of medications? Are they really a problem?

Yes—it's a serious problem, for even minor deficiencies can bring on major difficulties. For example:

- A "minor" deficiency of thiamin can induce depression, muscle weakness, generalized swelling of the body, and irritability.
- A "minor" deficiency of riboflavin can trigger reddening, burning, itching and tearing of the eyes, as well as dry, scaly, and itchy skin.
- A "minor" deficiency of vitamin B_6 can harm the heart and bring about sleep disturbances.
- A "minor" deficiency of vitamin B_{12} can lead to loss of appetite, nausea, vomiting, poor blood clotting, and fatigue.
- A "minor" deficiency of vitamin C can result in weakening of the immune system, swollen and tender joints, and bleeding gums.
- A "minor" deficiency of vitamin D can touch off muscle weakness and osteoporosis.
- A "minor" deficiency of vitamin E can weaken the immune system.
- A "minor" deficiency of calcium can provoke irregular heartbeat and high blood pressure.
- A "minor" deficiency of magnesium can induce breathing difficulties, muscle cramps, and premenstrual syndrome (PMS).
- A "minor" deficiency of potassium can force the heart to beat irregularly, and cause muscle weakness and fatigue.
- A "minor" deficiency of iron can trigger weakness and fatigue.
- A "minor" deficiency of zinc can hamper the immune system, paving the way for cancer and autoimmune diseases.
- A "minor" deficiency of biotin can set the stage for depression and skin and heart problems.

An In-Depth Look at Statins, Coenzyme Q$_{10}$, and Heart Health

One of the best-researched instances of drug-induced nutrient robbery involves the statin drugs and coenzyme Q$_{10}$ (CoQ$_{10}$). Since their introduction in the late 1980s, the statins have rapidly become the dominant class of drugs used to treat elevated cholesterol (hypercholesterolemia) and are among the most commonly prescribed drugs in the United States. There are several different statin drugs, including Lipitor (atorvastatin), Mevacor (lovastatin), Zocor (simvastatin), and Pravachol (pravastatin). Millions of Americans—especially the elderly—currently take statin drugs, and millions more will soon join them, because the new National Cholesterol Education Program guidelines suggest that they be prescribed even for people with low-normal cholesterol levels. This means that more people will soon be taking these drugs, they'll start them at a younger age, and they'll continue taking them for longer periods of time. Indeed, there's no "exit strategy" for the statins. Once you swallow your first pill, you can expect to take statins for the rest of your life—unless the side effects become too troublesome.

There's no doubt that the statins reduce cholesterol—and do so quite well. They work by slowing the action of an enzyme called HMG CoA reductase, which is a precursor of cholesterol. This means that the body produces less cholesterol, one of the major risk factors for heart disease and stroke. But this cholesterol precursor has another duty: It helps produce a substance called coenzyme Q$_{10}$. So while the statins reduce production of cholesterol, they also reduce manufacture of CoQ$_{10}$, which may be bad for the heart.

CoQ$_{10}$ is a vitamin-like substance that helps produce energy in the mitochondria, the tiny "energy factories" located inside cells. CoQ$_{10}$ is essential for heart health, for there are tremendous concentrations of mitochondria in the cells that make up the heart muscle and they require prodigious quantities of CoQ$_{10}$ to keep the heart beating. Without sufficient CoQ$_{10}$, the amount of blood pumped by the heart with each beat falls, leading to symptoms such as fatigue, muscle weakness, chest pain, and heart palpitations. If the problem is severe enough, heart failure and death can result. Key statin/CoQ$_{10}$ researchers have pointed out that the "overwhelming international evidence over at least 15 years" points to "an indispensability of CoQ$_{10}$ for human cardiac function."[1] Specifically, low levels of CoQ$_{10}$ in the blood and body tissues have been associated with heart failure, and "the severity of heart failure correlates with the severity of CoQ$_{10}$ deficiency."[2]

CoQ$_{10}$ has a second duty that makes it indispensable to the health of the entire cardiovascular system. It's a powerful antioxidant that slows the oxidation of LDL cholesterol, often called the "bad" cholesterol. When LDL is oxidized, it's more likely to damage the inner linings of the arteries and trigger cardiovascular disease, which can lead to heart attack, stroke, or other serious problems.

Clearly, you want to have ample stores of CoQ_{10} in the body. You can get small amounts of CoQ_{10} from many different foods, but the bulk of our supply is produced in the body. If you're taking statin drugs, your levels of the vital substance will automatically decrease. Numerous studies have examined the deleterious effects of statins on CoQ_{10}. Let's take a look at some of the key findings.

Statins Lower CoQ_{10} and Harm the Heart

The statin/CoQ_{10} connection in humans first came to light in 1990, when researchers noted that the blood levels of CoQ_{10} fell in five patients who were taking lovastatin. By itself, this finding may have passed without much comment, except that all five were also suffering from a potentially fatal disease of the heart muscle (cardiomyopathy). Their heart problems grew worse as their CoQ_{10} levels fell, but then improved when they were given supplemental CoQ_{10} to replace what the statin drug took away. This was the first study with humans to show that: statin drugs could lower CoQ_{10}; the shortfall could harm the heart; and both the deficit and the accompanying heart damage could easily be reversed.

The Greater the Statin Dose, the Lower the CoQ_{10}

Three years later, a group of British researchers examined the effects of a different statin drug, simvastatin, on CoQ_{10}. For their study, they compared groups of people who were either taking the drug and eating a special diet, were only eating the special diet, or were doing nothing. Those on simvastatin had significantly lower levels of CoQ_{10} in their blood. And the greater the drug dosage, the lower the blood levels of CoQ_{10}.

Statins Lower CoQ_{10} in the Platelets and the Blood

In 1994, a team of Italian researchers gave either simvastatin or simvastatin plus CoQ_{10} to 34 people with elevated cholesterol levels. Blood samples taken from each group revealed that the statin drug lowered CoQ_{10} levels in the blood and in the platelets (small cells within the blood that are essential for coagulation). However, the supplemental CoQ_{10} reversed the CoQ_{10} deficit in the blood and platelets.

Statins Increase LDL Oxidation

Finnish doctors examined the effects of lovastatin on CoQ_{10} and LDL oxidation in 29 men with elevated cholesterol. Lovastatin triggered a significant drop in CoQ_{10} in the blood. It also triggered increased oxidation of LDL, thus heightening the risk of heart attack, stroke, and other cardiovascular diseases.

Statin Drugs Harm the Heart

In 1999, a team of French researchers compared the effects of simvastatin to a nonstatin drug called fenofibrate. After 12 weeks, they noted that the statin weakened the heart muscle.

The Stamp of Approval

Many physicians don't feel a new idea is official until it's presented in the *Journal of the American Medical Association*. That happened in 2002, when the journal published the results of a study on simvastatin. Twenty milligrams per day of the statin pushed the blood levels of CoQ_{10} down by 22 percent.

These and other studies have made it clear that the statin drugs rob the body of CoQ_{10}—and the greater the dose, the more CoQ_{10} is lost. This might be acceptable in healthy, relatively young patients whose bodies are still producing good amounts of CoQ_{10}. But for people over the age of 40 whose ability to manufacture CoQ_{10} is diminished, and for those who already have heart disease and need large doses of CoQ_{10}, the statin drugs can be seriously detrimental. It's no wonder that several leading researchers have called upon the Food and Drug Administration (FDA) to put a warning label on statin drugs, reminding physicians that these medications rob the body of CoQ_{10}, which should be replaced with supplements.

This statin-induced nutrient robbery won't send you to the hospital right away. Depending on your age and heart health, months or even years may pass before you begin to feel the effects of CoQ_{10} depletion. But sooner or later, almost everyone taking these drugs will be affected—even those in their 30s and 40s who were put on statin drug therapy because their cholesterol was mildly or marginally elevated. And as the Baby Boomers roll into retirement, we'll undoubtedly see millions more taking these medications.

We're not saying that the statin drugs are bad. They have helped numerous people and should continue to be prescribed when necessary. But *people who take a statin should probably also take a CoQ_{10} supplement*, a fact that few people are aware of.

Common Antibiotics Can Be Dangerous Nutrient Thieves

Of course, statins aren't the only drugs that steal precious nutrients. Many other medicines, including some common ones whose use is considered routine, also participate in nutrient thievery. Take, for example, the ubiquitous antibiotics, routinely prescribed to treat flus, syphilis, gonorrhea, chlamydia, meningitis, tuberculosis, Lyme disease, herpes zoster (shingles) and herpes simplex, Kaposi's sarcoma, genital warts, and other infections. It's the rare person who has not taken antibiotics at some point in his or her life, and many people take them frequently or for extended periods of time.

As their name indicates, the antibiotics are designed to destroy bacteria. Unfortunately, these drugs are not always very discriminating, slaying helpful bacteria along with the harmful ones. The bacteria in our intestines are often the unintended victims of antibiotic therapy, leaving us bereft of their helpful actions, which include:

- Aiding in the production of various B vitamins which, in turn, help the body extract energy from foods
- Maintaining the body's acid-base balance at the right level for proper function of enzymes and other substances
- Slowing the growth of numerous toxins
- Eliminating harmful bacteria by crowding them out of the intestines
- Performing vital support functions for the numerous immune system cells that are located in the intestines

By interfering with our friendly intestinal bacteria, antibiotics can also reduce our supplies of vitamin K, which helps ensure proper clotting of the blood and guides calcium to the bones. This reduction in vitamin K can contribute to excessive bleeding and osteoporosis. If you take antibiotics for a short period of time and consume a nutritious diet based on a wide variety of foods, you'll probably replace the helpful intestinal bacteria and suffer no serious effects. But if you take antibiotics often or for an extended period of time, if your diet is not very nutritious, or if you have only borderline levels of these nutrients in your body, you may suffer from some of these side effects.

Certain antibiotics rob the body of vitamin C, which can lead to a weakened immune system and increased susceptibility to a variety of diseases. Might recurrent colds and flus be related to a deficit of vitamin C, the lack of which was originally caused by the very antibiotics used to treat them in the first place? It's entirely possible.

Antibiotics can also harm you by interfering with the absorption of nutrients from food. For example, tetracycline can bind to calcium in the digestive tract, making it difficult or impossible for the body to absorb this vital mineral. Neomycin can hamper the body's ability to absorb several nutrients by damaging the linings of the stomach and intestinal tract.

THE DRUG WITH THE DECEPTIVE NAME

Mineral oil sounds like a very useful substance, chock full of helpful minerals. It is, indeed, a helpful laxative, but it is not just a mineral "donor," as its name suggests. Instead, it robs you of beta-carotene, calcium, phosphorus, vitamin A, vitamin D, vitamin E, and vitamin K. Here's what a deficit of these nutrients can lead to:

- Beta-carotene: weakening of the immune system
- Calcium: osteoporosis, muscle cramps, heart palpitations, insomnia, nervous disorders
- Phosphorus: poor growth, weakness, bone pain
- Vitamin A: night blindness, dry and scaly skin, cancer
- Vitamin D: rheumatic pain, loss of hearing, increased bone fractures
- Vitamin E: dry skin, PMS, hot flashes, eczema, psoriasis, sterility, enlargement of the prostate
- Vitamin K: osteoporosis, easy bruising, and bleeding

Chemotherapy and Nutrient Robbery

Currently thousands and thousands of Americans are undergoing chemotheraphy for various types of cancer. Researchers have not conducted a large number of studies looking at the nutrient-depleting effects of the individual chemotherapeutic agents, but we know that many people undergoing chemo are suffering from multiple nutrient deficits. After all, depending on the type of cancer and specific chemotherapy drugs, patients may have difficulty eating due to loss of appetite, difficulty chewing and swallowing, changes in the way food tastes, aversions to certain foods, problems with the mouth and teeth, and nausea. This may force many people to cut back on their intake, to eat only their favorite foods, or to eat only the foods they can tolerate easily, without respect to a well-balanced diet. Chemotherapy can also induce vomiting and destroy cells lining the gastrointestinal tract, making it difficult for the body to absorb all the available nutrients in any given meal. There's also the problem of dysbiosis, or an imbalance in the bacteria in the intestines, causing gas, bloating, diarrhea, or constipation, and interfering with healthful eating and nutrient intake.

Thus, people undergoing chemotherapy may find themselves suffering from numerous nutrient deficiencies, which may be triggering side effects attributed to the chemo. It would be helpful to speak to your physician about a multivitamin and mineral supplement to restore some of what you're undoubtedly losing if you're on chemo.

Drugs Are Helpful, but . . .

This is not an antimedicine book. We're not opposed to the many medications physicians prescribe or to the over-the-counter medicines you may purchase on your own. Modern medicines perform many miracles every day, from controlling diabetes to containing virulent infections. However, we believe it is important for you to remember that all drugs have side effects—every single one of them, even the simple and ubiquitous aspirin—and that some of these side effects can be ameliorated or even eliminated by restoring the missing nutrients. For example:

- If you're taking penicillin or one of its chemical cousins, it may be wise to increase your potassium intake.
- If you're taking any of the tetracycline antibiotics, it may be wise to increase your calcium and magnesium.
- If you're taking nonsteroidal anti-inflammatories (NSAIDs), it may be wise to increase your folic acid intake.
- If you're taking corticosteroids, it may be wise to increase your calcium, folic acid, magnesium, potassium, selenium, vitamin C, vitamin D, and zinc intake.

- If you're taking cholestyramine or colestipol to lower your cholesterol, it may be wise to increase your beta-carotene, vitamin A, vitamin B_{12}, and vitamin E intake.

In this book, you'll learn about the drugs that rob you of nutrients, the deleterious effects of this robbery, and how to prevent or cure these side effects by selecting the right foods or supplements that can replace the missing nutrients. Let's begin with a quick look at the vitamins, minerals, and other substances that our popular pharmaceuticals are most likely to steal away.

CHAPTER 2

The Nutrients and Other Substances at Risk

More than 30 health-enhancing substances—including vitamins, minerals, and phyto-chemicals—are depleted by the medications included in this book. Sometimes the problem is severe, sometimes it is subtle; sometimes it comes on rapidly, and other times it doesn't strike for years.

This chapter briefly describes the health-enhancing substances robbed by medications. (These substances are collectively called nutrients for convenience, even though they're not all nutrients.) As you read through this chapter, you'll notice that some of the nutrients have a heading called "What the Research Shows," while others do not. We don't mean to imply that those with the discussion are superior to the others, it's just that we thought the research was more exciting for some substances than for others.

There are only a few things you have to know in order to read the descriptions. First, there's been a change in the Recommended Dietary Allowances (RDAs) and their Canadian equivalent, the Recommended Nutrient Intakes (RNIs). Both the RDAs and RNIs are being replaced by the Dietary Reference Intakes, or DRIs, which consist of four items:

1. *Estimated Average Requirement, or EAR:* The amount needed to meet half of your daily needs, assuming you're healthy
2. *Recommended Dietary Allowance, or RDA:* How much is needed to meet the daily needs of 97 percent of the healthy population
3. *Adequate Intake, or AI:* An estimate used when the RDA cannot be determined

4. *Tolerable Upper Intake Level, or UL:* The most you can take every day without risking ill effects

Confused? You're not alone. For the most part, you can ignore the EAR and continue to look for either the RDA or AI for your sex and age group. You might also glance at the UL to make sure you're not getting too much. For the nutrients in this chapter, we list the RDAs when they are available, or the AIs when they're not, as well as the ULs.

Second, you'll see a number of abbreviations as you read through the chapter: mg stands for milligrams, mcg for micrograms, IU for international units, oz for ounce and tbsp for tablespoon.

Finally, under the "Drugs That Interfere with . . ." heading at the end of each entry, the drugs are listed first by generic name. Then, in parentheses, one or two brand names are given.

BETA-CAROTENE/VITAMIN A

A Quick Look

Vitamin A is the "good vision" and anti-inflammation vitamin. Beta-carotene is the plant form of the vitamin, which is converted into active vitamin A inside the body.

The Whole Story

Vitamin A is actually a group of substances—including retinol and reti-nal—with similar activities in the body. Vitamin A's best-known duty is to en-sure that we can see at night. It's also vital for growth, reproduction, cell division, and a strong immune system, as well as the integrity of the skin and linings of the intestinal, respiratory, and urinary tracts. Keeping these barri-ers strong helps protect us from infections of various sorts.

Beta-carotene is one of many carotenes found in fruit and vegetables. It's called provitamin A because it's converted into the vitamin in the body as needed.

Studies looking at large populations have found that consuming more foods rich in beta-carotene and vitamin A lowers the risk of developing some types of cancer. However, when researchers have looked into whether taking supplements made up of these two nutrients would reduce the risk of can-cer, the results have been either mixed or negative. This suggests that beta-carotene and vitamin A boost health when we get them from foods, but not necessarily from supplements.

When You Run Short of Vitamin A

A deficiency can cause night blindness, inflammation of the eyes, blindness, increased susceptibility to infections, weight loss, loss of appetite, poor bone and tooth formation, and impaired growth.

Daily Requirement

The RDA for vitamin A is 3,000 IU per day for men ages 19 and up and 2,330 IU per day for women ages 19 and older. There is no daily requirement for beta-carotene.

Safety and Side Effects

The Tolerable Upper Intake Level (UL) of preformed vitamin A for men and women 19 years old and up is 10,000 IU per day. Excessive amounts of vitamin A can cause nausea, vomiting, loss of appetite and hair, pain in the bones and joints, weakness, and irritability.

There is no UL for beta-carotene.

Some Good Sources of Beta-Carotene

FOOD	SERVING SIZE	IU VITAMIN A FROM BETA-CAROTENE
Carrot, raw	1	20,250
Spinach, frozen, boiled	½ cup	7,395
Mango, raw	1 cup sliced	6,425
Cantaloupe, raw	1 cup	5,160
Apricot nectar, canned	½ cup	1,650

Some Good Sources of Vitamin A

FOOD	SERVING SIZE	IU VITAMIN A
Liver, beef, cooked	3 oz	30,325
Liver, chicken, cooked	3 oz	13,920
Cheese pizza	⅛ of a 12-inch diameter pie	380
Milk, whole	1 cup	305
Cheddar cheese	1 oz	300

Drugs That Interfere with Beta-Carotene

Cholestyramine (LoCHOLEST, Questran)	Mineral oil (Fleet Mineral Oil Enema, Milkinol)
Clofibrate (Atromid-S)	Neomycin (Mycifradin Sulfate Topical, Neo-Tabs Oral)
Colchicine	Octreotide (Sandostatin)
Colchicine plus probenecid (ColBenemid)	Omeprazole (Losec, Prilosec)
Colesevelam (WelChol)	Orlistat (Xenical)
Colestipol (Colestid)	Pantoprazole (Protonix)
Lansoprazole (Prevacid)	Rabeprazole (Aciphex)
Methotrexate (Folex PFS, Rheumatrex)	Simvastatin (Zocor)

Drugs That Interfere with Vitamin A

Aluminum hydroxide (Amphojel, Dialume)	Flunisolide (AeroBid-M, Nasalide)
Aluminum hydroxide plus magnesium carbonate (Gaviscon Liquid)	Fluticasone (Cutivate, Flonase)
Aluminum hydroxide plus magnesium hydroxide (Maalox, Mylanta)	Hydrocortisone (Bactine, Cortef)
Aluminum hydroxide plus magnesium hydroxide plus simethicone (Mylanta Liquid)	Methylprednisolone (Depoject Injection, Medrol Oral)
Aluminum hydroxide plus magnesium trisilicate (Gaviscon Tablet)	Mineral oil (Fleet Mineral Oil Enema, Milkinol)
Beclomethasone (Beconase, Propaderm)	Mometasone furoate (Elocom, Nasonex)
Betamethasone (Betatrex, Maxivate)	Neomycin (Mycifradin Sulfate Topical, Neo-Tabs Oral)
Budesonide (Entocort, Rhinocort)	Orlistat (Xenical)
Cholestyramine (LoCHOLEST, Questran)	Prednisolone (Delta-Cortef, Pediapred)
Colesevelam (WelChol)	Prednisone (Deltasone, Orasone)
Colestipol (Colestid)	Sucralfate (Carafate, Sulcrate)
Cortisone (Cortone)	Triamcinolone (Amcort, Tristoject)
Dexamethasone (Decadron, Maxidex)	

BIFIDOBACTERIUM BIFIDUM AND LACTOBACILLUS ACIDOPHILUS

The Whole Story

Bifidobacterium bifidum and *Lactobacillus acidophilus* are probiotics, or health-enhancing organisms found in the intestinal tract and other parts of the body.

The probiotics' best-known duty is to fix the accidental damage caused by antibiotics—that is, the destruction of the helpful bacteria in the intestines. Probiotics replace these bacteria and also help us digest food, manufacture vitamin K and other nutrients, and regulate cholesterol levels. In addition, they work with the immune system to help keep yeast and other organisms from growing unchecked and producing toxic substances. Some studies suggest that probiotics may even be able to ward off colon cancer.

When You Run Short of Bifidobacterium Bifidum and/or Lactobacillus Acidophilus

A deficiency of *Bifidobacterium bifidum* and/or *Lactobacillus acidophilus* may trigger digestive problems, a weakening of the immune system, and the growth of potentially harmful bacteria.

Daily Requirement

No daily requirement has been set for either *Bifidobacterium bifidum* or *Lactobacillus acidophilus*.

Safety and Side Effects

A Tolerable Upper Intake Level (UL) has not been set for *Bifidobacterium bifidum* or *Lactobacillus acidophilus*. Excessive amounts of *Bifidobacterium bifidum* and/or *Lactobacillus acidophilus* may cause mild gas or other gastrointestinal problems.

Some Good Sources of Bifidobacterium Bifidum and Lactobacillus Acidophilus

Foods such as Jerusalem artichokes, asparagus, garlic, and onions may stimulate the growth or activity of *Bifidobacterium bifidum*. *Lactobacillus acidophilus* is found in yogurt containing live lactobacillus cultures, kefir, and acidophilus milk.

Drugs That Interfere with Bifidobacterium Bifidum and Lactobacillus Acidophilus

Amikacin (Amikin)	Cefoperazone (Cefobid)
Amoxicillin (Amoxil, Novamoxin)	Cefotaxime (Claforan)
Ampicillin (Omnipen, Totacillin)	Cefotetan (Cefotan)
Azithromycin (Zithromax)	Cefoxitin (Mefoxin)
Carbenicillin (Geocillin)	Cefpodoxime (Vantin)
Cefaclor (Ceclor)	Cefprozil (Cefzil)
Cefadroxil (Duricef)	Ceftazidime (Ceptaz, Fortaz)
Cefamandole (Mandol)	Ceftibuten (Cedax)
Cefazolin (Ancef, Kefzol)	Ceftizoxime (Cefizox)
Cefdinir (Omnicef)	Ceftriaxone (Rocephin)
Cefditoren (Spectracef)	Cefuroxime (Ceftin, Kefurox)
Cefepime (Maxipime)	Cephalexin (Biocef, Keftab)
Cefonicid (Monocid)	Cephalothin (Ceporacin)

Cephapirin (Cefadyl)	Nafcillin (Nafcil Injection, Unipen Oral)
Cepharadine (Velosef)	Nalidixic acid (NegGram)
Cinoxacin (Cinobac)	Neomycin (Mycifradin Sulfate Topical, Neo-Tabs Oral)
Ciprofloxacin (Ciloxan, Cipro)	Nitrofurantoin (Furadantin, Macrobid)
Clarithromycin (Biaxin, Biaxin XL)	Norfloxacin (Chibroxin Ophthalmic, Noroxin Oral)
Clindamycin (Cleocin, Dalacin C)	Ofloxacin (Floxin, Ocuflox Ophthalmic)
Cloxacillin (Cloxapen, Nu-Cloxi)	Penicillin G benzathine (Bicillin L-A, Permapen)
Demeclocycline (Declomycin)	Penicillin G benzathine plus penicillin G procaine (Bicillin C-R)
Dicloxacillin (Dycill, Pathocil)	Pencillin G procaine (Pfizerpen-AS, Wycillin)
Dirithromycin (Dynabac)	Penicillin V potassium (Suspen, Truxcillin)
Doxycycline (Monodox, Vibramycin)	Piperacillin (Pipracil)
Erythromycin (Erythrocin, Staticin)	Piperacillin plus tazobactam sodium (Zosyn)
Gatofloxacin (Tequin)	Sparfloxacin (Zagam)
Gentamicin (Garamycin, Jenamicin)	Streptomycin
Kanamycin (Kantrex)	Sulfadiazine (Coptin, Microsulfon)
Levofloxacin (Levaquin, Quixin Ophthalmic)	Sulfisoxazole (Gantrisin)
Linezolid (Zyvox)	Tetracycline (Nu-Tetra, Topicycline Topical)
Lomefloxacin (Maxaquin)	Ticarcillin (Ticar)
Loracarbef (Lorabid)	Ticarcillin and clavulanate potassium (Timentin)
Meclocycline (Meclan Topical)	Tobramycin (Nebcin Injection, Tobrex Ophthlamic)
Metronidazole (Flagyl, MetroLotion)	Trimethoprim (Primsol, Trimpex)
Minocycline (Dynacin Oral, Minocin Oral)	Trovafloxacin (Trovan)
Moxifloxacin (Avelox)	

BIOTIN

A Quick Look

This B vitamin participates in many enzyme reactions and strengthens the immune system and skin.

The Whole Story

Biotin was the very first vitamin to be discovered back in 1901, and researchers didn't quite know what to make of it. They named it bios, which means "life," because it was vital to life, and then set it on the back burner. It was "discovered" several more times by various researchers and given names like protective factor X and vitamin H before it became apparent that all of these new discoveries were really the same old bios. Then it was given a new name: biotin.

Biotin, a member of the family of B vitamins, is necessary for a strong immune system and for healthy nerves, sex glands, bone marrow, skin, and hair. It also helps the body extract energy from carbohydrates, fat, and protein.

Because little biotin is stored in the body, you should eat biotin-rich foods every day.

When You Run Short of Biotin

A deficiency can cause depression, muscle pain, nausea, vomiting, and dry, itchy skin.

Daily Requirement

The Adequate Intake (AI) for biotin is 30 mcg per day for men and women ages 19 and over.

Safety and Side Effects

The Tolerable Upper Intake Level (UL) for biotin has not been set. There are no recognized signs of biotin "overdose," and supplemental doses of up to 200 mcg per day have not caused toxicity. However, consuming too much biotin can cause a deficiency of other B vitamins by interfering with their absorption.

Some Good Sources of Biotin

FOOD	SERVING SIZE	MCG BIOTIN
Beef liver, cooked	3½ oz	96
Soybeans, cooked	3½ oz	61
Rice bran	3½ oz	60
Peanut butter	3½ oz	39
Barley	3½ oz	31
Oatmeal	3½ oz	24

Drugs That Interfere with Biotin

Amikacin (Amikin)	Carbenicillin (Geocillin)
Amoxicillin (Amoxil, Novamoxin)	Cefaclor (Ceclor)
Ampicillin (Omnipen, Totacillin)	Cefadroxil (Duricef)
Azithromycin (Zithromax)	Cefamandole (Mandol)
Butabarbital (Butalan, Butisol)	Cefazolin (Ancef, Kefzol)
Butalbital plus acetaminophen plus caffeine (Esgic, Fioricet)	Cefdinir (Omnicef)
Butalbital plus aspirin plus caffeine (Fiorinal)	Cefditoren (Spectracef)
Carbamazepine (Nu-Carbamazepine, Tegretol)	Cefepime (Maxipime)

Cefonicid (Monocid)	Linezolid (Zyvox)
Cefoperazone (Cefobid)	Lomefloxacin (Maxaquin)
Cefotaxime (Claforan)	Loracarbef (Lorabid)
Cefotetan (Cefotan)	Meclocycline (Meclan Topical)
Cefoxitin (Mefoxin)	Minocycline (Dynacin Oral, Minocin Oral)
Cefpodoxime (Vantin)	Moxifloxacin (Avelox)
Cefprozil (Cefzil)	Nafcillin (Nafcil Injection, Unipen Oral)
Ceftazidime (Ceptaz, Fortaz)	Nalidixic acid (NegGram)
Ceftibuten (Cedax)	Norfloxacin (Chibroxin Ophthalmic, Noroxin Oral)
Ceftizoxime (Cefizox)	Ofloxacin (Floxin, Ocuflox Ophthalmic)
Ceftriaxone (Rocephin)	Oxcarbazepine (Trileptal)
Cefuroxime (Ceftin, Kefurox)	Penicillin G benzathine (Bicillin L-A, Permapen)
Cephalexin (Biocef, Keftab)	Penicillin G benzathine plus penicillin G procaine (Bicillin C-R)
Cephalothin (Ceporacin)	Penicillin G procaine (Pfizerpen-AS, Wycillin)
Cephapirin (Cefadyl)	Penicillin V potassium (Suspen, Truxcillin)
Cepharadine (Velosef)	Phenobarbital (Barbita, Solfoton)
Cinoxacin (Cinobac)	Phenytoin (Dilantin, Tremytoine)
Ciprofloxacin (Ciloxan, Cipro)	Piperacillin (Pipracil)
Clarithromycin (Biaxin, Biaxin XL)	Piperacillin plus tazobactam sodium (Zosyn)
Cloxacillin (Cloxapen, Nu-Cloxi)	Primidone (Mysoline, Sertan)
Demeclocycline (Declomycin)	Sparfloxacin (Zagam)
Dicloxacillin (Dycill, Pathocil)	Sulfadiazine (Coptin, Microsulfon)
Dirithromycin (Dynabac)	Sulfisoxazole (Gantrisin)
Doxycycline (Monodox, Vibramycin)	Tetracycline (Nu-Tetra, Topicycline Topical)
Erythromycin (Erythrocin, Staticin)	Ticarcillin (Ticar)
Ethosuximide (Zarontin)	Ticarcillin and clavulanate potassium (Timentin)
Fosphenytoin (Cerebyx)	Tobramycin (Nebcin Injection, Tobrex Ophthalmic)
Gatofloxacin (Tequin)	Trimethoprim (Primsol, Trimpex)
Gentamicin (Garamycin, Jenamicin)	Trovafloxacin (Trovan)
Kanamycin (Kantrex)	Zonisamide (Zonegran)
Levofloxacin (Levaquin, Quixin Ophthalmic)	

CALCIUM

A Quick Look

Calcium is a mineral that is banked in the bones and drawn on when necessary.

The Whole Story

Ninety-nine percent of the calcium in your body resides in your bones and teeth, with just a small amount floating through your bloodstream. But the calcium in your blood has many crucial duties. It helps:

- Control the blood pressure
- Promote blood clotting and wound healing
- Aid in muscle contraction and relaxation
- Send signals through the nervous system
- Synthesize hormones and enzymes
- Keep the heart beating properly

There must always be enough calcium in your bloodstream, ready to handle these myriad tasks. If there isn't, your body will "withdraw" some from its "account" in your bones to bring the blood levels back up to normal. Too much of this, of course, can cause thinning of the bones.

Your body absorbs larger or smaller amounts of calcium from your food according to your needs at the moment. If you have plenty, you may absorb only 10 percent of the calcium in your food. But if you're growing, pregnant, or lactating, any of which will increase your calcium needs, your body may absorb 50 percent or more of the calcium from your food.

When You Run Short of Calcium

A deficiency can cause problems with blood clotting, elevated blood pressure, and thinning of the bones.

What the Research Shows

Several researchers have studied the effects of calcium on high blood pressure. Although not all the studies agree, in general the results look promising. For example:

- A meta-analysis looking at the calcium–blood pressure connection was published in the *Journal of the American Medical Association* in 1996.[1] (A meta-analysis is a study of studies, a pooling of the results of many studies to produce a single, larger look at the situation.) Thirty-three different studies involving over 2,400 people were combined and analyzed. The authors concluded that calcium supplements produce a small reduction in systolic blood pressure. (Systolic pressure is the first or upper number in the blood pressure fraction, that is, 120 in 120/80.)
- Other researchers have examined the effects of calcium supplements during pregnancy. They found that there "was a modest reduction in high blood pressure with calcium supplementation" and that those who were at the greatest risk of developing hypertension and those who had lower levels of calcium to begin with benefited the most.[2]

Selecting Supplements

There are many calcium supplements on the market, and the difference between them goes beyond brand name or price.

The calcium in a calcium supplement comes attached to something else. For example, there's calcium carbonate, calcium citrate, calcium lactate, and so on, and each of these forms contains a different amount of elemental, or "pure," calcium. Calcium carbonate is 40 percent elemental calcium, calcium citrate is 21 percent, calcium lactate is 13 percent and calcium gluconate is a mere 9 percent. So, 1,000 mg calcium carbonate provides 400 mg elemental calcium, compared to the 90 mg offered by the same amount of calcium gluconate. Besides differences in the amount of elemental calcium, there are also differences in absorbability. If you take calcium supplements, ask your physician which is best for you.

Daily Requirement

The Adequate Intake (AI) for calcium is 1,000 mg per day for men and women ages 19 to 50 and 1,200 per day for men and women 51 years old and up.

Safety and Side Effects

The Tolerable Upper Intake Level (UL) of calcium for adults is 2,500 mg per day. Excessive amounts of calcium can damage the kidneys and cause other problems.

Some Good Sources of Calcium

FOOD	SERVING SIZE	MG CALCIUM
Milk, nonfat	1 cup	302
Yogurt, lowfat	8 oz	300
Figs, dried	10	270
Swiss cheese	1 oz	219
Salmon, canned with bones	3 oz	181
Spinach, cooked	½ cup	122
Tofu	½ cup	118
Broccoli, chopped	½ cup	89
Almonds, dry roasted	1 oz	80
Papaya	1 medium	72

Drugs That Interfere with Calcium

Alendronate (Fosamax)	Doxycycline (Monodox, Vibramycin)
Aluminum hydroxide (Amphojel, Dialume)	Ethacrynic acid (Edecrin)
Aluminum hydroxide plus magnesium carbonate (Gaviscon Liquid)	Ethosuximide (Zarontin)
Aluminum hydroxide plus magnesium hydroxide (Maalox, Mylanta)	Etidronate (Didronel)
Aluminum hydroxide plus magnesium hydroxide plus simethicone (Mylanta Liquid)	Famotidine (Alti-Famotidine, Pepcid)
Aluminum hydroxide plus magnesium trisilicate (Gaviscon Tablet)	Flucytosine (Ancobon)
Amifostine (Ethyol)	Flunisolide (AeroBid-M, Nasalide)
Amikacin (Amikin)	Fluticasone (Cutivate, Flonase)
Amiloride (Midamor)	Foscarnet (Foscavir)
Amphotericin B (Amphocin, Fungizone)	Fosphenytoin (Cerebyx)
Arsenic trioxide (Trisenox)	Frovatriptan (Frova)
Basiliximab (Simulect)	Furosemide (Apo-Furosemide, Lasix)
Beclomethasone (Beconase, Propaderm)	Gentamicin (Garamycin, Jenamicin)
Betamethasone (Betatrex, Maxivate)	Halobetasol (Ultravate)
Bisacodyl (Carter's Little Pills, Dulcolax)	Heparin (Hep-Lock)
Budesonide (Entocort, Rhinocort)	Hydrochlorothiazide (Apo-Hydro, Esidrix)
Bumetanide (Bumex, Burinex)	Hydrochlorothiazide plus triamterene (Dyazide, Maxzide)
Butabarbital (Butalan, Butisol)	Hydrocortisone (Bactine, Cortef)
Butalbital plus acetaminophen plus caffeine (Esgic, Fioricet)	Interferon Alfa-2a (Roferon-A)
Butalbital plus aspirin plus caffeine (Fiorinal)	Interferon Alfa-2b (Intron A)
Carbamazepine (Nu-Carbamazepine, Tegretol)	Isoniazid (Laniazid Oral, PMS-Isoniazid)
Carboplatin (Paraplatin, Paraplatin-AQ)	Kanamycin (Kantrex)
Cascara	Magnesium hydroxide (Phillips' Milk of Magnesia)
Cholestyramine (LoCHOLEST, Questran)	Magnesium oxide (Maox)
Cidofovir (Vistide)	Magnesium sulfate (Epsom Salts)
Cimetidine (Apo-Cimetidine, Tagamet)	Meclocycline (Meclan Topical)
Cisplatin (Platinol, Platinol-AQ)	Methotrexate (Folex PFS, Rheumatrex)
Colchicine	Methsuximide (Celotin)
Colestipol (Colestid)	Methylprednisolone (Depoject Injection, Medrol Oral)
Cortisone (Cortone)	Mineral oil (Fleet Mineral Oil Enema, Milkinol)
Dactinomycin (Cosmegen)	Minocycline (Dynacin Oral, Minocin Oral)
Deferoxamine (Desferal)	Mometasone furoate (Elocom, Nasonex)
Demeclocycline (Declomycin)	Mycophenolate (CellCept)
Denileukin diftitox (ONTAK)	Neomycin (Mycifradin Sulfate Topical, Neo-Tabs Oral)
Dexamethasone (Decadron, Maxidex)	Nizatidine (Apo-Nizatidine, Axid)
Diflorasone (Florone, Maxiflor)	Oxcarbazepine (Trileptal)
Digoxin (Digitek, Lanoxin)	Pamidronate (Aredia)

Pentamidine (NebuPent Inhalation, Pentacarinat Injection)	Streptomycin
Phenobarbital (Barbita, Solfoton)	Sucralfate (Carafate, Sulcrate)
Phenytoin (Dilantin, Tremytoine)	Tacrolimus (Prograf)
Plicamycin (Mithracin)	Tetracycline (Nu-Tetra, Topicycline Topical)
Potassium and sodium phosphates (K-Phos Neutral, Uro-KP-Neutral)	Tiludronate (Skelid)
Prednisolone (Delta-Cortef, Pediapred)	Tobramycin (Nebcin Injection, Tobrex Ophthlamic)
Prednisone (Deltasone, Orasone)	Torsemide (Demadex)
Primidone (Mysoline, Sertan)	Trandolapril (Mavik)
Ranitidine (Nu-Ranit, Zantac)	Trandolapril plus verapamil (Tarka)
Rifampin (Rimactane, Rofact)	Triamcinolone (Amcort, Tristoject)
Rifampin plus isoniazid (Rifamate)	Triamterene (Dyrenium)
Sodium bicarbonate (Neut)	Zalcitabine (Hivid)
Sodium phosphate (Fleet Enema, Fleet Phospho-Soda)	Zoledronic acid (Zometa)
Sodium polystyrene sulfonate (Kayexalate)	Zonisamide (Zonegran)

CARNITINE

The Whole Story

Carnitine is a vitamin-like compound that aids in the conversion of fat to energy inside body cells. Its name comes from the Latin "carnus," which refers to meat, because it was isolated from meat in 1905. Carnitine is not considered an essential nutrient because it's made in the body from two amino acids; however, we do get some from our food.

Carnitine is concentrated in the skeletal muscles, heart muscle, and other parts of the body that use fatty acids as their energy source. The body uses carnitine to keep the right amounts of cholesterol and triglycerides (fats) in the blood and to prevent too many fatty acids from accumulating in the muscles, liver, and heart.

Deficiencies of carnitine are rarely seen. However, problems with the liver or kidneys can lead to a shortfall. You may also run short if you're on a vegetarian diet and not getting enough of the amino acids needed to make carnitine.

When You Run Short of Carnitine

A deficiency may cause fatigue, muscle weakness, and confusion.

What the Research Shows

Carnitine is being investigated as a possible aid in treating dementia and for strengthening the immune system, warding off cardiovascular disease, and combating chronic fatigue syndrome. Although it's too early to draw definitive answers, some of the studies are intriguing, especially those concerning Alzheimer's disease. For example:

- In a study presented in the *Archives of Neurology*,[3] 30 people with mild to moderate probable Alzheimer's disease were given either 2.5 to 3.0 grams of carnitine or a placebo every day for six months. Those who took the carnitine showed "significantly less deterioration in timed cancellation tasks," one of the measurements of mental ability. The study's authors noted that carnitine "may retard the deterioration in some cognitive areas" in patients with Alzheimer's disease.
- In this double-blind, placebo-controlled study[4] comparing carnitine to placebo, 130 patients with Alzheimer's disease were given various tests, then took either carnitine or a placebo every day. They were reassessed a year later. The mental abilities of those taking carnitine had deteriorated at a slower rate than those taking the placebo.

Daily Requirement

There is no RDA for carnitine.

Safety and Side Effects

A Tolerable Upper Limit (UL) for carnitine has not been set. Generally speaking, carnitine supplements in the form of L-carnitine are well tolerated. Large doses of carnitine—3,000 mg per day or more—may cause a "fishy" body odor, diarrhea, abdominal cramps, nausea, and vomiting.

Some Good Sources of Carnitine

FOOD	SERVING SIZE	MG L-CARNITINE
Ground beef	3 oz	80
Pork	3 oz	24
Canadian bacon	3 oz	20
Milk, whole	1 cup	8
Cod	3 oz	5
Chicken, breast	3 oz	3
Avocado	1 medium	2
American cheese	1 oz	1
Whole wheat bread	2 slices	0.2
Asparagus	½ cup	0.2

Drugs That Interfere with Carnitine

Carbamazepine (Nu-Carbamazepine, Tegretol)	Phenytoin (Dilantin, Tremytoine)
Delavirdine (Rescriptor)	Primidone (Mysoline, Sertan)
Didanosine (Videx, Videx EC)	Stavudine (Zerit)
Doxorubicin (Adriamycin, Caelyx)	Valproic acid (Depacon, Depakote ER)
Doxorubicin liposomal (Doxil)	Zalcitabine (Hivid)
Lamivudine (Epivir)	Zidovudine (Apo-Zidovudine)
Nevirapine (Viramune)	Zidovudine plus lamivudine (AZT + 3TC)
Phenobarbital (Barbita, Solfoton)	Zidovudine plus lamivudine plus abacavir (Trizivir)

CHLORIDE

The Whole Story

Chloride is sodium's companion in the well-known duo of sodium chloride, or table salt. But chloride is also important on its own, as an essential mineral found in the hydrochloric acid secreted by the stomach, in the cerebrospinal fluid, red blood cells, bones, connective tissues, and elsewhere.

Chloride's duties include maintaining the proper amount of fluid in the body, forming stomach acid, aiding the red blood cells as they carry carbon dioxide to the lungs, and helping protect the body against bacteria that find their way into the stomach.

Most of us get plenty of chloride, because the standard American diet contains ample amounts of salt. But you may run short of chloride if you are suffering from diarrhea or vomiting, overly acidic blood (acidosis), or adrenal problems. A low-sodium diet, excessive sweating, or diuretics can also deplete your stores of this mineral.

When You Run Short of Chloride

A deficiency can cause a depressed appetite, shallow breathing, muscle cramps, and listlessness.

Daily Requirement

The Food and Nutrition Board had not set an Adequate Intake (AI) for chloride. Instead, it has determined an AI for salt, which contains both sodium and chloride. The AI for salt for men and women ages 19 to 50 is 3.8 grams per day; 3.3 grams per day for men and women ages 51 to 70; and 3.0 grams per day for those ages 71 and up. The average American consumes more than this every day.

Safety and Side Effects

There are no well-identified symptoms of chloride toxicity. However, salt (sodium chloride) has been linked to elevated blood pressure and other ailments among salt-sensitive people. The National Academy of Sciences' Institute of Medicine has set a Tolerable Upper Intake Level (UL) for salt at 5.8 grams per day. If you're salt sensitive, even this amount may be dangerous for you.

Some Good Sources of Chloride

The most prevalent source of chloride is the sodium chloride found in table salt and salty foods like hot dogs, pickles, pretzels, and potato chips.

Drugs That Interfere with Chloride

Bumetanide (Bumex, Burinex)	Furosemide (Apo-Furosemide, Lasix)
Ethacrynic acid (Edecrin)	Torsemide (Demadex)

CHROMIUM

The Whole Story

Only a small amount of chromium—about 6 mg—is found in the body, which is why it's called a trace mineral. All of its duties and modes of action have yet to be determined, but we do know that this mineral is part of the body's glucose tolerance factor, a substance that aids insulin as it rounds up blood sugar and transports it into certain cells. Chromium also activates several enzymes and is needed to metabolize carbohydrates and lipids. Some researchers believe that because this mineral stimulates insulin activity, it can also help build muscle and decrease fat stores.

When You Run Short of Chromium

A deficiency can cause weight loss, hamper your body's ability to utilize glucose, and increase the risk of coronary artery disease.

What the Research Shows

The results of several studies suggest that chromium may play a role in controlling diabetes and heart disease. For example:

- *Diabetes.* In one study, 180 people with type 2 diabetes were randomly assigned to receive 100 mcg elemental chromium, 500 mcg elemental chromium, or a placebo.[5] Four months later, those taking either dose of chromium scored significantly lower on their fasting and two-hour insulin level tests, indicating improvement in their disease. Those taking the higher amount of chromium were also found to have lower total cholesterol levels.

- *Heart disease.* Seventy-two men who were taking beta blockers to control heart disease were randomly given either chromium or a placebo every day for eight weeks.[6] The levels of HDL "good" cholesterol rose significantly in those taking the chromium.

Daily Requirement

The Adequate Intake (AI) for chromium is 35 mcg per day for men ages 19 to 50 and 30 mcg per day for men 51 years old and up. For women, the AI is 25 mcg per day for those ages 19 to 50 and 20 mcg per day for those 51 years old and up.

Safety and Side Effects

A Tolerable Upper Intake Level (UL) of chromium has not been established. Chromium supplements have been reported to cause mood swings, headaches, and sleep disturbances. Some experts feel that taking 300 mcg elemental chromium daily for several months might cause liver damage. Others feel that taking supplemental chromium for several years may cause the mineral to accumulate in body tissues and damage cellular DNA.

Some Good Sources of Chromium

FOOD	SERVING SIZE	MCG CHROMIUM
Broccoli	½ cup	11.0
Turkey ham, processed	3 oz	10.4
Waffle	1	6.7
English muffin	1	3.6
Potatoes, mashed	1 cup	2.7
Bagel	1	2.5
Orange juice	1 cup	2.2
Green beans	½ cup	1.1
Banana	1 medium	1.0

Drugs That Interfere with Chromium

Calcium carbonate (Alka-Mints, Tums)

COENZYME Q$_{10}$

A Quick Look

Coenzyme Q$_{10}$ is a biochemical assistant whose chief duty is to help the body's cells produce energy.

The Whole Story

Called CoQ$_{10}$ for short, coenzyme Q$_{10}$ is a natural substance necessary for energy production in the body's cells—especially those found in the heart, which have large numbers of mitochondria, those little "energy factories" that power our cells.

When we hit the age of 20 or so, our levels of CoQ$_{10}$ begin to drop. It's a slow decline that continues for years and may help explain why we have less energy as we grow older and why heart function begins to falter. CoQ$_{10}$ levels are also lower in people with certain forms of heart disease. In fact, as a general rule, it appears that the more severe the heart disease, the lower the CoQ$_{10}$ levels. And certain drugs can push these levels even lower.

Coenzyme Q$_{10}$ also has antioxidant properties, which means it can prevent free-radical damage to cells and tissues throughout the body. Specifically, it protects vitamin E, which, among other things, helps prevent the oxidation of cholesterol to its more dangerous form.

When You Run Short of Coenzyme Q$_{10}$

We don't have the kind of deficiency information for CoQ$_{10}$ that we have for vitamins and minerals. Thus, we can't say that when you run a little short of CoQ$_{10}$ you'll have certain symptoms, and when you run significantly short you'll develop a particular deficiency disease.

We can, however, look at studies of people who were given supplemental CoQ$_{10}$. The most definitive studies have been done with people suffering from heart disease, and many of these have shown that this substance is very much linked to heart health. For example:

- In a study of hospitalized patients, those with the lowest levels of CoQ$_{10}$ had the greatest risk of suffering from congestive heart failure or dying.[7]
- In another study, 144 people who had suffered a heart attack were given either 120 mg CoQ$_{10}$ per day or a placebo for four weeks.[8] The ones who took the CoQ$_{10}$ had fewer additional heart attacks and were less likely to die of a heart problem.

- A meta-analysis—a study that uses statistical methods to pool the results of several other studies—found that giving supplemental CoQ$_{10}$ to people with congestive heart failure improved several measures of their heart health.[9]
- In still another study, 322 people with congestive heart failure were given either CoQ$_{10}$ or a placebo every day for a year.[10] The ones who took the CoQ$_{10}$ were less likely to be hospitalized or develop the accumulation of fluid in the lungs seen with heart failure.

There is also intriguing evidence suggesting that supplemental CoQ$_{10}$ might be helpful in controlling blood pressure and keeping the heartbeat steady.

Daily Requirement

No daily requirement has been set. Typical supplemental dosages range from 30 to 225 mg per day.

Safety and Side Effects

In various studies, people have taken up to 200 mg CoQ$_{10}$ per day for as long as a year without any reported problems, with the exception of gastrointestinal difficulties in some people. Other reports note that CoQ$_{10}$ can cause loss of appetite, nausea, and diarrhea.

Some Good Sources of CoQ$_{10}$

Coenzyme Q$_{10}$ is manufactured in your body, but is also found in a variety of foods, including beef, chicken, trout, salmon, oranges, and broccoli.

Drugs That Interfere with CoQ$_{10}$

Acebutolol (Nu-Acebutolol, Sectral)	Carvedilol (Coreg)
Acetohexamide (Dymelor, Dimelor)	Chlorothiazide (Diuril)
Amiloride plus hydrochlorothiazide (Moduret, Nu-Amilzide)	Chlorpromazine (Thorazine)
Amitriptyline (Elavil, Vanatrip)	Chlorpropamide (Apo-Chlorpropamide, Diabinese)
Amoxapine (Asendin)	Clomipramine (Anafranil, Novo-Clopramine)
Atenolol (Apo-Atenol, Tenormin)	Clonidine (Catapres, Duraclon)
Atenolol plus chlorthalidone (Tenoretic)	Desipramine (Norpramin, PMS-Desipramine)
Atorvastatin (Lipitor)	Doxepin (Novo-Doxepin, Prudoxin)
Betaxolol (Betoptic S, Kerlone)	Enalapril plus hydrochlorothiazide (Vaseretic)
Bisoprolol (Monocor, Zebeta)	Enoxacin (Penetrex)
Candesartan plus hydrochlorothiazide (Atacand HCT)	Esmolol (Brevibloc)
Carteolol (Cartrol Oral, Ocupress Ophthalmic)	Fenofibrate (Apo-Fenofibrate, TriCor)

Fluphenazine (Modecate, Prolixin)	Nortriptyline (Aventyl Hydrochloride, Pamelor)
Fluvastatin (Lescol)	Penbutolol (Levatol)
Gemfibrozil (Apo-Gemfibrozil, Lopid)	Perphenazine (PMS-Perphenazine, Trilafon)
Glimepiride (Amaryl)	Pindolol (Visken)
Glipizide (Glucotrol)	Polythiazide (Renese)
Glyburide (DiaBeta, Glynase)	Pravastatin (Pravachol)
Glyburide plus metformin (Glucovance)	Prazosin plus polythiazide (Minizide)
Haloperidol (Haldol, Haldol Decanoate)	Prochlorperazine (Prorazin, Stemetil)
Hydralazine (Apo-Hydral, Apresoline)	Promethazine (Anergan, Prorex)
Hydralazine plus hydrochlorothiazide (Apresazide)	Propafenone (Rythmol)
Hydrochlorothiazide (Apo-Hydro, Esidrix)	Propranolol (Inderal, Nu-Propranolol)
Hydrochlorothiazide plus spironolactone (Aldactazide, Novo-Spirozine)	Propranolol plus hydrochlorothiazide (Inderide)
Hydrochlorothiazide plus triamterene (Dyazide, Maxzide)	Protriptyline (Triptil, Vivactil)
Imipramine (Novo-Pramine, Tofranil)	Repaglinide (Prandin)
Indapamide (Lozide, Lozol)	Simvastatin (Zocor)
Irbesartan plus hydrochlorothiazide (Avalide)	Sotalol (Betapace, Sotacor)
Labetalol (Normodyne, Tradnate)	Telmisartan plus hydrochlorothiazide (Micardis HCT, Micardis Plus)
Losartan plus hydrochlorothiazide (Hyzaar)	Thiethylperazine (Norzine, Torecan)
Lovastatin (Altocor, Mevacor)	Thioridazine (Mellaril)
Mesoridazine (Serentil)	Timolol (Apo-Timol, Blocadren Oral)
Methyclothiazide (Aquatensen, Enduron)	Tolazamide (Tolinase)
Methyldopa (Aldomet)	Tolbutamide (Apo-Tolbutamide, Orinase)
Methyldopa plus hydrochlorothiazide (Aldoril, PMS-Dopazide)	Trichlormethiazide (Metahydrin, Naqua)
Metolazone (Mykrox, Zaroxolyn)	Trifluoperazine (Stelazine)
Metoprolol (Betaloc, Lopressor)	Trimipramine (Apo-Trimip Rhotrimine)
Moexipril plus hydrochlorothiazide (Uniretic)	Valsartan plus hydrochlorothiazide (Diovan HCT)
Nadolol (Corgard, Novo-Nadolol)	

COPPER

A Quick Look

Because copper helps the body absorb iron and manufacture hemoglobin, this little-regarded mineral is absolutely vital to health.

The Whole Story

Way back in 400 B.C., the Greek physician Hippocrates used copper compounds to treat lung disease and other ailments. Copper continued to be used well into the eighteenth century, when it fell out of favor because it didn't seem to be curing many people—and could be dangerous.

In the early part of the twentieth century, medical researchers learned that copper, which is found throughout the body, especially in the brain, heart, kidneys, and liver, is important for health maintenance. As a member of many enzyme systems, copper helps the body build and maintain the myelin sheaths that protect nerve fibers; build collagen; and defend against free-radical damage. It's also necessary for the absorption of iron in the intestinal tract and for the production of hemoglobin, the protein that carries oxygen within the red blood cells.

When You Run Short of Copper

A deficiency can cause elevated blood pressure, damage to the blood vessels and skin, anemia, increased susceptability to infections, and bone damage.

Daily Requirement

The RDA for copper is 900 mcg per day for men and women ages 19 and up.

Safety and Side Effects

The Tolerable Upper Intake Level (UL) of copper for men and women ages 19 and up is 10,000 mcg per day. With Wilson's disease, a buildup of copper can damage the liver and nerve cells.

Some Good Sources of Copper

FOOD	SERVING SIZE	MCG COPPER
Beef liver, cooked	1 oz	1,265
Oysters, cooked	1 medium	670
Cashews	1 oz	629
Crab, meat, cooked	3 oz	624
Clams, cooked	3 oz	585
Sunflower seeds	1 oz	519
Lentils, cooked	1 cup	497
Hazelnuts	1 oz	496
Mushrooms, raw, sliced	1 cup	344
Almonds	1 oz	332

Drugs That Interfere with Copper

Delavirdine (Rescriptor)	Stavudine (Zerit)
Didanosine (Videx, Videx EC)	Zalcitabine (Hivid)
Ethambutol (Myambutol)	Zidovudine (Apo-Zidovudine)
Lamivudine (Epivir)	Zidovudine plus lamivudine (AZT + 3TC)
Nevirapine (Viramune)	Zidovudine plus lamivudine plus abacavir (Trizivir)
Penicillamine (Cuprimine, Depen)	

FOLIC ACID (FOLATE)

A Quick Look

Folic acid is a B vitamin that helps the body manufacture and maintain new cells and protects cells against potentially cancerous changes.

The Whole Story

Folic acid leapt to prominence in the first half of the twentieth century, when researchers discovered that it could prevent the anemia that often occurred during pregnancy.

Folic acid is necessary to make red blood cells. It also aids in the production of DNA and RNA, which, in turn, are used to manufacture new cells. Because pregnant and lactating women produce a great many new cells, their need for folic acid increases. If they don't get enough of this important vitamin, they can develop anemia. Women deficient in folic acid who become pregnant are also more likely to give birth to premature infants or to infants with low birthweight or neural tube defects (openings in the spinal cord or brain). Folic acid is also known as a guardian of the body's cells, because it helps protect them from DNA damage that could turn them cancerous.

Your need for folic acid increases if you have difficulty absorbing the vitamin, abuse alcohol, have liver disease, are on kidney dialysis, or have certain forms of anemia.

When You Run Short of Folic Acid

There are no dramatic symptoms indicating that you've run short of folic acid. You may lack a healthy appetite, lose weight, become irritable, or suffer from diarrhea. You might develop anemia, headaches, and heart palpitations, generalized weakness, and a sore tongue. But because these vague symptoms can be caused by a variety of other problems, the diagnosis of folate deficiency can be difficult to make.

What the Research Shows

Growing evidence suggests that folic acid may do more than help create and protect the body's cells. It may also help prevent:

- *Heart attack and stroke.* Elevated levels of an amino acid called homocysteine may increase the risk of heart attack and stroke by damaging the coronary arteries and/or encouraging blood clots. A lack of folic acid (or vitamin B_6 or vitamin B_{12}) can push homocysteine levels up, so some experts believe that taking folic acid can guard against heart attacks and strokes.
- *Cancer.* A number of studies looking at large population groups have found that low levels of folic acid in the diet are associated with an increased risk of cancer of the breast, colon, and pancreas. This is not surprising, because folic acid does help guard cells against potentially cancerous changes. Further research will show whether getting more folic acid in the diet or taking folic acid supplements will reduce the risk of developing these cancers.

Some Good Sources of Folic Acid

Folic acid is found in spinach and green leafy vegetables; dried peas and beans; some vegetables and fruits; and fortified grains and cereals.

FOOD	SERVING SIZE	MCG FOLIC ACID
Beef liver, braised	3 oz	185
Breakfast cereals, fortified	¾ cup	100
Spinach, frozen, boiled	½ cup	100
Great northern beans, boiled	½ cup	90
Asparagus, boiled	4 spears	85
Wheat germ, toasted	¼ cup	80
Orange juice	¾ cup	70
Turnip greens, frozen, boiled	½ cup	65
Vegetarian baked beans, canned	1 cup	60
Broccoli, chopped, frozen, cooked	½ cup	50

Daily Requirement

The RDA for folate is 400 mcg per day for adult men and women.

Safety and Side Effects

The Tolerable Upper Intake Level (UL) for adult men and women is 1,000 mcg folate. The vitamin is considered to be very nontoxic. However, taking more than 1,000 mcg folate per day may worsen nerve damage associated with a deficiency of vitamin B_{12}. Much higher doses of 15 mg per day may damage the central nervous system.

Drugs That Interfere with Folate

Aluminum hydroxide (Amphojel, Dialume)	Diflorasone (Florone, Maxiflor)
Aluminum hydroxide plus magnesium carbonate (Gaviscon Liquid)	Diflunisal (Dolobid, Apo-Diflunisal)
Aluminum hydroxide plus magnesium hydroxide (Maalox, Mylanta)	Doxycycline (Monodox, Vibramycin)
Aluminum hydroxide plus magnesium hydroxide plus simethicone (Mylanta Liquid)	Erythromycin (Erythrocin, Staticin)
Aluminum hydroxide plus magnesium trisilicate (Gaviscon Tablet)	Ethosuximide (Zarontin)
Amiloride (Midamor)	Ethotoin (Peganone)
Aminosalicylic acid (Paser, Sodium PAS)	Etodolac (Gen-Etodolac, Lodine)
Aspirin (Anacin, Novasen)	Famotidine (Alti-Famotidine, Pepcid)
Aspirin plus dipyridamole (Aggrenox)	Fenoprofen (Nalfon)
Balsalazide (Colazal)	Flunisolide (AeroBid-M, Nasalide)
Betamethasone (Betatrex, Maxivate)	Flurbiprofen (Ansaid, Froben)
Budesonide (Entocort, Rhinocort)	Fluticasone (Cutivate, Flonase)
Butabarbital (Butalan, Butisol)	Fosphenytoin (Cerebyx)
Butalbital plus acetaminophen plus caffeine (Esgic, Fioricet)	Glyburide plus metformin (Glucovance) Halobetasol (Ultravate)
Butalbital plus aspirin plus caffeine (Fiorinal)	Hydrochlorothiazide plus triamterene (Dyazide, Maxide)
Carbamazepine (Nu-Carbamazepine, Tegretol)	Hydrocodone plus aspirin (Azdone, Lortab ASA)
Carisoprodol plus aspirin (Soma Compound)	Hydrocortisone (Bactine, Cortef)
Carisoprodol plus aspirin plus codeine (Soma Compound with Codeine)	Ibuprofen (Advil, Motrin)
Celecoxib (Celebrex)	Indomethacin (Indocin, Nu-Indo)
Chloramphenicol (Diochloram, Pentamycetin)	Isoniazid (Laniazid Oral, PMS-Isoniazid)
Cholestyramine (LoCHOLEST, Questran)	Ketoprofen (Actron, Orudis)
Choline magnesium trisalicylate (Tricosal, Trilisate)	Ketorolac (Acular, Toradol)
Choline salicylate (Arthropan, Teejel)	Lansoprazole (Prevacid)
Cimetidine (Apo-Cimetidine, Tagamet)	Levonorgestrel (Norplant Implant, Plan B)
Colchicine	Magnesium hydroxide (Phillips' Milk of Magnesia)
Colesevelam (WelChol)	Meclofenamate (Meclomen)
Colestipol (Colestid)	Mefenamic acid (Ponstel)
Cortisone (Cortone)	Meloxicam (Mobic)
Cycloserine (Seromycin Pulvules)	Mephenytoin (Mesantoin)
Demeclocycline (Declomycin)	Mesalamine (Asacol Oral, Rowasa Rectal)
Dexamethasone (Decadron, Maxidex)	Metformin (Glucophage)
Diclofenac (Cataflam, Voltaren)	Methocarbamol plus aspirin (Robaxisal)
Diclofenac plus misoprostol (Arthrotec)	Methotrexate (Folex PFS, Rheumatrex)

Methsuximide (Celotin)	Prednisolone (Delta-Cortef, Pediapred)
Methylprednisolone (Depoject Injection, Medrol Oral)	Prednisone (Deltasone, Orasone)
Minocycline (Dynacin Oral, Minocin Oral)	Primidone (Mysoline, Sertan)
Mometasone furoate (Elocom, Nasonex)	Pseudoephedrine plus ibuprofen (Advil Cold & Sinus Caplets, Dimetapp Sinus Caplets)
Nabumetone (Relafen)	Rabeprazole (Aciphex)
Naproxen (Aleve, Naprosyn)	Ranitidine (Nu-Ranit, Zantac)
Nitrous oxide	Rofecoxib (Vioxx)
Nizatidine (Apo-Nizatidine, Axid)	Salsalate (Argesic-SA, Marthritic)
Norethindrone (Aygestin, Micronor)	Sevelamer (Renagel)
Olsalazine (Dipentum)	Sulfasalazine (Azulfidine, Salazopyrin)
Omeprazole (Losec, Prilosec)	Sulindac (Apo-Sulin, Clinoril)
Oxaprozin (Daypro)	Tetracycline (Nu-Tetra, Topicycline Topical)
Oxcarbazepine (Trileptal)	Tolmetin (Novo-Tolmetin, Tolectin)
Oxycodone plus aspirin (Oxycodan, Percodan)	Triamcinolone (Amcort, Tristoject)
Pentamidine (NebuPent Inhalation, Pentacarinat Injection)	Triamterene (Dyrenium)
Phenobarbital (Barbita, Solfoton)	Trimethoprim (Primsol, Trimpex)
Phenytoin (Dilantin, Tremytoine)	Valproic acid (Depacon, Depakote ER)
Piroxicam (Feldene, Nu-Pirox)	Zonisamide (Zonegran)

GLUTATHIONE

The Whole Story

Glutathione, the major antioxidant produced by the cells, may be more important to overall health than any other antioxidant. It plays a vital part in the body's defensive system, helping to deactivate toxins and carcinogens, keep the antioxidant vitamins C and E in their active forms, and assist immune system cells. Glutathione is also important in the manufacture and repair of DNA, synthesis of prostaglandins, production of protein, and transport of amino acids.

When You Run Short of Glutathione

A deficiency can trigger destruction of red blood cells, leading to anemia. The lack of this antioxidant is also associated with age-related macular degeneration (which can cause blindness), diabetes, Parkinson's disease, the preeclampsia seen with pregnancy, and other problems.

Daily Requirement

The Food and Nutrition Board has not set an RDA or Adequate Intake (AI) for glutathione. Glutathione itself isn't absorbed well in supplement form, so supplements will contain n-acetyl cysteine, a precursor to glutathione that is converted into the antioxidant by the body. A typical supplemental dose is 800 to 2,000 mg n-acetyl cysteine.

Safety and Side Effects

A Tolerable Upper Intake Level (UL) for glutathione has not been set.

Some Good Sources of Glutathione

Glutathione is found in vegetables, fruits, and meat.

Drugs That Interfere with Glutathione

Acetaminophen (Aspirin Free Anacin, Tylenol)	Hydrocodone plus acetaminophen (Hydrogesic, Vicodin)
Acetaminophen plus codeine (Tylenol with codeine)	Oxycodone plus acetaminophen (Endocet, Oxycocet)
Butalbital plus acetaminophen plus caffeine (Esgic, Fioricet)	Propoxyphene plus acetaminophen (Darvocet-N, Wygesic)

INOSITOL

The Whole Story

Inositol, a B vitamin manufactured by the body and (possibly) certain bacteria in the intestines, helps the body handle fats and build cell membranes.

Inositol is found in both plant and animal foods and can be synthesized by the body, so deficiencies are rare.

When You Run Short of Inositol

Low levels of inositol may be linked to eczema, hair loss, constipation, increased cholesterol levels, and eye problems. In animals, a deficiency can cause fatty liver, as well as intestinal and nerve problems.

Daily Requirement

There is no RDA or Adequate Intake (AI) for inositol.

Safety and Side Effects

The Tolerable Upper Intake Level (UL) for inositol has not been set.

Some Good Sources of Inositol

Inositol is found in fruits, vegetables, nuts, grains, organ meats, and other foods. Cantaloupe, oranges, green beans, grapefruit juice, and limes are all sources of inositol.

Drugs That Interfere with Inositol

Amikacin (Amikin)	Dirithromycin (Dynabac)
Amoxicillin (Amoxil, Novamoxin)	Doxycycline (Monodox, Vibramycin)
Ampicillin (Omnipen, Totacillin)	Erythromycin (Erythrocin, Staticin)
Azithromycin (Zithromax)	Gatofloxacin (Tequin)
Carbenicillin (Geocillin)	Gentamicin (Garamycin, Jenamicin)
Cefaclor (Ceclor)	Kanamycin (Kantrex)
Cefadroxil (Duricef)	Levofloxacin (Levaquin, Quixin Ophthalmic)
Cefamandole (Mandol)	Linezolid (Zyvox)
Cefazolin (Ancef, Kefzol)	Lithium (Carbolith, Duralith)
Cefdinir (Omnicef)	Lomefloxacin (Maxaquin)
Cefditoren (Spectracef)	Loracarbef (Lorabid)
Cefepime (Maxipime)	Meclocycline (Meclan Topical)
Cefonicid (Monocid)	Minocycline (Dynacin Oral, Minocin Oral)
Cefoperazone (Cefobid)	Moxifloxacin (Avelox)
Cefotaxime (Claforan)	Nafcillin (Nafcil Injection, Unipen Oral)
Cefotetan (Cefotan)	Nalidixic acid (NegGram)
Cefoxitin (Mefoxin)	Norfloxacin (Chibroxin Ophthalmic, Noroxin Oral)
Cefpodoxime (Vantin)	Ofloxacin (Floxin, Ocuflox Ophthalmic)
Cefprozil (Cefzil)	Penicillin G benzathine (Bicillin L-A, Permapen)
Ceftazidime (Ceptaz, Fortaz)	Penicillin G benzathine plus penicillin G procaine (Bicillin C-R)
Ceftibuten (Cedax)	Penicillin G procaine (Pfizerpen-AS, Wycillin)
Ceftizoxime (Cefizox)	Penicillin V potassium (Suspen, Truxcillin)
Ceftriaxone (Rocephin)	Piperacillin (Pipracil)
Cefuroxime (Ceftin, Kefurox)	Piperacillin plus tazobactam sodium (Zosyn)
Cephalexin (Biocef, Keftab)	Sparfloxacin (Zagam)
Cephalothin (Ceporacin)	Sulfadiazine (Coptin, Microsulfon)
Cephapirin (Cefadyl)	Sulfisoxazole (Gantrisin)
Cepharadine (Velosef)	Tetracycline (Nu-Tetra, Topicycline Topical)
Cinoxacin (Cinobac)	Ticarcillin (Ticar)
Ciprofloxacin (Ciloxan, Cipro)	Ticarcillin and clavulanate potassium (Timentin)
Clarithromycin (Biaxin, Biaxin XL)	Tobramycin (Nebcin Injection, Tobrex Ophthlamic)
Cloxacillin (Cloxapen, Nu-Cloxi)	Trimethoprim (Primsol, Trimpex)
Demeclocycline (Declomycin)	Trovafloxacin (Trovan)
Dicloxacillin (Dycill, Pathocil)	Zonisamide (Zonegran)

IRON

A Quick Look

Iron is an essential mineral that makes it possible for red blood cells to carry oxygen throughout the body.

The Whole Story

Iron plays a vital role in the body as part of the protein hemoglobin in red blood cells. The hemoglobin molecules transport oxygen from the lungs to the cells and help return carbon dioxide to the lungs to be exhaled. More than 60 percent of your body's iron resides in the hemoglobin; the rest of it is in the tissues, other proteins and enzymes, or in storage for later use.

The iron in food comes in two main forms: heme and nonheme. Heme iron, found in meat, poultry, and fish, is easily absorbed. The nonheme variety, found in plant foods, is not absorbed nearly as efficiently.

You might run short of iron if you're not taking in enough, you're losing too much from bleeding, and/or your need for the mineral increases. When that happens, you'll feel weak and tired, your performance at work or school will suffer, you'll feel cold, and your immune system will weaken. If you're pregnant, your baby will be at greater risk of premature delivery and low birthweight, and you'll be more likely to suffer from complications during delivery.

Your body is fairly good at regulating how much iron it takes in, simply absorbing more from your food when your stores run low. Unfortunately, the body is not very good at getting rid of iron—its best strategy is bleeding. This works well for menstruating women, but postmenopausal women and adult men lose very little iron and must be careful not to take in too much. An overload of iron may be stored in the heart, liver, and other organs, causing severe organ damage. That's why adult men and postmenopausal women should not take supplements containing iron except when prescribed by a physician.

Supplemental iron comes in two forms, ferrous and ferric. Ferrous iron is more readily absorbed.

When You Run Short of Iron

A deficiency can cause anemia, fatigue, shortness of breath, and dizziness.

But don't reach for an iron supplement if you feel you have a deficiency or are taking a medicine that interferes with your iron status. Check with your physician before taking iron supplements.

Daily Requirement

The RDA for iron is 8 mg per day for adult men, 18 mg per day for women ages 19 to 50, and 8 mg per day for women ages 51 and up.

Safety and Side Effects

The body excretes very little iron, so it has a moderate to high potential to cause toxic damage. Excessive amounts of iron can cause diabetes mellitus, cirrhosis of the liver, and heart damage.

The Tolerable Upper Intake Level (UL) is 45 mg iron per day for males and females ages 14 and up. For children up to the age of 14, the UL is 40 mg daily.

Some Good Sources of Iron

Here are some good sources of heme iron:

FOOD	SERVING SIZE	MG IRON
Chicken liver, cooked	3 oz	7.0
Oysters, breaded and fried	6	4.5
Beef chuck, braised	3 oz	3.2
Clams, breaded, fried	¾ cup	3.0
Beef tenderloin, roasted	3 oz	3.0

Here are some good sources of nonheme iron:

FOOD	SERVING SIZE	MG IRON
Ready-to-eat cereal, 100% fortified	¾ cup	18.0
Soybeans, mature, boiled	1 cup	8.8
Lentils, boiled	1 cup	6.6
Kidney beans, boiled	1 cup	5.2
Pinto beans, boiled	1 cup	4.6

Drugs That Interfere with Iron

Aluminum hydroxide (Amphojel, Dialume)	Aspirin plus dipyridamole (Aggrenox)
Aluminum hydroxide plus magnesium carbonate (Gaviscon Liquid)	Butalbital plus aspirin plus caffeine (Fiorinal)
Aluminum hydroxide plus magnesium hydroxide (Maalox, Mylanta)	Calcium carbonate (Alka-Mints, Tums)
Aluminum hydroxide plus magnesium hydroxide plus simethicone (Mylanta Liquid)	Carisoprodol plus aspirin (Soma Compound)
Aluminum hydroxide plus magnesium trisilicate (Gaviscon Tablet)	Carisoprodol plus aspirin plus codeine (Soma Compound with Codeine)
Aspirin (Anacin, Novasen)	Cholestyramine (LoCHOLEST, Questran)

Choline magnesium trisalicylate (Tricosal, Trilisate)	Meclocycline (Meclan Topical)
Choline salicylate (Arthropan, Teejel)	Methocarbamol plus aspirin (Robaxisal)
Cimetidine (Apo-Cimetidine, Tagamet)	Minocycline (Dynacin Oral, Minocin Oral)
Clofibrate (Atromid-S)	Neomycin (Mycifradin Sulfate Topical, Neo-Tabs Oral)
Colesevelam (WelChol)	Nizatidine (Apo-Nizatidine, Axid)
Colestipol (Colestid)	Omeprazole (Losec, Prilosec)
Demeclocycline (Declomycin)	Oxycodone plus aspirin (Oxycodan, Percodan)
Doxycycline (Monodox, Vibramycin)	Pantoprazole (Protonix)
Esomeprazole (Nexium)	Penicillamine (Cuprimine, Depen)
Famotidine (Alti-Famotidine, Pepcid)	Rabeprazole (Aciphex)
Hydrocodone plus aspirin (Azdone, Lortab ASA)	Ranitidine (Nu-Ranit, Zantac)
Indomethacin (Indocin, Nu-Indo)	Stanzolol (Winstrol)
Lansoprazole (Prevacid)	Tetracycline (Nu-Tetra, Topicycline Topical)
Magnesium hydroxide (Phillips' Milk of Magnesia)	

MAGNESIUM

A Quick Look

Magnesium is a biochemical handyman that plays a part in over 300 biochemical reactions.

The Whole Story

Every single cell in your body needs magnesium. It's used to produce energy, certain proteins, and lipids; it helps the muscles relax; and it is necessary for proper heart function. It also helps rid the body of excess ammonia, binds calcium to tooth enamel, and more.

About a third of the magnesium in your food is absorbed by your body, while the rest is excreted. The mineral can be crowded out of the intestinal absorption areas by calcium, and its absorption can also be slowed by dietary fat, phosphate, and other substances that bind to it during the digestion process and make it insoluble.

Roughly half of the magnesium in your body is inside your cells, and the other half is bound up with calcium and phosphorus in your bones. There isn't much in your bloodstream—only about 1 percent of all your magnesium—but your body makes sure that this 1 percent remains constant, drawing on the magnesium in your bones like a bank account when blood levels fall too low.

When You Run Short of Magensium

A deficiency can cause weakness, muscle tremors, personality changes, confusion, and lack of appetite. Over time, high blood pressure may develop, along with swollen gums, odd muscle movements, irregular heartbeat, and the death of parts of the heart muscle.

What the Research Shows

Scientific evidence suggests that magnesium may play a key role in controlling blood pressure and reducing the risk of heart disease and stroke.

- *Blood pressure.* A 1992 study presented in the journal *Circulation* followed 30,000 men for four years.[11] The researchers found that those with higher magnesium consumption had a lower risk of developing hypertension. The Joint National Committee on Prevention, Detection, Evaluation, and Treatment of High Blood Pressure states that getting adequate amounts of magnesium will help prevent hypertension.
- *Heart disease.* Studies looking at large groups of people have found that high levels of magnesium in the blood are associated with a lower risk of coronary artery disease. And surveys of dietary habits have found a similar link between magnesium intake and stroke: A greater intake of magnesium is associated with a lesser risk of stroke.

Daily Requirement

The RDA for magnesium is 400 mg per day for men ages 19 to 30 and 420 mg per day for men ages 31 and up. The RDA is 310 mg per day for women ages 19 to 30 and 320 mg per day for women ages 31 and up.

Safety and Side Effects

The Tolerable Upper Intake Level (UL) for *supplemental* magnesium for adult men and women is 350 mg per day. Taking too much supplemental magnesium can lead to weakness, lethargy, and diarrhea.

Some Good Sources of Magnesium

FOOD	SERVING SIZE	MG MAGNESIUM
Avocado, Florida	½ medium	103
Wheat germ, toasted	1 oz	90
Almonds, dry roasted	1 oz	86
Shredded wheat cereal	2 biscuits	80
Pumpkin seeds	½ oz	75

FOOD	SERVING SIZE	MG MAGNESIUM
Cashews, dry roasted	1 oz	73
Spinach, cooked	½ cup	65
Potato, baked with skin	2 medium	55
Soybeans, cooked	½ cup	54
Peanuts, dry roasted	1 oz	50

Drugs That Interfere with Magnesium

Acetazolamide (Apo-Acetazolamide, Diamox)	Dexamethasone (Decadron, Maxidex)
Alendronate (Fosamax)	Diflorasone (Florone, Maxiflor)
Aluminum hydroxide (Amphojel, Dialume)	Digoxin (Digitek, Lanoxin)
Aluminum hydroxide plus magnesium carbonate (Gaviscon Liquid)	Doxycycline (Monodox, Vibramycin)
Aluminum hydroxide plus magnesium hydroxide (Maalox, Mylanta)	Enalapril plus hydrochlorothiazide (Vaseretic)
Aluminum hydroxide plus magnesium hydroxide plus simethicone (Mylanta Liquid)	Enoxacin (Penetrex)
Aluminum hydroxide plus magnesium trisilicate (Gaviscon Tablet)	Ethacrynic acid (Edecrin)
Amikacin (Amikin)	Etidronate (Didronel)
Amiloride plus hydrochlorothiazide (Moduret, Nu-Amilzide)	Flucytosine (Ancobon)
Amphotericin B (Amphocin, Fungizone)	Flunisolide (AeroBid-M, Nasalide)
Arsenic trioxide (Trisenox)	Fluticasone (Cutivate, Flonase)
Atenolol plus chlorthalidone (Tenoretic)	Foscarnet (Foscavir)
Beclomethasone (Beconase, Propaderm)	Furosemide (Apo-Furosemide, Lasix)
Betamethasone (Betatrex, Maxivate)	Gemtuzumab Ozogamicin (Mylotarg)
Budesonide (Entocort, Rhinocort)	Gentamicin (Garamycin, Jenamicin)
Bumetanide (Bumex, Burinex)	Halobetasol (Ultravate)
Busulfan (Busulfex, Myleran)	Hydralazine (Apo-Hydral, Apresoline)
Calcium chloride (Calciject)	Hydralazine plus hydrochlorothiazide (Apresazide)
Candesartan plus hydrochlorothiazide (Atacand HCT)	Hydrochlorothiazide (Apo-Hydro, Esidrix)
Carboplatin (Paraplatin, Paraplatin-AQ)	Hydrochlorothiazide plus spironolactone (Aldactazide, Novo-Spirozine)
Chlorothiazide (Diuril)	Hydrochlorothiazide plus triamterene (Dyazide, Maxzide)
Chlorthalidone (Apo-Chlorthalidone, Thalitone)	Hydrocortisone (Bactine, Cortef)
Cholestyramine (LoCHOLEST, Questran)	Indapamide (Lozide, Lozol)
Cisplatin (Platinol, Platinol-AQ)	Irbesartan plus hydrochlorothiazide (Avalide)
Colchicine	Kanamycin (Kantrex)
Cortisone (Cortone)	Levonorgestrel (Norplant Implant, Plan B)
Cyclosporine (Neoral, Sandimmune)	Losartan plus hydrochlorothiazide (Hyzaar)
Demeclocycline (Declomycin)	Meclocycline (Meclan Topical)

Methyclothiazide (Aquatensen, Enduron)	Prednisone (Deltasone, Orasone)
Methyldopa plus hydrochlorothiazide (Aldoril, PMS-Dopazide)	Propranolol plus hydrochlorothiazide (Inderide)
Methylprednisolone (Depoject Injection, Medrol Oral)	Raloxifene (Evista)
Metolazone (Mykrox, Zaroxolyn)	Sodium phosphate (Fleet Enema, Fleet Phospho-Soda)
Minocycline (Dynacin Oral, Minocin Oral)	Spironolactone (Aldactone, Novospiroton)
Moexipril plus hydrochlorothiazide (Uniretic)	Streptomycin
Mometasone furoate (Elocom, Nasonex)	Tacrolimus (Prograf)
Mycophenolate (CellCept)	Telmisartan plus hydrochlorothiazide (Micardis HCT, Micardis Plus)
Neomycin (Mycifradin Sulfate Topical, Neo-Tabs Oral)	Tetracycline (Nu-Tetra, Topicycline Topical)
Norethindrone (Aygestin, Micronor)	Tobramycin (Nebcin Injection, Tobrex Ophthlamic)
Pamidronate (Aredia)	Torsemide (Demadex)
Penicillamine (Cuprimine, Depen)	Triamcinolone (Amcort, Tristoject)
Pentamidine (NebuPent Inhalation, Pentacarinat Injection)	Triamterene (Dyrenium)
Polythiazide (Renese)	Trichlormethiazide (Metahydrin, Naqua)
Potassium and sodium phosphates (K-Phos Neutral, Uro-KP-Neutral)	Valsartan plus hydrochlorothiazide (Diovan HCT)
Potassium chloride (Apo-K, Micro-K)	Voriconazole (VFEND)
Prazosin plus polythiazide (Minizide)	Zalcitabine (Hivid)
Prednisolone (Delta-Cortef, Pediapred)	Zoledronic Acid (Zometa)

MANGANESE

The Whole Story

Manganese, which gets its name from the Greek word for magic, is a trace element used in a number of enzyme systems. It helps the body metabolize carbohydrates, manufacture cholesterol, and build connective tissue, and it also serves as an antioxidant. Without manganese, insulin wouldn't work properly and the blood wouldn't clot as it should.

When You Run Short of Manganese

Other minerals can sometimes pinch hit for manganese, so the problems related to deficiency are not well known. In laboratory animals, a deficiency of manganese triggers brain abnormalities, reproduction difficulties, slow growth, and problems with bones and cartilage.

Daily Requirement

The Adequate Intake (AI) for manganese is 2.3 mg per day for men ages 19 and up and 1.8 mg per day for women ages 19 and older.

Safety and Side Effects

Manganese is considered to be safe, although we can't say with certainty how much you can take without suffering any side effects. If you inhale large amounts of the mineral—as miners might do—you may suffer from loss of appetite, impotence, headache, difficulty speaking, and other problems.

Some Good Sources of Manganese

FOOD	SERVING SIZE	MG MANGANESE
Raisin bran cereal	1 cup	1.88
Pineapple	½ cup diced	1.28
Pineapple juice	½ cup	1.24
Instant oatmeal	1 packet	1.20
Pecans	1 oz	1.12
Brown rice, cooked	½ cup	0.88
Spinach, cooked	½ cup	0.84
Almonds	1 oz	0.74
Whole wheat bread	1 slice	0.65
Peanuts	1 oz	0.59

Drugs That Interfere with Manganese

Calcium carbonate (Alka-Mints, Tums)

MELATONIN

A Quick Look

This hormone and sleep aid may one day prove to guard against cancer and premature aging.

The Whole Story

You don't get sleepy at night just because you're bored with that old rerun you've already seen six times, and you don't wake up in the morning just because the dog next door is barking. Inside the brain, in an area called the pineal gland, the hormone melatonin is being produced to regulate your sleep-wake cycle as well as the rise and fall of certain hormones.

Your blood levels of melatonin rise when it's dark, peak early in the morning, and recede during the day. Or to put it another way, more melatonin equals more sleepiness. That's why many people use this hormone to help them fall asleep, overcome jet lag, and adjust to shift changes (such as going from the morning shift to the graveyard shift).

Some studies (usually involving laboratory animals rather than humans) have suggested that melatonin may be helpful in slowing the aging process and reducing the risk of cancer. And because the hormone is produced in greater amounts once you hit puberty, some experts have suggested it could also be a libido enhancer. These are intriguing ideas, but we'll have to wait for large-scale human studies before we can say with certainty which are correct.

What the Research Shows

A spate of studies in the late 1990s suggested that melatonin might be a helpful adjunct to standard cancer treatment. That is, it might help you get through difficult chemotherapy regimens. For example:

- Eighty people with cancer of the breast, lung, or gastrointestinal tract were randomly given either chemotherapy by itself, or 20 mg per day of melatonin along with the chemotherapy.[12] Those who took the melatonin were significantly less likely to suffer from lack of energy or strength (asthenia).
- Two hundred and fifty people with cancer of the breast, lung, gastrointestinal tract, neck, or head were given either chemotherapy, or chemotherapy plus 20 mg of melatonin per day.[13] The group taking the melatonin had less weakness, inflammation of the mouth, and nerve and heart damage than those receiving chemotherapy alone.

Other studies have arrived at similar results. Perhaps, one day, melatonin will be routinely offered to people undergoing chemotherapy.

Daily Requirement

There is no daily requirement for melatonin. Supplemental dosages of melatonin may range from 0.5 to 5 mg per day.

Safety and Side Effects

We don't yet know how much melatonin can be taken without triggering side effects or for how long the hormone can be used. The typical dose of melatonin—1 to 3 mg per day—seems to be well tolerated by most people. Taking melatonin in the morning may make you less alert, and you should not use it if you're driving or doing anything else that requires you to be fully alert and focused. Melatonin can also cause headaches, dizziness, irritability, abdominal cramps, and transient feelings of depression.

Some Good Sources of Melatonin

Melatonin is manufactured in the body. Only minimal amounts of melatonin are found in food.

Drugs That Interfere with Melatonin

Acebutolol (Nu-Acebutolol, Sectral)	Fluticasone (Cutivate, Flonase)
Atenolol (Apo-Atenol, Tenormin)	Halobetasol (Ultravate)
Beclomethasone (Beconase, Propaderm)	Labetalol (Normodyne, Tradnate)
Betaxolol (Betoptic S, Kerlone)	Metoprolol (Betaloc, Lopressor)
Bisoprolol (Monocor, Zebeta)	Mometasone furoate (Elocom, Nasonex)
Budesonide (Entocort, Rhinocort)	Nadolol (Corgard, Novo-Nadolol)
Carteolol (Cartrol Oral, Ocupress Ophthalmic)	Pindolol (Visken)
Carvedilol (Coreg)	Propranolol (Inderal, Nu-Propranolol)
Diflorasone (Florone, Maxiflor)	Sotalol (Betapace, Sotacor)
Esmolol (Brevibloc)	Timolol (Apo-Timol, Blocadren Oral)
Flunisolide (AeroBid-M, Nasalide)	Valproic acid (Depacon, Depakote ER)
Fluoxetine (Prozac)	

NIACIN (VITAMIN B₃)

A Quick Look

Discovered as a cure for pellagra, niacin is a B vitamin that is used in nearly every cellular metabolic pathway in the body. Large amounts are sometimes given in the form of nicotinic acid to reduce cholesterol.

The Whole Story

Niacin was discovered in the early part of the twentieth century when a doctor from the U.S. Bureau of Health was sent to the southern United States to figure out why so many people were suffering from pellagra. Early symptoms of this disease include lack of appetite, weight loss, and weakness, which can progress to the three Ds: dementia, diarrhea, and dermatitis. The doctor soon realized that the problem was poor diet—specifically a diet that relied heavily on cornmeal, which contained little niacin.

Originally called vitamin B_3, niacin helps aid in the formation of cellular energy and the building of new compounds. It helps keep the skin, mouth, nerves, and intestines healthy and strong, and aids in the extraction of energy from carbohydrates, fat, and protein. Since the mid-1950s doctors have been using a form of niacin called nicotinic acid to reduce elevated cholesterol.

When You Run Short of Niacin

Besides the three Ds, symptoms of niacin deficiency include nausea, vomiting, headaches, and fatigue.

Daily Requirement

The RDA for niacin is 16 mg per day for men ages 19 and over and 14 mg per day for women ages 19 and up.

Safety and Side Effects

The Tolerable Upper Intake Level (UL) of niacin for men and women ages 19 and up is 35 mg niacin equivalent per day. Excessive amounts of the vitamin can cause flushing of the skin, abnormal glucose metabolism, nausea, and liver damage.

Some Good Sources of Niacin

FOOD	SERVING SIZE	MG NIACIN
Chicken breast, meat only	3 oz	11.8
Beef liver, braised	3 oz	9.1
Mackerel, canned	3 oz	8.9
Barley, pearl, dry	1 cup	7.4
Bulgur, dry, parboiled	1 cup	7.4
Salmon, canned	3 oz	6.5
Turkey, white meat	3 oz	5.8
Avocado, Florida	1	5.9
Peaches, dried	10 halves	5.7

Drugs That Interfere with Niacin

Amikacin (Amikin)	Dirithromycin (Dynabac)
Amoxicillin (Amoxil, Novamoxin)	Doxycycline (Monodox, Vibramycin)
Ampicillin (Omnipen, Totacillin)	Erythromycin (Erythrocin, Staticin)
Azithromycin (Zithromax)	Gatofloxacin (Tequin)
Carbenicillin (Geocillin)	Gentamicin (Garamycin, Jenamicin)
Cefaclor (Ceclor)	Isoniazid (Laniazid Oral, PMS-Isoniazid)
Cefadroxil (Duricef)	Kanamycin (Kantrex)
Cefamandole (Mandol)	Levofloxacin (Levaquin, Quixin Ophthalmic)
Cefazolin (Ancef, Kefzol)	Linezolid (Zyvox)
Cefdinir (Omnicef)	Lomefloxacin (Maxaquin)
Cefditoren (Spectracef)	Loracarbef (Lorabid)
Cefepime (Maxipime)	Meclocycline (Meclan Topical)
Cefonicid (Monocid)	Minocycline (Dynacin Oral, Minocin Oral)
Cefoperazone (Cefobid)	Moxifloxacin (Avelox)
Cefotaxime (Claforan)	Nafcillin (Nafcil Injection, Unipen Oral)
Cefotetan (Cefotan)	Nalidixic acid (NegGram)
Cefoxitin (Mefoxin)	Norfloxacin (Chibroxin Ophthalmic, Noroxin Oral)
Cefpodoxime (Vantin)	Ofloxacin (Floxin, Ocuflox Ophthalmic)
Cefprozil (Cefzil)	Penicillin G benzathine (Bicillin L-A, Permapen)
Ceftazidime (Ceptaz, Fortaz)	Penicillin G benzathine plus penicillin G procaine (Bicillin C-R)
Ceftibuten (Cedax)	Penicillin G procaine (Pfizerpen-AS, Wycillin)
Ceftizoxime (Cefizox)	Penicillin V potassium (Suspen, Truxcillin)
Ceftriaxone (Rocephin)	Piperacillin (Pipracil)
Cefuroxime (Ceftin, Kefurox)	Piperacillin plus tazobactam sodium (Zosyn)
Cephalexin (Biocef, Keftab)	Rifampin plus isoniazid (Rifamate)
Cephalothin (Ceporacin)	Sparfloxacin (Zagam)
Cephapirin (Cefadyl)	Sulfadiazine (Coptin, Microsulfon)
Cepharadine (Velosef)	Sulfisoxazole (Gantrisin)
Cinoxacin (Cinobac)	Tetracycline (Nu-Tetra, Topicycline Topical)
Ciprofloxacin (Ciloxan, Cipro)	Ticarcillin (Ticar)
Clarithromycin (Biaxin, Biaxin XL)	Ticarcillin and clavulanate potassium (Timentin)
Cloxacillin (Cloxapen, Nu-Cloxi)	Tobramycin (Nebcin Injection, Tobrex Ophthlamic)
Demeclocycline (Declomycin)	Trimethoprim (Primsol, Trimpex)
Dicloxacillin (Dycill, Pathocil)	Trovafloxacin (Trovan)

PHOSPHORUS

The Whole Story

Up to a pound or a pound and a half of your body weight is made up of phosphorus, most of which is combined with calcium to make your bones strong. Smaller amounts of the mineral are in your body's cells.

Phosphorus has many duties in the body. Besides keeping the bones and teeth strong, it's used to make DNA and RNA, help build muscles and strengthen cell walls, synthesize and metabolize proteins, ensure secretion of milk during breastfeeding, and maintain the proper amount of fluid in the body.

When You Run Short of Phosphorus

A deficiency can cause muscle weakness, loss of appetite, fatigue, irritability, bone pain, and rickets in children.

Daily Requirement

The RDA for phosphorus is 700 mg per day for men and women ages 19 and up.

Safety and Side Effects

The Tolerable Upper Intake Level (UL) of phosphorus for men and women ages 19 through 70 is 4,000 mg per day, and 3,000 mg per day for those 71 years and up. Excessive amounts can cause muscle spasms and upset calcium metabolism.

Some Good Sources of Phosphorus

FOOD	SERVING SIZE	MG PHOSPHORUS
Yogurt, plain nonfat	8 oz	383
Lentils, cooked	½ cup	356
Salmon, cooked	3 oz	252
Milk, skim	8 oz	247
Halibut, cooked	3 oz	242
Beef, cooked	3 oz	173
Turkey, cooked	3 oz	170
Chicken, cooked	3 oz	155
Cheese, mozzarella, part skim	1 oz	131
Peanuts	1 oz	101

Drugs That Interfere with Phosphorus

Acetazolamide (Apo-Acetazolamide, Diamox)	Indapamide (Lozide, Lozol)
Alendronate (Fosamax)	Irbesartan plus hydrochlorothiazide (Avalide)
Aluminum hydroxide (Amphojel, Dialume)	Isoniazid (Laniazid Oral, PMS-Isoniazid)
Aluminum hydroxide plus magnesium carbonate (Gaviscon Liquid)	Losartan plus hydrochlorothiazide (Hyzaar)
Aluminum hydroxide plus magnesium hydroxide (Maalox, Mylanta)	Magnesium hydroxide (Phillips' Milk of Magnesia)
Aluminum hydroxide plus magnesium hydroxide plus simethicone (Mylanta Liquid)	Magnesium oxide (Maox)
Aluminum hydroxide plus magnesium trisilicate (Gaviscon Tablet)	Magnesium sulfate (Epsom Salts)
Amiloride plus hydrochlorothiazide (Moduret, Nu-Amilzide)	Methyclothiazide (Aquatensen, Enduron)
Atenolol plus chlorthalidone (Tenoretic)	Methyldopa plus hydrochlorothiazide (Aldoril, PMS-Dopazide)
Basiliximab (Simulect)	Methylprednisolone (Depoject Injection, Medrol Oral)
Betamethasone (Betatrex, Maxivate)	Metolazone (Mykrox, Zaroxolyn)
Busulfan (Busulfex, Myleran)	Mineral oil (Fleet Mineral Oil Enema, Milkinol)
Calcium carbonate (Alka-Mints, Tums)	Moexipril plus hydrochlorothiazide (Uniretic)
Candesartan plus hydrochlorothiazide (Atacand HCT)	Mycophenolate (CellCept)
Chlorothiazide (Diuril)	Pamidronate (Aredia)
Chlorthalidone (Apo-Chlorthalidone, Thalitone)	Phenytoin (Dilantin, Tremytoine)
Cholestyramine (LoCHOLEST, Questran)	Plicamycin (Mithracin)
Cortisone (Cortone)	Polythiazide (Renese)
Dexamethasone (Decadron, Maxidex)	Prazosin plus polythiazide (Minizide)
Digoxin (Digitek, Lanoxin)	Prednisolone (Delta-Cortef, Pediapred)
Enalapril plus hydrochlorothiazide (Vaseretic)	Propranolol plus hydrochlorothiazide (Inderide)
Etidronate (Didronel)	Spironolactone (Aldactone, Novospiroton)
Fludrocortisone (Florinef)	Sucralfate (Carafate, Sulcrate)
Foscarnet (Foscavir)	Tacrolimus (Prograf)
Fosphenytoin (Cerebyx)	Telmisartan plus hydrochlorothiazide (Micardis HCT, Micardis Plus)
Furosemide (Apo-Furosemide, Lasix)	Theophylline (Elixophyllin, Uniphyl)
Hydralazine plus hydrochlorothiazide (Apresazide)	Trichlormethiazide (Metahydrin, Naqua)
Hydrochlorothiazide (Apo-Hydro, Esidrix)	Valsartan plus hydrochlorothiazide (Diovan HCT)
Hydrochlorothiazide plus spironolactone (Aldactazide, Novo-Spirozine)	Zoledronic acid (Zometa)

POTASSIUM

A Quick Look

Potassium works with other minerals to regulate your body fluids and keep the heart beating properly.

The Whole Story

Most of the potassium in the body is inside the cells, with smaller amounts in the fluid surrounding them. Together with sodium and chloride, potassium helps ensure that body fluids are properly balanced and distributed. Potassium also plays a role in muscle contraction, the manufacture of protein, and maintaining proper blood pressure and a regular heart rhythm. Although potassium is readily absorbed from food, the kidneys excrete any excess to make sure that it doesn't build up inside the body.

A lack of potassium is called hypokalemia, thanks to the British chemist who discovered potassium back in 1807 and named it kalium, which is Latin for "alkali" (nonacidic).

When You Run Short of Potassium

If you should run short of potassium, you may suffer from alterations in blood pressure, irregular heartbeat, fragile bones, diarrhea, muscle twitching, and possibly a heart attack.

Daily Requirement

The Adequate Intake (AI) for potassium for men and women ages 19 and up is 4,700 mg per day.

Safety and Side Effects

It's difficult to "overdose" on potassium from food, but it can happen with supplements. Excessive amounts can cause muscle fatigue, nausea and vomiting, irregular heartbeat, and heart attack. Large doses of potassium—in the range of 6,000 to 10,000 mg per day—have been linked to hemorrhages and obstructions in the gastrointestinal tract.

Some Good Sources of Potassium

FOOD	SERVING SIZE	MG POTASSIUM
Figs, dried	10	1,332
Avocado, California	1 medium	1,208
Papaya	1 medium	780
Banana	1 medium	550
Dates	10	541
Bulgur, parboiled	1 cup	459
Milk, skim	1 cup	408
Guava	1	256
Cantaloupe	¼ melon	251
Orange juice, fresh	½ cup	236

Drugs That Interfere with Potassium

Acetazolamide (Apo-Acetazolamide, Diamox)	Carisoprodol plus aspirin plus codeine (Soma Compound with Codeine)
Albuterol (Apo-Salvent, Proventil)	Cascara
Amikacin (Amikin)	Caspofungin (Cancidas)
Amiloride plus hydrochlorothiazide (Moduret, Nu-Amilzide)	Celecoxib (Celebrex)
Ammonium chloride	Chlorothiazide (Diuril)
Amoxicillin (Amoxil, Novamoxin)	Chlorthalidone (Apo-Chlorthalidone, Thalitone)
Amphotericin B (Amphocin, Fungizone)	Choline magnesium trisalicylate (Tricosal, Trilisate)
Ampicillin (Omnipen, Totacillin)	Choline salicylate (Arthropan, Teejel)
Arsenic trioxide (Trisenox)	Cidofovir (Vistide)
Aspirin (Anacin, Novasen)	Cisplatin (Platinol, Platinol-AQ)
Aspirin plus dipyridamole (Aggrenox)	Cloxacillin (Cloxapen, Nu-Cloxi)
Atenolol plus chlorthalidone (Tenoretic)	Colchicine
Basiliximab (Simulect)	Colchicine plus probenecid (ColBenemid)
Beclomethasone (Beconase, Propaderm)	Cortisone (Cortone)
Betamethasone (Betatrex, Maxivate)	Cyclophosphamide (Cytoxan, Neosar)
Bisacodyl (Carter's Little Pills, Dulcolax)	Cyclosporine (Neoral, Sandimmune)
Budesonide (Entocort, Rhinocort)	Denileukin diftitox (ONTAK)
Bumetanide (Bumex, Burinex)	Dexamethasone (Decadron, Maxidex)
Busulfan (Busulfex, Myleran)	Dicloxacillin (Dycill, Pathocil)
Butalbital plus aspirin plus caffeine (Fiorinal)	Diflorasone (Florone, Maxiflor)
Candesartan plus hydrochlorothiazide (Atacand HCT)	Digoxin (Digitek, Lanoxin)
Carbenicillin (Geocillin)	Digoxin immune fab (Digibind, Digi-Fab)
Carboplatin (Paraplatin, Paraplatin-AQ)	Disopyramide (Norpace, Rythmodan)
Carisoprodol plus aspirin (Soma Compound)	Enalapril plus hydrochlorothiazide (Vaseretic)

Enoxacin (Penetrex)	Methocarbamol plus aspirin (Robaxisal)
Epoprostenol (Flolan)	Methyclothiazide (Aquatensen, Enduron)
Ethacrynic acid (Edecrin)	Methyldopa plus hydrochlorothiazide (Aldoril, PMS-Dopazide)
Etidronate (Didronel)	Methylprednisolone (Depoject Injection, Medrol Oral)
Fenofibrate (Apo-Fenofibrate, TriCor)	Metolazone (Mykrox, Zaroxolyn)
Fenoldopam (Corlopam)	Mineral oil (Fleet Mineral Oil Enema, Milkinol)
Ferric gluconate (Ferrlecit)	Moexipril plus hydrochlorothiazide (Uniretic)
Fluconazole (Apo-Fluconazole, Diflucan)	Mometasone furoate (Elocom, Nasonex)
Flucytosine (Ancobon)	Mycophenolate (CellCept)
Fludrocortisone (Florinef)	Nafcillin (Nafcil Injection, Unipen Oral)
Flunisolide (AeroBid-M, Nasalide)	Neomycin (Mycifradin Sulfate Topical, Neo-Tabs Oral)
Fluticasone (Cutivate, Flonase)	Ondansetron (Zofran)
Fondaparinux (Arixtra)	Oxaliplatin (Eloxatin)
Foscarnet (Foscavir)	Oxycodone plus aspirin (Oxycodan, Percodan)
Fosphenytoin (Cerebyx)	Pamidronate (Aredia)
Furosemide (Apo-Furosemide, Lasix)	Penicillin G benzathine (Bicillin L-A, Permapen)
Gemfibrozil (Apo-Gemfibrozil, Lopid)	Pencillin G benzathine plus penicillin G procaine (Bicillin C-R)
Gemtuzumab ozogamicin (Mylotarg)	Penicillin G procaine (Pfizerpen-AS, Wycillin)
Gentamicin (Garamycin, Jenamicin)	Penicillin V potassium (Suspen, Truxcillin)
Halobetasol (Ultravate)	Piperacillin (Pipracil)
Hydralazine (Apo-Hydral, Apresoline)	Piperacillin plus tazobactam sodium (Zosyn)
Hydralazine plus hydrochlorothiazide (Apresazide)	Plicamycin (Mithracin)
Hydrochlorothiazide (Apo-Hydro, Esidrix)	Polythiazide (Renese)
Hydrocodone plus aspirin (Azdone, Lortab ASA)	Prazosin plus polythiazide (Minizide)
Hydrocortisone (Bactine, Cortef)	Prednisolone (Delta-Cortef, Pediapred)
Imatinib (Gleevec)	Prednisone (Deltasone, Orasone)
Inamrinone	Propranolol plus hydrochlorothiazide (Inderide)
Indapamide (Lozide, Lozol)	Salsalate (Argesic-SA, Marthritic)
Irbesartan plus hydrochlorothiazide (Avalide)	Sodium bicarbonate (Neut)
Itraconazole (Sporanox)	Sodium chloride
Kanamycin (Kantrex)	Sodium phosphate (Fleet Enema, Fleet Phospho-Soda)
Leflunomide (Arava)	Sodium polystyrene sulfonate (Kayexalate)
Levalbuterol (Xopenex)	Streptomycin
Levodopa (Dopar, Larodopa)	Tacrolimus (Prograf)
Levodopa and carbidopa (Sinemet, Lodosyn)	Telmisartan plus hydrochlorothiazide (Micardis HCT, Micardis Plus)
Losartan plus hydrochlorothiazide (Hyzaar)	Ticarcillin (Ticar)
Magnesium oxide (Maox)	Ticarcillin and clavulanate potassium (Timentin)
Mannitol (Osmitrol)	Tobramycin (Nebcin Injection, Tobrex Ophthlamic)
Methazolamide (MZM, Neptazane)	Torsemide (Demadex)

Triamcinolone (Amcort, Tristoject)	Valsartan plus hydrochlorothiazide (Diovan HCT) Voriconazole (VFEND)
Trichlormethiazide (Metahydrin, Naqua)	Zoledronic acid (Zometa)

RIBOFLAVIN (VITAMIN B₂)

A Quick Look

This member of the B vitamin family helps turn your food into energy that your body can use.

The Whole Story

Riboflavin—also known as vitamin B₂—helps the body release energy from food, prevent oxidative damage, manufacture hormones, keep the vision sharp, strengthen the immune system, manufacture blood cells, and maintain a healthy nervous system. Originally called vitamin G because it was important for growth, riboflavin is a fluorescent yellow substance that gives urine a bright yellow color.

When You Run Short of Riboflavin

A deficiency can cause cracks at the corners of the mouth; inflammation and soreness of the lips, mouth, and tongue; vision problems; and burning and itching of the eyes. A severe deficiency may trigger greasy scaling of the skin, depression, and other problems.

What the Research Shows

Riboflavin is being used to treat migraine headaches. Positive experience with patients is backed up by scientific studies such as one presented in the journal *Neurology* in 1998.[14] In this double-blind study, 55 people with migraines were randomly given either 400 mg riboflavin or a placebo every day for three months. Those taking the vitamin reported having fewer migraines, fewer days during which they had the headaches, and shorter migraines than those taking the placebo.

Daily Requirement

The RDA for riboflavin is 1.3 mg per day for men ages 19 and up and 1.1 mg per day for women ages 19 and over.

Safety and Side Effects

A Tolerable Upper Intake Level (UL) for riboflavin has not been set. There are no known toxic effects from high doses of riboflavin, although taking large doses for a long time may interfere with the metabolism of other B vitamins.

Some Good Sources of Riboflavin

FOOD	SERVING SIZE	MG RIBOFLAVIN
Liver, braised	3 oz	3.5
Turkey heart, cooked	1 cup	1.3
Chicken, roasted	½	0.5
Gefilte fish	3 oz	0.3
Sardines, canned	3 oz	0.3
Sweet potato, peeled, mashed	½	0.2
Spinach, raw, chopped	½ cup	0.1
Turnip greens, chopped, cooked	½ cup	0.1

Drugs That Interfere with Riboflavin

Amikacin (Amikin)	Ceftizoxime (Cefizox)
Amitriptyline (Elavil, Vanatrip)	Ceftriaxone (Rocephin)
Amoxapine (Asendin)	Cefuroxime (Ceftin, Kefurox)
Amoxicillin (Amoxil, Novamoxin)	Cephalexin (Biocef, Keftab)
Ampicillin (Omnipen, Totacillin)	Cephalothin (Ceporacin)
Azithromycin (Zithromax)	Cephapirin (Cefadyl)
Carbenicillin (Geocillin)	Cepharadine (Velosef)
Cefaclor (Ceclor)	Chlorpromazine (Thorazine)
Cefadroxil (Duricef)	Cinoxacin (Cinobac)
Cefamandole (Mandol)	Ciprofloxacin (Ciloxan, Cipro)
Cefazolin (Ancef, Kefzol)	Clarithromycin (Biaxin, Biaxin XL)
Cefdinir (Omnicef)	Clomipramine (Anafranil, Novo-Clopramine)
Cefditoren (Spectracef)	Cloxacillin (Cloxapen, Nu-Cloxi)
Cefepime (Maxipime)	Demeclocycline (Declomycin)
Cefonicid (Monocid)	Desipramine (Norpramin, PMS-Desipramine)
Cefoperazone (Cefobid)	Dicloxacillin (Dycill, Pathocil)
Cefotaxime (Claforan)	Dirithromycin (Dynabac)
Cefotetan (Cefotan)	Doxepin (Novo-Doxepin, Prudoxin)
Cefoxitin (Mefoxin)	Doxorubicin (Adriamycin, Caelyx)
Cefpodoxime (Vantin)	Doxorubicin liposomal (Doxil)
Cefprozil (Cefzil)	Doxycycline (Monodox, Vibramycin)
Ceftazidime (Ceptaz, Fortaz)	Erythromycin (Erythrocin, Staticin)
Ceftibuten (Cedax)	Fluphenazine (Modecate, Prolixin)

Gatofloxacin (Tequin)	Penicillin G procaine (Pfizerpen-AS, Wycillin)
Gentamicin (Garamycin, Jenamicin)	Penicillin V potassium (Suspen, Truxcillin)
Imipramine (Novo-Pramine, Tofranil)	Perphenazine (PMS-Perphenazine, Trilafon)
Kanamycin (Kantrex)	Piperacillin (Pipracil)
Levofloxacin (Levaquin, Quixin Ophthalmic)	Piperacillin plus tazobactam sodium (Zosyn)
Levonorgestrel (Norplant Implant, Plan B)	Prochlorperazine (Prorazin, Stemetil)
Linezolid (Zyvox)	Promethazine (Anergan, Prorex)
Lomefloxacin (Maxaquin)	Protriptyline (Triptil, Vivactil)
Loracarbef (Lorabid)	Sparfloxacin (Zagam)
Meclocycline (Meclan Topical)	Sulfadiazine (Coptin, Microsulfon)
Mesoridazine (Serentil)	Sulfisoxazole (Gantrisin)
Metoclopramide (Octamide, Relgan)	Tetracycline (Nu-Tetra, Topicycline Topical)
Minocycline (Dynacin Oral, Minocin Oral)	Thiethylperazine (Norzine, Torecan)
Moxifloxacin (Avelox)	Thioridazine (Mellaril)
Nafcillin (Nafcil Injection, Unipen Oral)	Ticarcillin (Ticar)
Nalidixic acid (NegGram)	Ticarcillin and clavulanate potassium (Timentin)
Norethindrone (Aygestin, Micronor)	Tobramycin (Nebcin Injection, Tobrex Ophthlamic)
Norfloxacin (Chibroxin Ophthalmic, Noroxin Oral)	Trifluoperazine (Stelazine)
Nortriptyline (Aventyl Hydrochloride, Pamelor)	Trimethoprim (Primsol, Trimpex)
Ofloxacin (Floxin, Ocuflox Ophthalmic)	Trimipramine (Rhotrimine, Surmontil)
Penicillin G benzathine (Bicillin L-A, Permapen)	Trovafloxacin (Trovan)
Penicillin G benzathine plus penicillin G procaine (Bicillin C-R)	

SAMe

A Quick Look

Made in the body and found in most body tissues and fluids, SAMe (pronounced "sammy") may provide relief from osteoarthritis and depression.

The Whole Story

SAMe (S-adenosyl-L-methionine) is a naturally occurring substance that the body makes from the amino acid methionine. SAMe helps the body build hormones and proteins and has other duties.

In Europe, SAMe is used to treat osteoarthritis and depression. It hasn't achieved medicinal status in the United States, as it has in some European countries, but that hasn't stopped people from using it to soothe their aching joints or their depression.

SAMe has received a thumbs-up from the Arthritis Foundation, which notes that "SAMe is an effective anti-inflammatory and analgesic" for osteoarthritis. It relieves symptoms as well as the standard pain pills (non-steroidal anti-inflammatory drugs [NSAIDs]) but is less likely to trigger gastrointestinal side effects.[15]

For depression, SAMe has performed well compared to placebo and some of the tricyclic antidepressants. This is encouraging news, but it remains to be seen how SAMe will fare when pitted head-to-head against the newer SSRIs (selective serotonin reuptake inhibitors) like Prozac.

Daily Requirement

Neither an RDA nor an Adequate Intake (AI) for SAMe has been established. Typical supplemental dosages range from 200 to 1,600 mg per day.

Safety and Side Effects

The Tolerable Upper Intake Level (UL) for SAMe has not been set. Although SAMe is generally well tolerated, it may trigger anxiety, headache, flatulence, diarrhea, and nausea in some people.

Some Good Sources of SAMe

Additional SAMe is obtained from supplements, not food.

Drugs That Interfere with SAMe

Levodopa (Dopar, Larodopa)	Levodopa and carbidopa (Sinemet, Lodosyn)

SELENIUM

A Quick Look

Selenium is an essential trace mineral with antioxidant properties.

The Whole Story

A newcomer to the nutrient list, selenium wasn't recognized as essential to human health until the 1970s. We still don't fully understand how this mineral operates in the body. But we do know that it forms part of the antioxidant enzyme called glutathione peroxidase and helps protect cells and their internal energy factories (mitochondria) from damaging oxygen radicals. This trace mineral—so-called because it's required only in small amounts—also aids in the proper function of the thyroid and the male reproductive system.

The best sources of selenium are seafood, red meat, eggs, and whole grains. The amount of selenium found in vegetables will vary according to how much of the mineral is in the soil.

When You Run Short of Selenium

A lack of selenium may cause heart damage, cataracts, and slow growth.

What the Research Shows

Studies suggest that selenium may play a key role in the prevention of cancer, heart disease, and arthritis.

- *Cancer.* Some, but not all, studies of large population groups suggest that the risk of dying from lung, prostate, colorectal, and other cancers is lower among those who have higher selenium intakes or greater amounts of the mineral in their blood.
- *Heart disease.* Some studies have linked low levels of selenium with heart disease. For example, when researchers studied some 3,000 Danish men for three years, they learned that the men with the lowest levels of selenium had a 70 percent greater risk of having a heart attack.[16]
- *Rheumatoid arthritis.* Some studies have found lower levels of selenium in the blood of people with rheumatoid arthritis. The link between selenium and this form of arthritis may be free radicals, which the body strives to keep under very tight control. It may be that these free radicals go wild and attack the joints, causing or worsening rheumatoid arthritis, and that selenium helps by destroying the errant free radicals.

Daily Requirement

The RDA for selenium is 55 mcg per day for men and women ages 19 and older.

Safety and Side Effects

The Tolerable Upper Intake Level (UL) is 400 mcg per day for adult men and women. Excessive amounts can cause hair loss, vomiting, diarrhea, irritability, and fatigue.

Some Good Sources of Selenium

Although, as noted, the amount of selenium in foods varies according to the amount in the soil, you can use this list as a general guide.

FOOD	SERVING SIZE	MCG SELENIUM
Brazil nuts, unblanched, dried	1 oz	840
Tuna, canned in oil, drained	3½ oz	78
Liver, beef or calves'	3 oz	48
Cod, cooked in dry heat	3 oz	40
Turkey breast, oven roasted	3½ oz	31
Spaghetti with meat sauce	1 cup	25
Beef chuck roast, lean, oven roasted	3 oz	23
Bread, whole wheat, enriched	2 slices	20
Oatmeal, cooked	1 cup	16
Egg, whole, raw	1 large	15

Drugs That Interfere with Selenium

Betamethasone (Betatrex, Maxivate)	Hydrocortisone (Bactine, Cortef)
Budesonide (Entocort, Rhinocort)	Methylprednisolone (Depoject Injection, Medrol Oral)
Cortisone (Cortone)	Mometasone furoate (Elocom, Nasonex)
Dexamethasone (Decadron, Maxidex)	Prednisolone (Delta-Cortef, Pediapred)
Diflorasone (Florone, Maxiflor)	Prednisone (Deltasone, Orasone)
Flunisolide (AeroBid-M, Nasalide)	Triamcinolone (Amcort, Tristoject)
Fluticasone (Cutivate, Flonase)	Valproic acid (Depacon, Depakote ER)
Halobetasol (Ultravate)	

SODIUM

The Whole Story

Normally we're concerned about consuming too much sodium in the form of sodium chloride, or table salt. But sodium is an important mineral needed to maintain the body's fluid balance, transmit nerve signals, allow muscles to contract, and absorb and metabolize carbohydrates. It also plays a role in regulating blood pressure.

Consuming too much sodium can contribute to hypertension in salt-sensitive people.

When You Run Short of Sodium

A lack of sodium can trigger nausea, vomiting, headache, fatigue, muscle cramps, fainting, and disorientation. Severe deficiencies can lead to seizures, brain damage, and coma.

Several drugs deplete you of sodium, but we don't recommend that you take a sodium supplement or eat extra table salt. This can be harmful to people who are salt-sensitive and possibly push blood pressure to dangerous levels, so be sure to speak to your physician before increasing your sodium intake.

Daily Requirement

The Adequate Intake (AI) for sodium is 1.5 grams per day for men and women ages 19 through 50 and 1.3 grams per day for those ages 51 and older.

Safety and Side Effects

The Tolerable Upper Intake Level (UL) of sodium for adult men and women is 2.3 grams per day. Excessive amounts may trigger elevated blood pressure in salt-sensitive people.

Sources of Sodium

Sodium is found naturally in modest amounts in many foods and in higher amounts in salty foods, processed meats, fast foods, soup, canned vegetables, and many snack foods.

Drugs That Interfere with Sodium

Acetazolamide (Apo-Acetazolamide, Diamox)	Carisoprodol plus aspirin plus codeine (Soma Compound with Codeine)
Amikacin (Amikin)	Cascara
Amiloride (Midamor)	Celecoxib (Celebrex)
Amiloride plus hydrochlorothiazide (Moduret, Nu-Amilzide)	Chlorothiazide (Diuril)
Amitriptyline (Elavil, Vanatrip)	Choline magnesium trisalicylate (Tricosal, Trilisate)
Ammonium chloride	Choline salicylate (Arthropan, Teejel)
Amphotericin B (Amphocin, Fungizone)	Cisplatin (Platinol, Platinol-AQ)
Aspirin (Anacin, Novasen)	Clomipramine (Anafranil, Novo-Clopramine)
Aspirin plus dipyridamole (Aggrenox)	Colchicine
Atenolol plus chlorthalidone (Tenoretic)	Colchicine plus probenecid (ColBenemid)
Bisacodyl (Carter's Little Pills, Dulcolax)	Cyclophosphamide (Cytoxan, Neosar)
Bumetanide (Bumex, Burinex)	Desipramine (Norpramin, PMS-Desipramine)
Butalbital plus aspirin plus caffeine (Fiorinal)	Doxepin (Novo-Doxepin, Prudoxin)
Candesartan plus hydrochlorothiazide (Atacand HCT)	Enalapril plus hydrochlorothiazide (Vaseretic)
Captopril (Capoten, Novo-Captopril)	Esomeprazole (Nexium)
Carbamazepine (Nu-Carbamazepine, Tegretol)	Ethacrynic acid (Edecrin)
Carboplatin (Paraplatin, Paraplatin-AQ)	Flucytosine (Ancobon)
Carisoprodol plus aspirin (Soma Compound)	Fosinopril (Monopril)

Furosemide (Apo-Furosemide, Lasix)	Mycophenolate (CellCept)
Gentamicin (Garamycin, Jenamicin)	Neomycin (Mycifradin Sulfate Topical, Neo-Tabs Oral)
Glimepiride (Amaryl)	Nortriptyline (Aventyl Hydrochloride, Pamelor)
Glipizide (Glucotrol)	Omeprazole (Losec, Prilosec)
Glyburide (DiaBeta, Glynase)	Oxcarbazepine (Trileptal)
Glyburide plus metformin (Glucovance)	Oxycodone plus aspirin (Oxycodan, Percodan)
Haloperidol (Haldol, Haldol Decanoate)	Polythiazide (Renese)
Hydralazine plus hydrochlorothiazide (Apresazide)	Prazosin plus polythiazide (Minizide)
Hydrochlorothiazide (Apo-Hydro, Esidrix)	Propranolol plus hydrochlorothiazide (Inderide)
Hydrochlorothiazide plus spironolactone (Aldactazide, Novo-Spirozine)	Protriptyline (Triptil, Vivactil)
Hydrochlorothiazide plus triamterene (Dyazide, Maxzide)	Sodium phosphate (Fleet Enema, Fleet Phospho-Soda)
Hydrocodone plus aspirin (Azdone, Lortab ASA)	Spironolactone (Aldactone, Novospiroton)
Imipramine (Novo-Pramine, Tofranil)	Telmisartan plus hydrochlorothiazide (Micardis HCT, Micardis Plus)
Indapamide (Lozide, Lozol)	Tobramycin (Nebcin Injection, Tobrex Ophthlamic)
Interferon Alfa 2a (Roferon-A)	Torsemide (Demadex)
Irbesartan plus hydrochlorothiazide (Avalide)	Trichlormethiazide (Metahydrin, Naqua)
Losartan plus hydrochlorothiazide (Hyzaar)	Trimethoprim (Primsol, Trimpex)
Methocarbamol plus aspirin (Robaxisal)	Trimipramine (Rhotrimine, Surmontil)
Methyclothiazide (Aquatensen, Enduron)	Valproic acid (Depacon, Depakote ER)
Methyldopa plus hydrochlorothiazide (Aldoril, PMS-Dopazide)	Valsartan plus hydrochlorothiazide (Diovan HCT)
Metolazone (Mykrox, Zaroxolyn)	Zalcitabine (Hivid)
Moexipril plus hydrochlorothiazide (Uniretic)	

THIAMIN (VITAMIN B₁)

A Quick Look

Also known as vitamin B_1, thiamin helps the body extract energy from food.

The Whole Story

In the beginning, there was only vitamin B. Then researchers discovered that what they thought was one substance was actually many. As the various members of the B family of vitamins were isolated, they were named B_1, B_2, B_3 and so on. Today, B_1 is generally called thiamin.

Thiamin helps the body break down and convert carbohydrates, fats, and protein into energy and is necessary for proper nerve function.

The classic thiamin deficiency disease is beriberi, which literally means "I can't, I can't..." in Sinhalese, the language of Sri Lanka. Symptoms of beriberi include irritability, loss of appetite, weakness, poor coordination, tingling sensations throughout the body, and pain in the calves. Beriberi often arises in areas where the diet is based on white rice, which has been stripped of its bran and germ layer (and therefore its thiamin). Thiamin is not stored in any significant amount in the body, so thiamin-rich foods should be eaten every day.

When You Run Short of Thiamin

A deficiency can cause beriberi, depression, fatigue, poor appetite, and gastrointestinal problems.

Daily Requirement

The RDA for thiamin is 1.2 mg per day for men ages 19 and up and 1.1 mg per day for women ages 19 and over.

Safety and Side Effects

There are no known toxic effects of consuming up to 200 mg per day of supplemental thiamin, although excessive amounts of this vitamin may interfere with the absorption of other B vitamins. A Tolerable Upper Intake Level (UL) for thiamin has not been set.

Some Good Sources of Thiamin

FOOD	SERVING SIZE	MG THIAMIN
Sunflower seeds, dried	1 oz	0.7
Orange juice, frozen, reconstituted	¾ cup	0.6
Bulgur, parboiled	1 cup dried	0.5
Spinach noodles, cooked	1 cup	0.4
Pine nuts, dried	1 oz	0.4
Hickory nuts, dried	1 oz	0.3
Yellow corn, boiled	1 ear	0.2
Potato, baked	7 oz	0.2

Drugs That Interfere with Thiamin

Amikacin (Amikin)	Fluorouracil (Adrucil, Carac)
Amoxicillin (Amoxil, Novamoxin)	Fosphenytoin (Cerebyx)
Ampicillin (Omnipen, Totacillin)	Furosemide (Apo-Furosemide, Lasix)
Azithromycin (Zithromax)	Gatofloxacin (Tequin)
Bumetanide (Bumex, Burinex)	Gentamicin (Garamycin, Jenamicin)
Carbenicillin (Geocillin)	Kanamycin (Kantrex)
Cefaclor (Ceclor)	Lansoprazole (Prevacid)
Cefadroxil (Duricef)	Levofloxacin (Levaquin, Quixin Ophthalmic)
Cefamandole (Mandol)	Linezolid (Zyvox)
Cefazolin (Ancef, Kefzol)	Lomefloxacin (Maxaquin)
Cefdinir (Omnicef)	Loracarbef (Lorabid)
Cefditoren (Spectracef)	Meclocycline (Meclan Topical)
Cefepime (Maxipime)	Minocycline (Dynacin Oral, Minocin Oral)
Cefonicid (Monocid)	Moxifloxacin (Avelox)
Cefoperazone (Cefobid)	Nafcillin (Nafcil Injection, Unipen Oral)
Cefotaxime (Claforan)	Nalidixic acid (NegGram)
Cefotetan (Cefotan)	Nizatidine (Apo-Nizatidine, Axid)
Cefoxitin (Mefoxin)	Norfloxacin (Chibroxin Ophthalmic, Noroxin Oral)
Cefpodoxime (Vantin)	Ofloxacin (Floxin, Ocuflox Ophthalmic)
Cefprozil (Cefzil)	Omeprazole (Losec, Prilosec)
Ceftazidime (Ceptaz, Fortaz)	Pantoprazole (Protonix)
Ceftibuten (Cedax)	Penicillin G benzathine (Bicillin L-A, Permapen)
Ceftizoxime (Cefizox)	Penicillin G benzathine plus penicillin G procaine (Bicillin C-R)
Ceftriaxone (Rocephin)	Penicillin G procaine (Pfizerpen-AS, Wycillin)
Cefuroxime (Ceftin, Kefurox)	Penicillin V potassium (Suspen, Truxcillin)
Cephalexin (Biocef, Keftab)	Phenytoin (Dilantin, Tremytoine)
Cephalothin (Ceporacin)	Piperacillin (Pipracil)
Cephapirin (Cefadyl)	Piperacillin plus tazobactam sodium (Zosyn)
Cepharadine (Velosef)	Rabeprazole (Aciphex)
Cimetidine (Apo-Cimetidine, Tagamet)	Ranitidine (Nu-Ranit, Zantac)
Cinoxacin (Cinobac)	Sparfloxacin (Zagam)
Ciprofloxacin (Ciloxan, Cipro)	Sulfadiazine (Coptin, Microsulfon)
Clarithromycin (Biaxin, Biaxin XL)	Sulfisoxazole (Gantrisin)
Cloxacillin (Cloxapen, Nu-Cloxi)	Tetracycline (Nu-Tetra, Topicycline Topical)
Demeclocycline (Declomycin)	Theophylline (Elixophyllin, Uniphyl)
Dicloxacillin (Dycill, Pathocil)	Ticarcillin (Ticar)
Digoxin (Digitek, Lanoxin)	Ticarcillin and clavulanate potassium (Timentin)
Dirithromycin (Dynabac)	Tobramycin (Nebcin Injection, Tobrex Ophthlamic)
Doxycycline (Monodox, Vibramycin)	Torsemide (Demadex)
Erythromycin (Erythrocin, Staticin)	Trimethoprim (Primsol, Trimpex)
Ethacrynic acid (Edecrin)	Trovafloxacin (Trovan)
Famotidine (Alti-Famotidine, Pepcid)	Zonisamide (Zonegran)

TYROSINE

The Whole Story

Tyrosine is a nonessential amino acid, which means that we don't need to get it from our food because it's synthesized in our bodies. Tyrosine is used to make dopamine, serotonin, and other mood-regulating substances. It also participates in the manufacture and regulation of adrenal, pituitary, and thyroid hormones, as well as in the making of enkephalins, part of the body's built-in pain relief system.

When You Run Short of Tyrosine

A deficiency of tyrosine had been linked to depression, sluggish thyroid, low body temperature, and low blood pressure.

Daily Requirement

There is no daily requirement for tyrosine. Typical supplemental dosages range up to 1,000 mg per day.

Safety and Side Effects

The Tolerable Upper Intake Level (UL) for tyrosine has not been determined.

Some Good Sources of Tyrosine

Tyrosine is found in soy and soy products, turkey, chicken, peanuts, almonds, fish, bananas, milk, cheese, cottage cheese, pumpkin seeds, and other foods.

Drugs That Interfere with Tyrosine

Estradiol and ethynodiol diacetate (Demulen, Zovia)	Ethinyl estradiol and norethindrone (Brevicon, Loestrin, Modicon)
Ethinyl estradiol and desogestrel (Apri, Cyclessa, Marvelon)	Ethinyl estradiol and norgestimate (Ortho-Cyclen, Tri-Cyclen)
Ethinyl estradiol and levonorgestrel (Levlen, PREVEN, Triphasil)	Ethinyl estradiol and norgestrel (Cryselle, Ogestrel, Ovral)

VITAMIN B$_6$

A Quick Look

A member of the B family of vitamins, B$_6$ helps keep the red blood cells, immune system, and other part of the body in good working order.

The Whole Story

Also known as pyridoxine, vitamin B$_6$ is actually a group of related compounds with a wide variety of biochemical duties. Among other things, it helps:

- Synthesize proteins
- Extract energy from carbohydrates, protein, and fats
- Manufacture the hemoglobin the red blood cells need to carry oxygen
- Keep the nervous system running smoothly
- Keep the thymus, spleen, and lymph nodes healthy
- Keep your blood sugar (glucose) in the proper range
- Transport and distribute selenium in the body
- Convert the amino acid tryptophan into the vitamin niacin

When You Run Short of Vitamin B$_6$

A lack of vitamin B$_6$ causes depression, scaly skin, anemia, and a weakened immune system. These rather vague symptoms can be difficult to connect to a deficiency because they can also be caused by many other illnesses and conditions. Studies looking at large groups of people have linked low levels of vitamin B$_6$ in the blood to an increased risk of cardiovascular disease.

What the Research Shows

Vitamin B$_6$ has been proposed as a treatment for the symptoms of PMS, for carpal tunnel syndrome, asthma, and other ailments. Some of the more exciting research findings have to do with the vitamin's link to better heart health. For example:

- A paper appearing in the *Journal of the American Medical Association* presented results from the large-scale Nurses Health Study, which tracked the health of some eighty-thousand women for more than a decade.[17] Those who got the largest amounts of vitamin B$_6$ and folic acid from their foods and supplements had the lowest risk of suffering a heart attack. The researchers noted that ". . . intake of folate and vitamin B$_6$

above the current recommended dietary allowance may be important in the primary prevention of [coronary heart disease] among women."
- The Atherosclerosis Risk in Communities Study tracked middle-aged men and women for slightly over three years and found that having more vitamin B$_6$ in the blood led to a lower risk of heart disease.[18]

These and other studies suggest that the vitamin may be an important part of any healthy-heart program.

Daily Requirement

The RDA for vitamin B$_6$ is 1.3 mg per day for males ages 19 to 50 and 1.7 for males ages 51 and up; for women the numbers are 1.3 mg per day for those ages 19 to 50 and 1.5 for those over 50.

Safety and Side Effects

The Tolerable Upper Intake Level (UL) of vitamin B$_6$ for men and women ages 19 and up is 100 mg per day. Taking in too much of the vitamin via supplements can damage the nerves in the arms and legs.

Some Good Sources of Vitamin B$_6$

FOOD	SERVING SIZE	MG VITAMIN B$_6$
Potato, flesh and skin, baked	1 medium	0.70
Banana	1 medium	0.68
Garbanzo beans, canned	½ cup	0.57
Chicken breast, cooked, meat only	½ breast	0.52
Oatmeal, instant, fortified	1 packet	0.42
Pork loin, lean meat only, cooked	3 oz	0.42
Mackerel, cooked	3 oz	0.40
Snapper, cooked	3 oz	0.40
Wheat germ, toasted	¼ cup	0.30
Walnuts	1 oz	0.10

Drugs That Interfere with Vitamin B$_6$

Amikacin (Amikin)	Budesonide (Entocort, Rhinocort)
Amoxicillin (Amoxil, Novamoxin)	Bumetanide (Bumex, Burinex)
Ampicillin (Omnipen, Totacillin)	Carbenicillin (Geocillin)
Azithromycin (Zithromax)	Cefaclor (Ceclor)
Beclomethasone (Beconase, Propaderm)	Cefadroxil (Duricef)
Betamethasone (Betatrex, Maxivate)	Cefamandole (Mandol)

Cefazolin (Ancef, Kefzol)	Gentamicin (Garamycin, Jenamicin)
Cefdinir (Omnicef)	Hydralazine (Apo-Hydral, Apresoline)
Cefditoren (Spectracef)	Hydralazine plus hydrochlorothiazide (Apresazide)
Cefepime (Maxipime)	Hydrochlorothiazide plus triamterene (Dyazide, Maxzide)
Cefonicid (Monocid)	Hydrocortisone (Bactine, Cortef)
Cefoperazone (Cefobid)	Isoniazid (Laniazid Oral, PMS-Isoniazid)
Cefotaxime (Claforan)	Kanamycin (Kantrex)
Cefotetan (Cefotan)	Levofloxacin (Levaquin, Quixin Ophthalmic)
Cefoxitin (Mefoxin)	Levonorgestrel (Norplant Implant, Plan B)
Cefpodoxime (Vantin)	Linezolid (Zyvox)
Cefprozil (Cefzil)	Lomefloxacin (Maxaquin)
Ceftazidime (Ceptaz, Fortaz)	Loracarbef (Lorabid)
Ceftibuten (Cedax)	Meclocycline (Meclan Topical)
Ceftizoxime (Cefizox)	Methyldopa plus hydrochlorothiazide (Aldoril, PMS-Dopazide)
Ceftriaxone (Rocephin)	Methylprednisolone (Depoject Injection, Medrol Oral)
Cefuroxime (Ceftin, Kefurox)	Minocycline (Dynacin Oral, Minocin Oral)
Cephalexin (Biocef, Keftab)	Mometasone furoate (Elocom, Nasonex)
Cephalothin (Ceporacin)	Moxifloxacin (Avelox)
Cephapirin (Cefadyl)	Nafcillin (Nafcil Injection, Unipen Oral)
Cepharadine (Velosef)	Nalidixic acid (NegGram)
Cinoxacin (Cinobac)	Neomycin (Mycifradin Sulfate Topical, Neo-Tabs Oral)
Ciprofloxacin (Ciloxan, Cipro)	Norethindrone (Aygestin, Micronor)
Clarithromycin (Biaxin, Biaxin XL)	Norfloxacin (Chibroxin Ophthalmic, Noroxin Oral)
Cloxacillin (Cloxapen, Nu-Cloxi)	Ofloxacin (Floxin, Ocuflox Ophthalmic)
Cortisone (Cortone)	Penicillamine (Cuprimine, Depen)
Cycloserine (Seromycin Pulvules)	Penicillin G benzathine (Bicillin L-A, Permapen)
Demeclocycline (Declomycin)	Penicillin G benzathine plus penicillin G procaine (Bicillin C-R)
Dexamethasone (Decadron, Maxidex)	Penicillin G procaine (Pfizerpen-AS, Wycillin)
Dicloxacillin (Dycill, Pathocil)	Penicillin V potassium (Suspen, Truxcillin)
Dirithromycin (Dynabac)	Phenelzine (Nardil)
Doxycycline (Monodox, Vibramycin)	Phenobarbital (Barbita, Solfoton)
Enalapril plus hydrochlorothiazide (Vaseretic)	Piperacillin (Pipracil)
Enoxacin (Penetrex)	Piperacillin plus tazobactam sodium (Zosyn)
Erythromycin (Erythrocin, Staticin)	Prednisolone (Delta-Cortef, Pediapred)
Ethacrynic acid (Edecrin)	Prednisone (Deltasone, Orasone)
Fluorouracil (Adrucil)	Primidone (Mysoline, Sertan)
Flunisolide (AeroBid-M, Nasalide)	Raloxifene (Evista)
Fluticasone (Cutivate, Flonase)	Rifampin plus isoniazid (Rifamate)
Furosemide (Apo-Furosemide, Lasix)	Sparfloxacin (Zagam)
Gatofloxacin (Tequin)	Sulfadiazine (Coptin, Microsulfon)

Sulfasalazine (Azulfidine, Salazopyrin)	Tobramycin (Nebcin Injection, Tobrex Ophthlamic)
Sulfisoxazole (Gantrisin)	Torsemide (Demadex)
Tetracycline (Nu-Tetra, Topicycline Topical)	Triamcinolone (Amcort, Tristoject)
Theophylline (Elixophyllin, Uniphyl)	Trimethoprim (Primsol, Trimpex)
Ticarcillin (Ticar)	Trovafloxacin (Trovan)
Ticarcillin and clavulanate potassium (Timentin)	

VITAMIN B$_{12}$

A Quick Look

Vitamin B$_{12}$ is necessary for healthy nerves and red blood cells.

The Whole Story

In the 1800s, researchers in England discovered a form of anemia that reduced the production of red blood cells, damaged the nervous system, and caused death within two to five years. They called this disease pernicious anemia ("pernicious" means "gradually causing a harmful effect"). But the cause of this anemia wasn't found until the 1940s, when medical researchers isolated a substance—in liver—that cured the anemia. It was named vitamin B$_{12}$, but is also called cobalamin because it contains cobalt.

We need to get vitamin B$_{12}$ from our food, but the body can't absorb the B$_{12}$ unless it's released from the food by stomach acid and then combined with a substance produced by the stomach called intrinsic factor. If you lack sufficient intrinsic factor, you may develop pernicious anemia because your body can't take up enough B$_{12}$, even if your food contains good amounts of this vitamin.

When You Run Short of Vitamin B$_{12}$

A lack of B$_{12}$ interrupts the maturation of red blood cells in the bone marrow and causes fever, loss of appetite, weight loss, weakness, and numbness and tingling in the extremities. Symptoms of nerve destruction can occur about three years after the onset of pernicious anemia, and a prolonged B$_{12}$ deficiency can cause paralysis and signs of dementia.

Daily Requirement

The Adequate Intake (AI) for vitamin B$_{12}$ is 2.4 mcg per day for adult men and women.

Safety and Side Effects

Vitamin B$_{12}$ is felt to be very safe. According to the National Academy of Sciences' Institute of Medicine, "no adverse effects have been associated with excess vitamin B$_{12}$ intake from food and supplements in healthy individuals."[19] A Tolerable Upper Intake Level (UL) for vitamin B$_{12}$ has not been set.

Some Good Sources of Vitamin B$_{12}$

Meat and other foods from animals are the only foods that contain good amounts of vitamin B$_{12}$. This means that strict vegetarians who eat no foods of animal origin are at risk of developing a deficiency.

FOOD	SERVING SIZE	MCG VITAMIN B$_{12}$
Beef liver, cooked	3 oz	60.0
Fortified breakfast cereal	$^3/_4$ cup	6.0
Rainbow trout, cooked	3 oz	5.3
Sockeye salmon, cooked	3 oz	4.9
Beef, cooked	3 oz	2.1
Haddock, cooked	3 oz	1.2
Milk	1 cup	0.9
Yogurt	8 oz	0.9
Egg	1 large	0.5
American cheese	1 oz	0.4

Drugs That Interfere with Vitamin B$_{12}$

Amikacin (Amikin)	Cefoxitin (Mefoxin)
Aminosalicylic acid (Paser, Sodium PAS)	Cefpodoxime (Vantin)
Amoxicillin (Amoxil, Novamoxin)	Cefprozil (Cefzil)
Ampicillin (Omnipen, Totacillin)	Ceftazidime (Ceptaz, Fortaz)
Azithromycin (Zithromax)	Ceftibuten (Cedax)
Carbenicillin (Geocillin)	Ceftizoxime (Cefizox)
Cefaclor (Ceclor)	Ceftriaxone (Rocephin)
Cefadroxil (Duricef)	Cefuroxime (Ceftin, Kefurox)
Cefamandole (Mandol)	Cephalexin (Biocef, Keftab)
Cefazolin (Ancef, Kefzol)	Cephalothin (Ceporacin)
Cefdinir (Omnicef)	Cephapirin (Cefadyl)
Cefditoren (Spectracef)	Cepharadine (Velosef)
Cefepime (Maxipime)	Chloramphenicol (Diochloram, Pentamycetin)
Cefonicid (Monocid)	Cholestyramine (LoCHOLEST, Questran)
Cefoperazone (Cefobid)	Cimetidine (Apo-Cimetidine, Tagamet)
Cefotaxime (Claforan)	Cinoxacin (Cinobac)
Cefotetan (Cefotan)	Ciprofloxacin (Ciloxan, Cipro)

Clarithromycin (Biaxin, Biaxin XL)	Neomycin (Mycifradin Sulfate Topical, Neo-Tabs Oral)
Clofibrate (Atromid-S)	Nevirapine (Viramune)
Cloxacillin (Cloxapen, Nu-Cloxi)	Nitrous oxide
Colchicine	Nizatidine (Apo-Nizatidine, Axid)
Colchicine plus probenecid (ColBenemid)	Norethindrone (Aygestin, Micronor)
Colesevelam (WelChol)	Norfloxacin (Chibroxin Ophthalmic, Noroxin Oral)
Colestipol (Colestid)	Ofloxacin (Floxin, Ocuflox Ophthalmic)
Cycloserine (Seromycin Pulvules)	Omeprazole (Losec, Prilosec)
Delavirdine (Rescriptor)	Pantoprazole (Protonix)
Demeclocycline (Declomycin)	Penicillin G benzathine (Bicillin L-A, Permapen)
Dicloxacillin (Dycill, Pathocil)	Penicillin G benzathine plus penicillin G procaine (Bicillin C-R)
Didanosine (Videx, Videx EC)	Penicillin G procaine (Pfizerpen-AS, Wycillin)
Dirithromycin (Dynabac)	Penicillin V potassium (Suspen, Truxcillin)
Doxycycline (Monodox, Vibramycin)	Phenobarbital (Barbita, Solfoton)
Erythromycin (Erythrocin, Staticin)	Phenytoin (Dilantin, Tremytoine)
Esomeprazole (Nexium)	Piperacillin (Pipracil)
Famotidine (Alti-Famotidine, Pepcid)	Piperacillin plus tazobactam sodium (Zosyn)
Fosphenytoin (Cerebyx)	Potassium chloride (Apo-K, Micro-K)
Gatofloxacin (Tequin)	Primidone (Mysoline, Sertan)
Gentamicin (Garamycin, Jenamicin)	Rabeprazole (Aciphex)
Glyburide plus metformin (Glucovance)	Ranitidine (Nu-Ranit, Zantac)
Isoniazid (Laniazid Oral, PMS-Isoniazid)	Sparfloxacin (Zagam)
Kanamycin (Kantrex)	Stavudine (Zerit)
Lamivudine (Epivir)	Sulfadiazine (Coptin, Microsulfon)
Lansoprazole (Prevacid)	Sulfasalazine (Azulfidine, Salazopyrin)
Levofloxacin (Levaquin, Quixin Ophthalmic)	Sulfisoxazole (Gantrisin)
Levonorgestrel (Norplant Implant, Plan B)	Tetracycline (Nu-Tetra, Topicycline Topical)
Linezolid (Zyvox)	Ticarcillin (Ticar)
Lomefloxacin (Maxaquin)	Ticarcillin and clavulanate potassium (Timentin)
Loracarbef (Lorabid)	Tobramycin (Nebcin Injection, Tobrex Ophthlamic)
Meclocycline (Meclan Topical)	Trimethoprim (Primsol, Trimpex)
Metformin (Glucophage)	Trovafloxacin (Trovan)
Methotrexate (Folex PFS, Rheumatrex)	Valproic acid (Depacon, Depakote ER)
Methyldopa (Aldomet)	Zalcitabine (Hivid)
Minocycline (Dynacin Oral, Minocin Oral)	Zidovudine (Apo-Zidovudine)
Moxifloxacin (Avelox)	Zidovudine plus lamivudine (AZT + 3TC)
Nafcillin (Nafcil Injection, Unipen Oral)	Zidovudine plus lamivudine plus abacavir (Trizivir)
Nalidixic acid (NegGram)	

VITAMIN C

A Quick Look

The "anti-scurvy" vitamin is an important antioxidant and immune-system booster.

The Whole Story

Since ancient times, sailors and others who were denied fresh fruit for several months developed a disease called scurvy. Weak and listless, those with scurvy developed bone and muscle aches, dry skin, bruises, and little red spots on their skin. Their gums swelled and bled, and they bled into their muscles. Wounds refused to heal, the whites of their eyes turned yellow-brown, their bones thinned, and they soon died.

The cure for scurvy was found and forgotten several times before the British Navy realized in the 1700s that giving their sailors lime juice could solve the problem. But it wasn't until the early part of the twentieth century that the curative factor in the lime juice was isolated and named vitamin C.

Also known as ascorbic acid, vitamin C helps the body build a number of substances, including collagen, blood vessels, tendons, ligaments, skin, muscles, bones, teeth, hormones, and neurotransmitters. It's necessary for the repair of injuries and metabolism of fats and is also believed to strengthen the immune system by increasing the production white blood cells and encouraging certain immune-system cells to attack germs. More recently, vitamin C has gained prominence as an antioxidant that deactivates dangerous free radicals and protects vitamins A and E from oxidation.

Because relatively little vitamin C is stored in the body, it's necessary to eat at least one vitamin C-rich food every day.

When You Run Short of Vitamin C

A deficiency may cause anemia, spontaneous bruising, loose teeth, and swollen and bleeding gums.

What the Research Shows

Ever since the 1970s, when Nobel Prize–winning scientist Linus Pauling published research indicating that vitamin C may help fight the common cold, this vitamin has been "hot." Although not all studies agree, and the whys and wherefores have not been completely worked out, it does appear that vitamin C can be useful in combatting a number of ailments. For example:

- *Immune system health.* Fifty-seven senior citizens hospitalized for respiratory infections were randomly given either 200 mg of vitamin C per day, or a placebo.[20] Two and four weeks after beginning the study, the patients were checked for breathlessness, cough, and X-ray evidence of chest infection. Overall, those taking the vitamin fared better than those on the placebo.
- *Heart health.* Sixteen hundred Finnish men were enrolled in a study looking at the link between vitamin C and heart disease.[21] In this group of men, who ranged in age from 42 to 60, lower levels of vitamin C in the blood were linked to a greater incidence of heart attacks.
- *Cataracts.* The link between vitamin C and cataracts was measured in over 50,000 women participating in the Nurses Health Study.[22] Among these women, who ranged in age from 45 to 67, the risk of developing cataracts was 45 percent lower in those who had been taking vitamin C supplements for at least 10 years.

Vitamin C has also been studied as a treatment for cancer and asthma, as an antioxidant, and as a means of improving your ability to exercise and engage in athletics.

Daily Requirement

The RDA for vitamin C is 90 mg per day for adult men and 75 mg per day for adult women.

Safety and Side Effects

The Tolerable Upper Intake Level (UL) of vitamin C for men and women ages 19 years old and up is 2,000 mg per day. Excessive amounts of the vitamin may cause heart damage, oxalate kidney stones, and a buildup of iron.

Some Good Sources of Vitamin C

FOOD	SERVING SIZE	MG VITAMIN C
Papaya	1 medium	188
Guava, raw	1 medium	165
Red pepper, raw	1 medium	141
Cantaloupe	½ melon	113
Black currants	½ cup	101
Green pepper	1	97
Kiwifruit	1	75
Orange	1	70
Broccoli, cooked	½ cup	49
Cauliflower, cooked	½ cup	34

Drugs That Interfere with Vitamin C

Aspirin (Anacin, Novasen)	Fluticasone (Cutivate, Flonase)
Aspirin plus dipyridamole (Aggrenox)	Furosemide (Apo-Furosemide, Lasix)
Beclomethasone (Beconase, Propaderm)	Halobetasol (Ultravate)
Betamethasone (Betatrex, Maxivate)	Hydrocodone plus aspirin (Azdone, Lortab ASA)
Budesonide (Entocort, Rhinocort)	Hydrocortisone (Bactine, Cortef)
Bumetanide (Bumex, Burinex)	Levonorgestrel (Norplant Implant, Plan B)
Butalbital plus aspirin plus caffeine (Fiorinal)	Methocarbamol plus aspirin (Robaxisal)
Carisoprodol plus aspirin (Soma Compound)	Methylprednisolone (Depoject Injection, Medrol Oral)
Carisoprodol plus aspirin plus codeine (Soma Compound with Codeine)	Minocycline (Dynacin Oral, Minocin Oral)
Choline magnesium trisalicylate (Tricosal, Trilisate)	Mometasone furoate (Elocom, Nasonex)
Choline salicylate (Arthropan, Teejel)	Norethindrone (Aygestin, Micronor)
Cortisone (Cortone)	Oxycodone plus aspirin (Oxycodan, Percodan)
Demeclocycline (Declomycin)	Prednisolone (Delta-Cortef, Pediapred)
Dexamethasone (Decadron, Maxidex)	Prednisone (Deltasone, Orasone)
Diflorasone (Florone, Maxiflor)	Tetracycline (Nu-Tetra, Topicycline Topical)
Doxycycline (Monodox, Vibramycin)	Torsemide (Demadex)
Ethacrynic acid (Edecrin)	Triamcinolone (Amcort, Tristoject)
Flunisolide (AeroBid-M, Nasalide)	

VITAMIN D

A Quick Look

Vitamin D, the "sunshine vitamin" that can be made by the body when the skin is exposed to sunlight, regulates calcium usage and bone metabolism.

The Whole Story

Vitamin D functions both as a vitamin and a hormone. It helps with the absorption of calcium from food and the maintenance of the proper amounts of calcium and phosphorus in the blood. Vitamin D also works with other vitamins, minerals, and hormones for proper bone formation, and can help ward off osteoporosis (the thinning and hollowing of the bones).

The classic vitamin D deficiency disease in children is rickets, characterized by malformed bones—especially bowed legs that seem to be giving way under the strain of supporting the body. Osteomalacia (which means "soft bones") is the adult form of rickets, and is characterized by bones that are weak, porous, and easily fractured.

A lack of vitamin D can be the result of either too little of the vitamin in the diet or not enough exposure to the sun. Our bodies have the ability to make vitamin D when ultraviolet light strikes the skin and reacts with a substance called 7-dehydrocholesterol. But those who get little vitamin D in their diets *and* are not exposed to much sunlight can develop a deficiency. In Boston, for example, between November and February there isn't usually enough sunlight to ensure that those who live there will manufacture enough vitamin D. Luckily, this is not usually a problem, because most milk is fortified with vitamin D. Fatty fish is another excellent source.

When You Run Short of Vitamin D

A deficiency can cause the bone problems called osteomalacia in adults and rickets in children.

Daily Requirement

The Adequate Intake (AI) for vitamin D is 200 IU per day for men and women ages 19 to 50; 400 IU per day for men and women ages 51 to 69; and 600 IU per day for men and women age 70 years and older.

Safety and Side Effects

The Tolerable Upper Intake Level (UL) of vitamin D for adult men and women is 2,000 IU. Taking in too much vitamin D can lead to nausea, vomiting, weakness, weight loss, irregular heartbeat, and confusion and other mental changes.

Some Good Sources of Vitamin D

With the exception of fatty fish, there aren't many good food sources of vitamin D, so the vitamin is often added to milk, breakfast cereals, and other foods.

FOOD	SERVING SIZE	IU VITAMIN D
Salmon, cooked	3½ oz	360
Mackerel, cooked	3½ oz	345
Sardines, canned in oil, drained	3½ oz	270
Eel, cooked	3½ oz	200
Milk, vitamin D fortified	1 cup	98

Drugs That Interfere with Vitamin D

Aluminum hydroxide (Amphojel, Dialume)	Hydrochlorothiazide (Apo-Hydro, Esidrix)
Aluminum hydroxide plus magnesium carbonate (Gaviscon Liquid)	Hydrocortisone (Bactine, Cortef)
Aluminum hydroxide plus magnesium hydroxide (Maalox, Mylanta)	Isoniazid (Laniazid Oral, PMS-Isoniazid)
Aluminum hydroxide plus magnesium hydroxide plus simethicone (Mylanta Liquid)	Magnesium hydroxide (Phillips' Milk of Magnesia)
Aluminum hydroxide plus magnesium trisilicate (Gaviscon Tablet)	Mephenytoin (Mesantoin)
Beclomethasone (Beconase, Propaderm)	Methsuximide (Celotin)
Betamethasone (Betatrex, Maxivate)	Methylprednisolone (Depoject Injection, Medrol Oral)
Budesonide (Entocort, Rhinocort)	Mineral oil (Fleet Mineral Oil Enema, Milkinol)
Butabarbital (Butalan, Butisol)	Mometasone furoate (Elocom, Nasonex)
Butalbital plus acetaminophen plus caffeine (Esgic, Fioricet)	Neomycin (Mycifradin Sulfate Topical, Neo-Tabs Oral)
Butalbital plus aspirin plus caffeine (Fiorinal)	Nizatidine (Apo-Nizatidine, Axid)
Carbamazepine (Nu-Carbamazepine, Tegretol)	Orlistat (Xenical)
Cascara	Oxcarbazepine (Trileptal)
Cholestyramine (LoCHOLEST, Questran)	Phenobarbital (Barbita, Solfoton)
Cimetidine (Apo-Cimetidine, Tagamet)	Phenytoin (Dilantin, Tremytoine)
Colesevelam (WelChol)	Prednisolone (Delta-Cortef, Pediapred)
Colestipol (Colestid)	Prednisone (Deltasone, Orasone)
Cortisone (Cortone)	Primidone (Mysoline, Sertan)
Dexamethasone (Decadron, Maxidex)	Ranitidine (Nu-Ranit, Zantac)
Diflorasone (Florone, Maxiflor)	Rifabutin (Mycobutin)
Ethosuximide (Zarontin)	Rifampin (Rimactane, Rofact)
Ethotoin (Peganone)	Rifampin plus isoniazid (Rifamate)
Famotidine (Alti-Famotidine, Pepcid)	Rifapentine (Priftin)
Flunisolide (AeroBid-M, Nasalide)	Sevelamer (Renagel)
Fluticasone (Cutivate, Flonase)	Sucralfate (Carafate, Sulcrate)
Fosphenytoin (Cerebyx)	Triamcinolone (Amcort, Tristoject)
Halobetasol (Ultravate)	Valproic acid (Depacon, Depakote ER)
Heparin (Hep-Lock)	

VITAMIN E

A Quick Look

Originally known as the fertility vitamin, vitamin E is now better known as a powerful antioxidant.

The Whole Story

Although we refer to it as a single entity, vitamin E is actually a family of eight substances. One of these, alpha-tocopherol, is believed to be the most abundant form of E found in foods and the most active form found in the body.

Vitamin E was first noticed as the unknown substance in food that laboratory animals needed to be able to bear young. If laboratory animals were fed a diet deficient in E, they suffered from irreversible damage to their reproductive systems and fetuses were reabsorbed or spontaneously aborted. Because of this, vitamin E was given the scientific name tocopherol, which means "to bring forth children."

Vitamin E is also a powerful antioxidant that protects cells throughout your body from those harmful by-products of metabolism called free radicals. The free radicals—whose numbers are increased when you smoke or are exposed to stress and other toxic substances—cause cellular damage that can lead to cancer, heart disease, and other degenerative diseases. Free radicals are also believed to be a major cause of aging.

Laboratory studies suggest that vitamin E is good for the heart. It appears to slow the conversion of LDL "bad" cholesterol to its more dangerous oxidized form, helps prevent unnecessary clots from forming in the blood, and helps keep blood cells from sticking to the artery walls. All of these actions reduce the risk of coronary heart disease and heart attack. The vitamin is also necessary for healthy red blood cells.

Vitamin E deficiency can be difficult to diagnosis because it may show itself in several different ways, each of which can be confused with other problems.

When You Run Short of Vitamin E

A deficiency can cause infertility, destruction of red blood cells, muscle damage, and nerve problems.

What the Research Shows

Vitamin E is one of the "hottest" of the nutrients, with many experts suggesting that it can help prevent heart disease, Alzheimer's disease, and other ailments. Some of the evidence is encouraging:

- *Heart disease.* Several studies looking at large population groups—including the Nurses Health Study and the Health Professionals Follow-up Study—have found that taking vitamin E supplements for two years or more reduced the risk of coronary heart disease by about 40 percent.

However, other studies in which people were given vitamin E supplements have come back with mixed or negative results, suggesting that vitamin E by itself may not be the key factor. It may be that the vitamin works best when combined with other nutrients.

- *Alzheimer's.* The Alzheimer's Disease Cooperative Study looked to see how much time would pass before participants suffered an "outcome of interest" (not being able to perform basic tasks of daily living, developing severe dementia, being institutionalized, or dying).[23] Among those taking the placebo, 440 days passed before one of these things happened. But among those taking vitamin E, many more days—670 on average—passed before the "outcome of interest" appeared.

Daily Requirement

The RDA for vitamin E is 22 IU per day for men and women ages 19 and up.

Safety and Side Effects

The Tolerable Upper Intake Level (UL) of supplemental vitamin E for adult men and women is 1,500 IU alpha-tocopherol. This level was chosen primarily because too much vitamin E can thin the blood and increase the risk of unnecessary bleeding. Excessive amounts may also decrease the level of thyroid hormone while increasing the blood fat (triglyceride) levels.

Some Good Sources of Vitamin E

FOOD	SERVING SIZE	IU VITAMIN E
Wheat germ oil	1 tbsp	26.2
Almonds, dry roasted	1 oz	7.5
Safflower oil	1 tbsp	4.7
Corn oil	1 tbsp	2.9
Soybean oil	1 tbsp	2.5
Mango, raw	1 fruit	2.3
Broccoli, chopped, frozen, boiled	½ cup	1.5
Dandelion greens, boiled	½ cup	1.3
Pistachio nuts, dry roasted	1 oz	1.2
Kiwifruit	1 medium	0.85

Drugs That Interfere with Vitamin E

Cholestyramine (LoCHOLEST, Questran)	Mineral oil (Fleet Mineral Oil Enema, Milkinol)
Clofibrate (Atromid-S)	Neomycin (Mycifradin Sulfate Topical, Neo-Tabs Oral)
Colesevelam (WelChol)	Orlistat (Xenical)
Colestipol (Colestid)	Sevelamer (Renagel)
Fenofibrate (Apo-Fenofibrate, TriCor)	Simvastatin (Zocor)
Gemfibrozil (Apo-Gemfibrozil, Lopid)	Sucralfate (Carafate, Sulcrate)

VITAMIN K

A Quick Look

The "koagulation vitamin" helps the blood to clot and keeps the bones strong.

The Whole Story

In 1929, a Danish researcher made an interesting discovery: When chickens were put on a fat-free diet, blood leaked out of their arteries. And this blood coagulated very slowly. The scientist quickly learned that the chicks were bleeding because they were missing a blood-clotting substance found in the fatty parts of food, a substance he named the "koagulation vitamin." Today we call it vitamin K.

Like several other vitamins, K is really a family of related substances: K_1 (phylloquinone), K_2 (a group of compounds called the menaquinones), and K_3 (a synthetic variant of the vitamin called menadione).

Vitamin K is fat-soluble and thus is found in the fatty parts of foods such as soybean and other plant oils, butter, beef liver, chicken egg yolk, certain cheeses, and fermented soybean products. It's also found in green leafy vegetables. Vitamin K_2 is also made by intestinal organisms. Only small amounts of vitamin K are stored in the body, so it's a good idea to eat K-rich foods every day.

In addition to helping the blood clot, vitamin K plays an important role in keeping the bones strong by activating a protein that holds calcium in the bones. It may also keep the artery linings healthy and flexible by preventing the unnecessary deposition of calcium.

A series of relatively new studies suggest that vitamin K may also be helpful in combating cancer. Specifically, vitamin K_2 encourages the suicide (apoptosis) of pancreatic and ovarian cancer cells.

When You Run Short of Vitamin K

A deficiency of vitamin K can cause bleeding.

Daily Requirement

The Adequate Intake (AI) for vitamin K is 120 mcg per day for men above the age of 19 and 90 mcg per day for women above the age of 19.

Safety and Side Effects

The Tolerable Upper Intake Level (UL) for vitamin K has not been set.

According to the Food and Nutrition Board, "No adverse effects associated with vitamin K consumption from food or supplements have been reported in humans or animals." This statement refers to vitamins K_1 and K_2, not the synthetic K_3 and its derivatives. You should, however, check with your physician if you are taking medications such as blood thinners that may be affected by the vitamin.

Some Good Sources of Vitamin K

FOOD	SERVING SIZE	MCG VITAMIN K
Kale, raw, chopped	1 cup	547
Broccoli, cooked, chopped	1 cup	420
Parsley, raw, chopped	1 cup	324
Swiss chard, raw, chopped	1 cup	299
Spinach, raw, chopped	1 cup	120
Leaf lettuce, raw, shredded	1 cup	118
Watercress, raw, chopped	1 cup	85
Soybean oil	1 tbsp	26.1
Canola oil	1 tbsp	19.7
Mayonnaise	1 tbsp	11.9

Drugs That Interfere with Vitamin K

Amikacin (Amikin)	Butalbital plus aspirin plus caffeine (Fiorinal)
Amoxicillin (Amoxil, Novamoxin)	Carbenicillin (Geocillin)
Ampicillin (Omnipen, Totacillin)	Cefaclor (Ceclor)
Azithromycin (Zithromax)	Cefadroxil (Duricef)
Beclomethasone (Beconase, Propaderm)	Cefamandole (Mandol)
Betamethasone (Betatrex, Maxivate)	Cefazolin (Ancef, Kefzol)
Budesonide (Entocort, Rhinocort)	Cefdinir (Omnicef)
Butabarbital (Butalan, Butisol)	Cefditoren (Spectracef)
Butalbital plus acetaminophen plus caffeine (Esgic, Fioricet)	Cefepime (Maxipime)

Cefonicid (Monocid)

Cefoperazone (Cefobid)

Cefotaxime (Claforan)

Cefotetan (Cefotan)

Cefoxitin (Mefoxin)

Cefpodoxime (Vantin)

Cefprozil (Cefzil)

Ceftazidime (Ceptaz, Fortaz)

Ceftibuten (Cedax)

Ceftizoxime (Cefizox)

Ceftriaxone (Rocephin)

Cefuroxime (Ceftin, Kefurox)

Cephalexin (Biocef, Keftab)

Cephalothin (Ceporacin)

Cephapirin (Cefadyl)

Cepharadine (Velosef)

Cholestyramine (LoCHOLEST, Questran)

Cinoxacin (Cinobac)

Ciprofloxacin (Ciloxan, Cipro)

Clarithromycin (Biaxin, Biaxin XL)

Clindamycin (Cleocin, Dalacin C)

Cloxacillin (Cloxapen, Nu-Cloxi)

Colesevelam (WelChol)

Colestipol (Colestid)

Cortisone (Cortone)

Demeclocycline (Declomycin)

Dexamethasone (Decadron, Maxidex)

Dicloxacillin (Dycill, Pathocil)

Dirithromycin (Dynabac)

Doxycycline (Monodox, Vibramycin)

Erythromycin (Erythrocin, Staticin)

Ethosuximide (Zarontin)

Flunisolide (AeroBid-M, Nasalide)

Fluticasone (Cutivate, Flonase)

Fosphenytoin (Cerebyx)

Gatofloxacin (Tequin)

Gentamicin (Garamycin, Jenamicin)

Griseofulvin (Fulvicin)

Kanamycin (Kantrex)

Levofloxacin (Levaquin, Quixin Ophthalmic)

Linezolid (Zyvox)

Lomefloxacin (Maxaquin)

Loracarbef (Lorabid)

Meclocycline (Meclan Topical)

Methsuximide (Celotin)

Methylprednisolone (Depoject Injection, Medrol Oral)

Metronidazole (Flagyl, MetroLotion)

Mineral oil (Fleet Mineral Oil Enema, Milkinol)

Minocycline (Dynacin Oral, Minocin Oral)

Mometasone furoate (Elocom, Nasonex)

Moxifloxacin (Avelox)

Nafcillin (Nafcil Injection, Unipen Oral)

Nalidixic acid (NegGram)

Neomycin (Mycifradin Sulfate Topical, Neo-Tabs Oral)

Norfloxacin (Chibroxin Ophthalmic, Noroxin Oral)

Ofloxacin (Floxin, Ocuflox Ophthalmic)

Orlistat (Xenical)

Penicillin G benzathine (Bicillin L-A, Permapen)

Penicillin G benzathine plus penicillin G procaine (Bicillin C-R)

Penicillin G procaine (Pfizerpen-AS, Wycillin)

Penicillin V potassium (Suspen, Truxcillin)

Phenobarbital (Barbita, Solfoton)

Phenytoin (Dilantin, Tremytoine)

Piperacillin (Pipracil)

Piperacillin plus tazobactam sodium (Zosyn)

Prednisolone (Delta-Cortef, Pediapred)

Prednisone (Deltasone, Orasone)

Primidone (Mysoline, Sertan)

Sevelamer (Renagel)

Sparfloxacin (Zagam)

Sucralfate (Carafate, Sulcrate)

Sulfadiazine (Coptin, Microsulfon)

Sulfisoxazole (Gantrisin)

Tetracycline (Nu-Tetra, Topicycline Topical)

Ticarcillin (Ticar)

Ticarcillin and clavulanate potassium (Timentin)

Tobramycin (Nebcin Injection, Tobrex Ophthlamic)

Triamcinolone (Amcort, Tristoject)

Trimethoprim (Primsol, Trimpex)

Trovafloxacin (Trovan)

ZINC

A Quick Look

Zinc is key to many bodily functions, from making babies to keeping hair on your head.

The Whole Story

In days not too long past, if a couple was having trouble getting pregnant, a friend might whisper to the husband, "Eat oysters."

What's the link between oysters and babies? Oysters are good sources of zinc, a mineral necessary for male potency. Indeed, zinc is concentrated in the prostate gland and prostate secretions, as well as in the brain, liver, kidneys, eyes, and muscles.

The couple of grams of zinc in the human body have a variety of duties. Zinc participates in well over 100 enzyme reactions that help metabolize carbohydrates, synthesize proteins and nucleic acids, and transport carbon dioxide. The mineral helps the body store and use vitamin A, keeps the bones strong and the immune system healthy, and is necessary for wound healing and normal taste sensations. Zinc is also necessary for growth and development.

Alcoholics are likely to be low in zinc because alcohol interferes with the absorption of the mineral and encourages zinc excretion via the urine. Chronic diarrhea can also deplete zinc stores. Vegetarians should pay close attention to their zinc status, because it's harder for the body to absorb zinc from plant foods than it is from animal foods.

When You Run Short of Zinc

A lack of zinc can cause a variety of symptoms, including loss of hair, delayed sexual maturity, poor growth and development, impotence, loss of appetite, diarrhea, and poor wound healing.

What the Research Shows

Zinc has been suggested as a natural cure for colds and acne and a way to improve fertility, enhance athletic performance, and strengthen the immune system in senior citizens. It may also help those with macular degeneration, an incurable disease that damages a part of the retina called the macula and severely impairs vision.

The research on the effects of zinc on colds and macular degeneration has produced some good results. For example:

- *Colds.* For a double-blind study presented in the *Annals of Internal Medicine* in 2000, 50 people suffering from the common cold were randomly given either 12.8 mg zinc or a placebo several times a day for as long as they had symptoms.[24] Among those taking the zinc, symptoms lasted an average of 4.5 days, compared to 8.1 days for those who got the placebo.
- *Colds.* In an earlier study published in the *Annals of Internal Medicine*, 100 people suffering from colds were given either 13.3 mg zinc or a placebo several times a day until their symptoms disappeared.[25] The time it took for the symptoms to vanish was 4.4 days for those taking zinc and 7.6 days for those taking the placebo.
- *Macular degeneration.* In a 2001 double-blind study, over 3,600 people suffering from age-related macular degeneration were randomly given antioxidants, zinc, antioxidants plus zinc, or a placebo.[26] All took their supplements for a little over six years. Compared to placebo, the zinc reduced the risk of developing advanced macular degeneration by 25 percent. Zinc plus antioxidants lowered the risk by 28 percent.

Daily Requirement

The RDA for zinc is 11 mg per day for men ages 19 and up and 8 mg per day for women ages 19 and over.

Safety and Side Effects

The Tolerable Upper Intake Level (UL) of zinc for adult men and women is 40 mg per day. Taking in excessive amounts of zinc can harm the immune system and reduce your levels of the HDL "good" cholesterol.

Some Good Sources of Zinc

FOOD	SERVING SIZE	MG ZINC
Oysters, battered, fried	6	16.0
Beef shank, lean meat, cooked	3 oz	8.9
Chicken leg, roasted	1	2.7
Pork tenderloin, lean, cooked	3 oz	2.5
Yogurt, plain, low-fat	1 cup	2.2
Baked beans, vegetarian, canned	½ cup	1.7
Cashews, dry roasted	1 oz	1.6
Pecans, dry roasted	1 oz	1.4
Swiss cheese	1 oz	1.1
Milk	1 cup	0.9

Drugs That Interfere with Zinc

Aluminum hydroxide (Amphojel, Dialume)	Flunisolide (AeroBid-M, Nasalide)
Aluminum hydroxide plus magnesium carbonate (Gaviscon Liquid)	Fluticasone (Cutivate, Flonase)
Aluminum hydroxide plus magnesium hydroxide (Maalox, Mylanta)	Fosinopril (Monopril)
Aluminum hydroxide plus magnesium hydroxide plus simethicone (Mylanta Liquid)	Furosemide (Apo-Furosemide, Lasix)
Aluminum hydroxide plus magnesium trisilicate (Gaviscon Tablet)	Gatofloxacin (Tequin)
Amiloride plus hydrocholorothiazide (Moduret, Nu-Amilzide)	Halobetasol (Ultravate)
Aspirin (Anacin, Novasen)	Hydralazine (Apo-Hydral, Apresoline)
Aspirin plus dipyridamole (Aggrenox)	Hydralazine plus hydrochlorothiazide (Apresazide)
Atenolol plus chlorthalidone (Tenoretic)	Hydrochlorothiazide (Apo-Hydro, Esidrix)
Beclomethasone (Beconase, Propaderm)	Hydrochlorothiazide plus spironolactone (Aldactazide, Novo-Spirozine)
Benazepril (Lotensin)	Hydrochlorothiazide plus triamterene (Dyazide, Maxzide)
Betamethasone (Betatrex, Maxivate)	Hydrocortisone (Bactine, Cortef)
Budesonide (Entocort, Rhinocort)	Indapamide (Lozide, Lozol)
Bumetanide (Bumex, Burinex)	Irbesartan plus hydrochlorothiazide (Avalide)
Candesartan plus hydrochlorothiazide (Atacand HCT)	Lamivudine (Epivir)
Captopril (Capoten, Novo-Captopril)	Lansoprazole (Prevacid)
Chlorothiazide (Diuril)	Levofloxacin (Levaquin, Quixin Ophthalmic)
Chlorthalidone (Apo-Chlorthalidone, Thalitone)	Levonorgestrel (Norplant Implant, Plan B)
Cholestyramine (LoCHOLEST, Questran)	Lisinopril (Prinivil, Zestril)
Cimetidine (Apo-Cimetidine, Tagamet)	Lomefloxacin (Maxaquin)
Ciprofloxacin (Ciloxan, Cipro)	Losartan plus hydrochlorothiazide (Hyzaar)
Cortisone (Cortone)	Magnesium hydroxide (Phillips' Milk of Magnesia)
Delavirdine (Rescriptor)	Methyclothiazide (Aquatensen, Enduron)
Demeclocycline (Declomycin)	Methyldopa plus hydrochlorothiazide (Aldoril, PMS-Dopazide)
Dexamethasone (Decadron, Maxidex)	Methylprednisolone (Depoject Injection, Medrol Oral)
Didanosine (Videx, Videx EC)	Metolazone (Mykrox, Zaroxolyn)
Diflorasone (Florone, Maxiflor)	Minocycline (Dynacin Oral, Minocin Oral)
Doxycycline (Monodox, Vibramycin)	Moexipril (Univasc)
Enalapril (Vasotec)	Moexipril plus hydrochlorothiazide (Uniretic)
Enalapril plus felodipine (Lexxel)	Mometasone furoate (Elocom, Nasonex)
Enalapril plus hydrochlorothiazide (Vaseretic)	Moxifloxacin (Avelox)
Enoxacin (Penetrex)	Nevirapine (Viramune)
Ethacrynic acid (Edecrin)	Nizatidine (Apo-Nizatidine, Axid)
Ethambutol (Myambutol)	Norethindrone (Aygestin, Micronor)
Famotidine (Alti-Famotidine, Pepcid)	Norfloxacin (Chibroxin Ophthalmic, Noroxin Oral)

Ofloxacin (Floxin, Ocuflox Ophthalmic)	Telmisartan plus hydrochlorothiazide (Micardis HCT, Micardis Plus)
Omeprazole (Losec, Prilosec)	Tetracycline (Nu-Tetra, Topicycline Topical)
Penicillamine (Cuprimine, Depen)	Torsemide (Demadex)
Perindopril erbumine (Aceon)	Trandolapril (Mavik)
Polythiazide (Renese)	Trandolapril plus verapamil (Tarka)
Prazosin plus polythiazide (Minizide)	Triamcinolone (Amcort, Tristoject)
Prednisolone (Delta-Cortef, Pediapred)	Triamterene (Dyrenium)
Prednisone (Deltasone, Orasone)	Trichlormethiazide (Metahydrin, Naqua)
Propranolol plus hydrochlorothiazide (Inderide)	Trovafloxacin (Trovan)
Quinapril (Accupril)	Valsartan plus hydrochlorothiazide (Diovan HCT)
Rabeprazole (Aciphex)	Zalcitabine (Hivid)
Ramipril (Altace)	Zidovudine (Apo-Zidovudine)
Ranitidine (Nu-Ranit, Zantac)	Zidovudine plus lamivudine (AZT + 3TC)
Sparfloxacin (Zagam)	Zidovudine plus lamivudine plus Abacavir (Trizivir)
Stavudine (Zerit)	

CHAPTER 3 | **Drugs That Rob You of Nutrients, A to Z**

Now comes the heart of the book, the listing of drugs and the nutrients they rob you of. The drugs are listed alphabetically by generic name—that's the usually-difficult-to-pronounce name health professionals use. The generic name is the drug's official name, and it often tells you something about the drug. For example, just by looking at the generic name simvastatin, you can tell that the drug is a member of the statin family of drugs, which are used to reduce cholesterol.

Immediately after the generic name is a pronunciation guide. Oddly enough, there are different ways to pronounce some of these generic names, so don't be surprised if your physician or pharmacist has a slightly different pronunciation than we give.

Just below the generic name is a listing of some of the brand names used in the United States and Canada. Brand names, also called trade names, are the popular and usually-easier-to-pronounce names most layfolk know. There may be only one brand name for a drug, or there may be many. Our listings are not exhaustive, so we may not have listed the brand name of the drug you're taking. Don't be alarmed if you don't see your brand name; just look for the generic name that matches the one for your medicine.

We've stretched the traditional definition of nutrients to include vitamins, minerals, and other substances your body needs to maintain good health. And when we say that they rob you of nutrients, we mean that they may deplete your reserves, hinder the absorption of, interfere with the metabolism of, increase your need for, or cause you to excrete more of the nutrient(s).

We searched through a wide variety of sources to develop our list of drugs and the nutrients they deplete. We consulted studies published in scientific journals, textbooks of pharmacology and other disciplines, books discussing drug-nutrient-herb interactions, and drug guidebooks. We looked for drugs that had been directly studied and shown to deplete nutrients, as well as "related" drugs—that is, drugs that had the same mechanism(s) of action in the body and would thus deplete the same nutrients in the same way.

Our goal is to make you aware of the fact that drugs can deplete you of nutrients, that this can trigger some side effects, and that it may be possible to avoid these problems by replacing the missing substances via food or supplements.

We don't want to alarm you unnecessarily by giving you the impression that nutrients will start disappearing from your body as soon as you swallow your first dose of a medicine. It may take a while before the depletion becomes a problem. And if you happen to have a lot of the depleted nutrient stored in your body and/or get plenty of it in your diet, it may not be a problem for you.

But we feel that it's better to alert you and your doctor to potential drug-induced nutrient thievery than to overlook possibilities. Why suffer through unnecessary side effects or be forced to take yet another medication or get off the original medicine altogether, when restocking your internal stores of nutrients may be all that's required?

One final note: The discussions that follow look only at the way various drugs may rob you of nutrients. They're not meant to be exhaustive examinations of the drugs, they're not intended be to guides to using the drugs, and they do not give the full set of warnings you should receive before taking a drug. Neither do they alert you to all the potential problems that arise when you mix supplements and/or food with drugs or change your dietary or supplement regimens. Some drugs work by interfering with a certain nutrient in your body, so taking in more of that nutrient can interfere with these drugs' actions. There's also the possibility that taking a supplement to replenish a deficiency caused by one drug may interfere with or heighten the actions of a second drug you're taking.

That's why it is imperative that you discuss *any* changes in your medications, diet, or supplement regimen with your physician *before* you make them. Even a small change in your medicines, diet, or supplements can affect your health, so you *must* consult with your physician before making any changes—any whatsoever—to your diet or supplements, your medications or lifestyle.

The form of each nutrient—for example, whether it's calcium citrate or calcium carbonate—can make a difference. Even the time of day you take a medicine, whether you take it with or without food, whether you can take it with nutrients, or should separate medicines and nutrients, can make a difference, so check everything carefully with your physician. What you take, when you take it, how you take it—check it all.

That's so important it needs to be said again: *Don't change your medication, diet, or supplement regimens without talking it over with your physician.* If you do take supplements, find out which form of each is best for you. And find out exactly when and how to take your medicines and supplements. Even a simple, normally harmless vitamin pill can alter the way your body absorbs or responds to a drug, so you must review all changes with your doctor *before* you make them.

ACEBUTOLOL (a-se-BYOO-toe-lole)

Brand Names: Apo-Acebutolo, Gen-Acebutolol, Monitan, Novo-Acebutolol, Nu-Acebutolol, Sectral

About Acebutolol

Acebutolol is a beta-blocker, which means that it works by blockading specialized beta-receptors in the heart and elsewhere.

To understand what that means, forget about the doctor-speak. Instead, think about an old-fashioned battle, with the general standing on a hill watching the fight below. From way up on his perch, he can see that it's time for the artillery to begin firing, but he's too far away to give the command himself. So he sends a runner down the hill to the artillery captain to pass on his orders. The cannon roars and the battle is won. The general made a brilliant decision, but without the runner to relay his instructions, that decision would have been worthless.

Sometimes a general gives bad instructions, perhaps ordering the artillery to fire fast and furiously at the wrong time, which exhausts the ammunition stores, and the battle is lost. At times like these, it would be great if the general's messenger was kept from relaying the errant instructions.

Similarly, the brain—the body's "general"—gives commands that must be relayed to other parts of the body, where various battles are taking place. And sometimes the brain sends orders that are counterproductive. It may tell the heart to keep beating vigorously even when there's no need to speed blood through the blood vessels. It may make the blood pressure rise when it's actually time for the heart to slow down and relax a bit.

At times like these, wouldn't it be nice to prevent the "messenger" from delivering the errant message? That's what beta-blocker drugs do: They prevent too many "beat faster" or other deleterious messages from getting to the heart by preventing the messengers from getting through. Because they do this by occupying specialized structures called beta-receptors, they're called beta-blockers.

Acebutolol is one of these beta-blockers. By standing in the way and preventing the "beat faster" messages from getting through to the heart, it helps to lower elevated blood pressure, ease angina, and normalize certain kinds of irregular heartbeat.

Possible Side Effects

The drug's more common side effects include fatigue, confusion, headache, dizziness, stomach upsets, and difficulty breathing.

Which Nutrients Are Robbed

Taking this medicine may deplete your supply of, increase your need for, or interfere with the activity of:

- Coenzyme Q_{10} • Melatonin

Additional Ways This Drug May Upset Your Nutritional Balance

Acebutolol can cause low blood sugar, nausea, vomiting, and abdominal pain, all of which can upset your eating habits and interfere with good nutrition. It may also trigger diarrhea, which can hamper nutrient absorption.

Restoring Your Nutritional Balance

To compensate for the nutrient loss caused by this drug, speak to your physician about taking 30–100 mg coenzyme Q_{10} and 1–3 mg melatonin per day.

You can also eat foods that contain the depleted nutrient:

- Coenzyme Q_{10}: beef, chicken, trout, salmon, oranges, broccoli

Consult with your physician before making any changes to your diet or supplemental regimen.

ACETAMINOPHEN, ACETAMINOPHEN PLUS CODEINE
(uh-seet-uh-MIN-oh-fen, KOE-deen)

Brand Names: Abenol, Aspirin Free Anacin, Cetafen Extra, Empracet-30, Genapap, Liquiprin for Children, Phenaphen with Codeine, Tempra, Tylenol

About Acetaminophen, Acetaminophen plus Codeine

Acetaminophen, a popular, readily available nonprescription remedy, is used for the mild to moderate pain of headaches, muscle aches, arthritis, backaches, toothaches, menstrual cramps, and other painful conditions. It also helps to relieve fever. The drug works by slowing the production of the prostaglandins that play a role in triggering pain and fever.

Acetaminophen is considered to be as effective as aspirin at quelling pain, and many people think the two medications are interchangeable. But while both drugs relieve pain and fever, only aspirin relieves inflammation and "thins" the blood by preventing platelets from clumping together unnecessarily.

In certain cases—perhaps following surgery or a tooth extraction—you may be given acetaminophen plus codeine. Codeine is a narcotic agonist, which means that it plugs into narcotic receptor sites in the central nervous system and eases pain. This combination of drugs may seem innocent because acetaminophen is taken so casually, but remember that codeine is a narcotic that can cause dependence or addiction.

Possible Side Effects

In rare cases, acetaminophen may cause anemia, skin rash, hepatitis, or toxic injury to the kidneys. Codeine's more common side effects include drowsiness and constipation.

Which Nutrients Are Robbed

Taking this medicine may deplete your supply of, increase your need for, or interfere with the activity of:

• Glutathione

Restoring Your Nutritional Balance

To compensate for the nutrient loss caused by this drug, speak to your physician about taking 800–2,000 mg n-acetyl cysteine (a precursor to glutathione) per day.

Consult with your physician before making any changes to your diet or supplemental regimen.

ACETAZOLAMIDE (uh-set-uh-ZOLE-uh-mide)

Brand Names: Acetazolam, Apo-Acetazolamide, Diamox, Diamox Sequels

About Acetazolamide

There's a story—no vouching for its authenticity—about a man who made a fast climb up to a very high elevation in the mountains, where he set out to build a cabin. He cut a piece of wood board to use for one of the cabin walls and was dismayed to find that it was too short. So he measured again, cut a little more off the edge of the board and was astonished to find that it was *still* too short. He kept measuring and cutting, but no matter how much he shaved off the end, the board was always too short.

This poor fellow may have been suffering from acute mountain sickness, which is caused by a rapid increase in elevation that doesn't allow enough time for the body to adjust. The early symptoms include headache, dizziness, nausea, vomiting, and drowsiness. Later symptoms include difficulty in concentrating, irritability, audio and visual disturbances, a rapid heart rate, and accumulation of fluid in the lungs.

To prevent acute mountain sickness, your doctor may recommend that you take acetazolamide before and during a climb and for a few days after you reach a high altitude. Acetazolamide can also be used to treat acute mountain sickness that has already set in. The drug works by reducing the formation of cerebrospinal fluid and decreasing the fluid's pH (or acid/base balance).

Acetazolamide is also used as a diuretic, an anticonvulsant, and to treat certain seizures.

Possible Side Effects

The drug's more common side effects include weakness, nausea and vomiting, increased urination, and numbness or tingling of the hands, feet, mouth, lips, and/or anus.

Which Nutrients Are Robbed

Taking this medicine may deplete your supply of, increase your need for, or interfere with the activity of:

- Magnesium
- Potassium
- Phosphorus
- Sodium

Additional Ways This Drug May Upset Your Nutritional Balance

Acetazolamide can cause loss of appetite, nausea, vomiting, and a metallic taste, all of which can upset your eating habits and possibly interfere with good nutrition. It may also trigger diarrhea, which can hamper nutrient absorption.

Restoring Your Nutritional Balance

To compensate for the nutrient loss caused by this drug, speak to your physician about taking 500–1,000 mg magnesium, 700 mg phosphorus, and 100–300 mg potassium per day. Also ask your physician to consider the potential effects of sodium depletion.

You can also eat foods that contain the depleted nutrients:

- Magnesium: Florida avocado, toasted wheat germ, almonds, shredded wheat cereal, pumpkin seeds
- Phosphorus: plain nonfat yogurt, lentils, salmon, milk, halibut
- Potassium: dried figs, California avocado, papaya, banana, dates

Consult with your physician before making any changes to your diet or supplemental regimen.

ACETOHEXAMIDE (uh-set-oh-HEKS-uh-mide)

Brand Names: Dymelor, Dimelor

About Acetohexamide

Diabetes is a serious disease, capable of killing if left untreated. In simple terms, diabetes is a delivery problem. That is, the hormone insulin, which is supposed to deliver blood sugar (glucose) to certain cells, doesn't work as well as it should—or doesn't work at all.

Your blood glucose level rises after you eat or drink something that contains carbohydrates. But blood sugar can't enter many cells by itself; it needs to hook up with insulin, which acts like a key to open the locks (insulin receptor sites) on cell membranes. Without sufficient insulin, or if the insulin isn't able to do its job because the cells don't respond properly, blood glucose levels build up to dangerously high levels and wreak havoc on many areas of the body, including the kidneys, nerves, blood vessels, and eyes.

Some 15 million Americans either don't make enough insulin (type 1 diabetes) or have cells that resist insulin's efforts (type 2 diabetes). Either way, the glucose levels in the blood rise to unhealthy levels, causing widespread damage throughout the body.

Acetohexamide, which is used to treat mild to moderate cases of type 2 diabetes, attacks the problem by stimulating the pancreas to release more insulin. In type 2 diabetes, your pancreas makes a normal amount of insulin, but the body's cells tend to ignore it. Acetohexamide tries to solve this problem of "ignored insulin" by getting more insulin into action.

Possible Side Effects

The drug's side effects include weakness, tingling in the feet and hands, nausea and vomiting, and low blood sugar.

Which Nutrients Are Robbed

Taking this medicine may deplete your supply of, increase your need for, or interfere with the activity of:

- Coenzyme Q_{10}

Additional Ways This Drug May Upset Your Nutritional Balance

Acetohexamide can cause loss of appetite, stomach upset, and nausea and vomiting, all of which can upset your eating habits and possibly interfere with good nutrition.

Restoring Your Nutritional Balance

To compensate for the nutrient loss caused by this drug, speak to your physician about taking 30–100 mg coenzyme Q_{10} per day.

You can also eat foods that contain the depleted nutrient:

- Coenzyme Q_{10}: beef, chicken, trout, salmon, oranges, broccoli

Consult with your physician before making any changes to your diet or supplemental regimen.

ALBUTEROL (al-BYOO-ter-ole)

Brand Names: AccuNeb, Alti-Salbutamol, Apo-Salvent, Novo-Salmol, Proventil, Ventolin, Volmax, VoSpire ER

About Albuterol

Asthma attacks make it difficult for about 18 million Americans to take their next breath. There are many reasons or triggers for the disease, which causes the airways to narrow, swell, and become filled with mucous, leaving little room for air to flow in and out.

The muscles surrounding the breathing tubes play an important role in asthma. Just like arteries, the breathing tubes have muscles that contract and relax on command, allowing the airways to become wider or narrower according to your needs. With asthma, these muscles contract for no reason, making the passageways smaller. Inflammation sets in, causing swelling that further narrows the passageways. Then the secretion of thick mucus blocks the airways even more.

But these muscles don't decide to contract on their own. They're stimulated when certain substances plug into specialized receptor sites along the airways. Drugs like albuterol help combat asthma by giving the air tubes the order to relax, stop squeezing, and open wider. With more room in the airways, breathing is easier.

Albuterol is also used to treat chronic obstructive lung disease and to prevent spasms of the airways during exercise.

Possible Side Effects

The drug's side effects include irregular heartbeat, dizziness, stomach upset, muscle cramps, and weakness.

Which Nutrients Are Robbed

Taking this medicine may deplete your supply of, increase your need for, or interfere with the activity of:

- Potassium

Additional Ways This Drug May Upset Your Nutritional Balance

Albuterol can cause nausea, vomiting, and changes in taste, all of which can upset your eating habits and possibly interfere with good nutrition. It may also trigger diarrhea, which can hamper nutrient absorption.

Restoring Your Nutritional Balance

To compensate for the nutrient loss caused by this drug, speak to your physician about taking 100–300 mg potassium per day.

You can also eat foods that contain the depleted nutrient:

- Potassium: dried figs, California avocado, papaya, banana, dates

Consult with your physician before making any changes to your diet or supplemental regimen.

ALENDRONATE (uh-LEN-droe-nate)

Brand Name: Fosamax

About Alendronate

Perhaps the most obvious sign of osteoporosis is the "dowager's hump" you may see on some older women. Several of the vertebrae in the upper spine have collapsed due to osteoporosis, the thinning and hollowing of the bones. This causes the spine to curve and produce what appears to be a small hump where the back meets the neck. While dowager's humps aren't all that common, osteoporosis certainly is. The disease affects about 10 million Americans, 8 million of whom are women.

Think of osteoporosis as a disease of imbalance. Your bones are not static; they're not built once and then left alone. Instead, your body continually remodels them, breaking them down and rebuilding them all through your life. This is a good idea, for it allows your bones to grow in length and width when you're young. It also allows them to grow in width and strength when you're older, if you stress them by doing weight-bearing exercises such as walking.

There are two bone crews in your body, one to break the bones down and one to rebuild them. When you're young, hormones and other factors make the bone-building crew work harder than the bone-breakdown crew. As a result, your bones grow. When you're older, the bone-building crew slows down, but the bone-breakdown crew keeps going full steam ahead. As a result, your bones begin to thin once you're past your 30s. If the thinning becomes severe, you may suffer the bone fractures seen with osteoporosis.

Alendronate helps to prevent the breakdown of bone tissue. The drug is incorporated inside the bone matrix, and normal bone forms on top of the alendronate. Alendronate has been shown to increase bone density and reduce the risk of fractures.

Alendronate is used to prevent and treat osteoporosis, as well as for Paget's disease (which causes overgrowth of the bones).

Possible Side Effects

The drug's more common side effects include low blood levels of calcium and phosphorus, abdominal pain, muscle pain and cramping, ulcers, and acid reflux.

Which Nutrients Are Robbed

Taking this medicine may deplete your supply of, increase your need for, or interfere with the activity of:

- Calcium
- Phosphorus
- Magnesium

Additional Ways This Drug May Upset Your Nutritional Balance

Alendronate can cause abdominal pain, acid reflux, nausea, esophageal ulcer, abdominal distension, vomiting, and gastric ulcer, all of which can upset your eating habits and possibly interfere with good nutrition. It may also trigger diarrhea, which can hamper nutrient absorption.

Restoring Your Nutritional Balance

To compensate for the nutrient loss caused by this drug, speak to your physician about taking 1,200 mg calcium, 500–1,000 mg magnesium, and 700 mg phosphorus per day.

You can also eat foods that contain the depleted nutrients:

- Calcium: milk, dried figs, Swiss cheese, yogurt, tofu
- Magnesium: Florida avocado, toasted wheat germ, almonds, shredded wheat cereal, pumpkin seeds
- Phosphorus: plain nonfat yogurt, lentils, salmon, milk, halibut

Consult with your physician before making any changes to your diet or supplemental regimen.

ALUMINUM ANTACIDS Aluminum Hydroxide, Aluminum Hydroxide plus Magnesium Carbonate, Aluminum Hydroxide plus Magnesium Hydroxide, Aluminum Hydroxide plus Magnesium Trisilicate, Aluminum Hydroxide plus Magnesium Hydroxide plus Simethicone (uh-LOO-mi-num hye-DROKS-ide, mag-NEE-zee-um KAR-bun-nate, hye-DROKS-ide, trye-SIL-i-kate, sye-METH-i-kone)

Brand Names: Aluminum hydroxide: ALternaGel, Alu-Cap, Alu-Tab, Amphojel, Basaljel, Dialume; *Aluminum hydroxide plus magnesium carbonate:* Gaviscon Extra Strength, Gaviscon Liquid; *Aluminum hydroxide plus magnesium hydroxide:* Diovol, Gelusil, Maalox, Maalox TC (Therapeutic Concentrate), Mylanta, Univol; *Aluminum hydroxide plus magnesium trisilicate:* Gaviscon Tablet; *Aluminum hydroxide plus magnesium hydroxide plus simethicone:* Diovol Plus, Maalox Fast Release Liquid, Maalox Max, Mylanta Regular Strength, Mylanta Double Strength, Mylanta Extra Strength Liquid, Mylanta Liquid

About Aluminum Antacids

The process of extracting nutrients from the foods we eat isn't neat and clean. Stomach acid is a very powerful substance that burns food down to a mealy mass from which nutrients are plucked. Large amounts of stomach acid are required to begin breaking down the food, and sometimes that acid escapes from the stomach and backs up into the esophagus ("food tube"). This is bad news, for while the stomach has a special mucosal lining that shields it against the acid, the esophagus does not, making it ill-equipped to handle this caustic liquid. The result is heartburn, or acid regurgitation, which, besides pain, can cause bleeding, esophageal ulcers, narrowing of the esophagus, and precancerous changes in esophageal cells.

Antacids are popular over-the-counter (nonprescription) remedies for heartburn. As you'll recall from high school chemistry, acids and bases cancel each other out. Antacids, which are weak bases, are designed to neutralize or counteract the stomach acid, which can keep it from burning the esophagus. And some studies have suggested that antacids do more than just neutralize acid, helping to heal ulcers by other means, although exactly how this works is not yet fully understood.

There are several types of antacids, most of which have aluminum hydroxide and/or magnesium hydroxide as principal ingredients.

Possible Side Effects

The more common side effects seen with aluminum hydroxide include a chalky taste in the mouth, stomach cramps, constipation, and fecal impaction. Side effects of magnesium hydroxide include low blood pressure, high blood levels of magnesium, abdominal cramps, and muscle weakness.

Which Nutrients Are Robbed

Taking these medicines may deplete your supply of, increase your need for, or interfere with the activity of:

- Vitamin A
- Folic acid
- Vitamin D
- Calcium
- Chromium
- Iron
- Magnesium
- Phosphorus
- Zinc

Additional Ways This Drug May Upset Your Nutritional Balance

Aluminum hydroxide can cause nausea and vomiting, which can upset your eating habits and possibly interfere with good nutrition.

Restoring Your Nutritional Balance

To compensate for the nutrient loss caused by these drugs, speak to your physician about taking 5,000 IU vitamin A, 400–800 mcg folic acid, 400 IU vitamin D, 1,200 mg calcium, 1,000 mcg chromium, 500–1,500 mg magnesium, and 50–200 mg zinc per day. Also ask your physician to consider the potential effects of iron and phosphorus depletion.

You can also eat foods that contain the depleted nutrients:

- Vitamin A: beef liver, chicken liver, cheese pizza, whole milk, cheddar cheese
- Folic acid: beef liver, fortified breakfast cereals, spinach, great northern beans, asparagus
- Vitamin D: salmon, mackerel, sardines, eel, fortified milk
- Calcium: milk, dried figs, Swiss cheese, yogurt, tofu
- Chromium: broccoli, green beans, potatoes, grape juice, orange juice
- Magnesium: Florida avocado, toasted wheat germ, almonds, shredded wheat cereal, pumpkin seeds
- Zinc: oysters, beef shank, chicken, pork tenderloin, plain yogurt

Consult with your physician before making any changes to your diet or supplemental regimen.

AMIFOSTINE (am-i-FOSS-teen)

Brand Name: Ethyol

About Amifostine

Treatments for cancer can be brutal. For the most part, we don't have smart medicines that gently and discreetly zero in on cancer cells alone, then destroy them without damaging any nearby tissues. Instead, we use not-so-smart drugs that search for cancer cells and anything else that resembles them, killing all such cells indiscriminately. We see the same problem in radiation treatment, because we can't yet focus it precisely enough to destroy only the cancer cells without including nearby healthy cells.

Fortunately, we're developing new ways to protect healthy tissues from the ravages of cancer treatment, including the drug amifostine. Inside the body, amifostine is converted into another substance, thiol, which is absorbed into healthy cells. The thiol binds with certain anticancer drugs or their metabolites and deactivates them, thus warding off damage to healthy cells. (Thiol is taken into cancerous cells, too, but at a much slower rate.) Amifostine may also encourage the growth of bone marrow in patients with bone marrow diseases and guard against dryness of the mouth in people receiving postsurgical radiation treatment for head and neck cancer.

Possible Side Effects

The drug's more common side effects include nausea and vomiting (may be severe), low blood pressure, dizziness, flushing, chills, sneezing, and excessive sleepiness.

Which Nutrients Are Robbed

Taking this medicine may deplete your supply of, increase your need for, or interfere with the activity of:

- Calcium

Additional Ways This Drug May Upset Your Nutritional Balance

Amifostine can cause nausea and vomiting, which may be severe. This can upset your eating habits and possibly interfere with good nutrition.

Restoring Your Nutritional Balance

To compensate for the nutrient loss caused by this drug, speak to your physician about taking 1,200 mg calcium per day.

You can also eat foods that contain the depleted nutrient:

- Calcium: milk, dried figs, Swiss cheese, yogurt, tofu

Consult with your physician before making any changes to your diet or supplemental regimen.

AMIKACIN (am-i-KAY-sin)

Brand Name: Amikin

About Amikacin

Amikacin is a survivor of the bacterial wars—so far.

Bacteria that invade your body don't passively wait to be destroyed by drugs or your immune system, and neither do they run and hide. Instead, they fight back. One of their strategies is to develop new enzymes that they squirt at medicines or immune system cells to destroy or disable their enemies. Clever bacteria have figured out how to destroy or defend against a great many antibacterials, which is why medicines like penicillin and streptomycin are no longer as useful as they used to be.

Fortunately, drugs like amikacin have not succumbed to all of these bacterial counterattacks. Amikacin is immune to many of the enzymes that deactivate its chemical cousin medicines. In fact, it's specifically used to treat infections of the bone, respiratory tract, or blood that are resistant to other antibiotics.

Possible Side Effects

The drug's more common side effects include changes in the structure and function of the nervous system (neurotoxicity) and damage to hearing and the kidneys.

Which Nutrients Are Robbed

Taking this medicine may deplete your supply of, increase your need for, or interfere with the activity of:

- Biotin
- Inositol
- Thiamin
- Riboflavin
- Niacin
- Vitamin B_6
- Vitamin B_{12}

- Vitamin K
- Calcium
- Magnesium
- Potassium
- Sodium
- *Bifidobacterium bifidum*
- *Lactobacillus acidophilus*

Restoring Your Nutritional Balance

To compensate for the nutrient loss caused by this drug, speak to your physician about taking 500–1,000 mcg biotin, 250–1,000 mg inositol, 25–100 mg thiamin, 25–100 mg riboflavin, 50–100 mg niacin, 50–100 mg vitamin B_6, 500–1,000 mcg vitamin B_{12}, 60–80 mcg vitamin K, 1,200 mg calcium, 500–1,000 mg magnesium, 100–300 mg potassium, 15 billion live *Bifidobacterium bifidum* organisms, and 15 billion live *Lactobacillus acidophilus* organisms per day. And ask your physician to consider the potential effects of sodium depletion.

You can also eat foods that contain the depleted nutrients:

- Biotin: beef liver, soybeans, rice bran, peanut butter, barley
- Inositol: cantaloupe, oranges, green beans, grapefruit juice, limes
- Thiamin: braised liver, turkey heart, roasted chicken, gefilte fish, sardines
- Riboflavin: dried sunflower seeds, orange juice, bulgur, spinach noodles, pine nuts
- Niacin: chicken breast, beef liver, mackerel, barley, bulgur
- Vitamin B_6: potato, banana, garbanzo beans, chicken breast, fortified oatmeal
- Vitamin B_{12}: beef liver, rainbow trout, sockeye salmon, beef, haddock
- Vitamin K: kale, broccoli, parsley, Swiss chard, spinach
- Calcium: milk, dried figs, Swiss cheese, yogurt, tofu
- Magnesium: Florida avocado, toasted wheat germ, almonds, shredded wheat cereal, pumpkin seeds
- Potassium: dried figs, California avocado, papaya, banana, dates
- *Bifidobacterium bifidum*: Jerusalem artichokes, asparagus, garlic, and onions may stimulate the growth or activity of this probiotic
- *Lactobacillus acidophilus*: yogurt containing live lactobacillus cultures, kefir, acidophilus milk

Consult with your physician before making any changes to your diet or supplemental regimen.

AMILORIDE (uh-MIL-oh-ride)

Brand Name: Midamor

About Amiloride

If fluid is pooling in your legs or elsewhere, as may be the case in conges-tive heart failure, or if your doctor wants to reduce the amount of fluid in your bloodstream to lower your blood pressure, you may be given a diuretic. These so-called water pills encourage the kidneys to filter more fluid out of the bloodstream, and send it to the bladder for disposal.

This approach works well, except for one small problem: The expelled wa-ter takes the mineral potassium and other substances along with it. If you lose too much potassium, you may develop a condition called hypokalemic meta-bolic alkalosis. Alkalosis means that the blood is too alkaline (not acidic enough), a condition that can cause irritability, muscle cramps, twitching, and spasms.

Diuretic-induced alkalosis can be avoided if your doctor gives you a potassium-sparing diuretic such as amiloride. Amiloride interferes with the process that filters potassium out of the blood, allowing the mineral to re-main in the blood. Amiloride may be used to treat hypertension, heart fail-ure, or other problems by itself or in combination with other diuretics, preventing the potassium loss that would be caused by the other water pills.

Possible Side Effects

The drug's more common side effects include impotence, stomach upset, muscle cramps, cough, constipation, fatigue, and dizziness.

Which Nutrients Are Robbed

Taking this medicine may deplete your supply of, increase your need for, or interfere with the activity of:

- Folic acid
- Magnesium
- Calcium
- Sodium

Additional Ways This Drug May Upset Your Nutritional Balance

Amiloride can cause nausea, vomiting, abdominal pain, gas pain, and ap-petite changes, all of which can upset your eating habits and possibly inter-fere with good nutrition. It may also trigger diarrhea, which can hamper nutrient absorption.

This drug can also trigger hyperkalemia, which means too much potassium in the blood. It might also cause a buildup of zinc in the body.

Restoring Your Nutritional Balance

To compensate for the nutrient loss caused by this drug, speak to your physician about taking 400–800 mcg folic acid and 1,200 mg calcium per day. And ask your physician to consider the potential effects of sodium depletion.

There is some concern that potassium-sparing diuretics such as amiloride may cause the body to retain magnesium, so ask your physician to monitor your magnesium level.

A Note on Potassium: "Regular" diuretics lower potassium levels, while potassium-sparing diuretics do not—they may increase levels instead. It is not uncommon for doctors to prescribe two different diuretics. That's why you should speak to your physician about your potassium levels, and whether it is appropriate for you to take supplements or eat potassium-rich foods.

You can also eat foods that contain the depleted nutrients:

- Folic acid: beef liver, fortified breakfast cereals, spinach, great northern beans, asparagus
- Calcium: milk, dried figs, Swiss cheese, yogurt, tofu

Consult with your physician before making any changes to your diet or supplemental regimen.

AMILORIDE PLUS HYDROCHLOROTHIAZIDE (uh-MIL-oh-ride, hye-droe-klor-oh-THYE-uh-zide)

Brand Names: Alti-Amiloride HCTZ, Apo-Amilzide, Moduret, Moduretic, Novamilor, Nu-Amilzide

About Amiloride plus Hydrochlorothiazide

Amiloride is a diuretic with potassium-sparing properties. This means that it stimulates the kidneys to draw water out of the bloodstream and send it to the bladder for excretion. But unlike many other diuretics, it does this without causing the body to lose large amounts of potassium in the urine. A lack of potassium in the blood can be a very dangerous condition, so protecting this mineral from being lost through the urine is quite a plus.

Unfortunately, amiloride is not always powerful enough to do the trick for people suffering from congestive heart failure, elevated blood pressure, or other conditions in which doctors want to draw off some body fluid. So amiloride is often combined with other drugs, such as the powerful diuretic hydrochlorothiazide.

Like amiloride, hydrochlorothiazide flushes water out of the body, but it does cause the loss of potassium. By combining amiloride and hydrochlorothiazide, excess fluid can be drained from the body without washing away too much potassium at the same time.

Possible Side Effects

Amiloride's more common side effects include impotence, stomach upset, muscle cramps, cough, fatigue, and dizziness. Side effects seen with hydrochlorothiazide include low blood pressure, sensitivity to light, allergic reactions, reduced blood potassium, and elevated blood calcium levels.

Which Nutrients Are Robbed

Taking this medicine may deplete your supply of, increase your need for, or interfere with the activity of:

- Magnesium
- Sodium
- Phosphorus
- Zinc
- Potassium
- Coenzyme Q_{10}

Additional Ways This Drug May Upset Your Nutritional Balance

Amiloride can cause nausea, vomiting, abdominal pain, gas pain, and appetite changes, while hydrochlorothiazide can cause loss of appetite. These side effects can upset your eating habits and possibly interfere with good nutrition. Amiloride may also trigger diarrhea, which can hamper nutrient absorption.

Amiloride can also trigger hyperkalemia (too much potassium).

Restoring Your Nutritional Balance

To compensate for the nutrient loss caused by this drug, speak to your physician about taking 500–1,000 mg magnesium, 700 mg phosphorus, 50–200 mg zinc, and 30–100 mg coenzyme Q_{10} per day. And ask your physician to consider the potential effects of sodium depletion.

A Note on Potassium: "Regular" diuretics lower potassium levels, while potassium-sparing diuretics do not—they may increase levels instead. It is not uncommon for doctors to prescribe two different diuretics. That's why you should speak to your physician about your potassium levels, and whether it is appropriate for you to take supplements or eat potassium-rich foods.

You can also eat foods that contain the depleted nutrients:

- Magnesium: Florida avocado, toasted wheat germ, almonds, shredded wheat cereal, pumpkin seeds
- Phosphorus: plain nonfat yogurt, lentils, salmon, milk, halibut
- Zinc: oysters, beef shank, chicken, pork tenderloin, plain yogurt
- Coenzyme Q_{10}: beef, chicken, trout, salmon, oranges, broccoli

Consult with your physician before making any changes to your diet or supplemental regimen.

AMINOSALICYLIC ACID (uh-mee-noe-sal-i-SIL-ik ASS-id)

Brand Names: Aminosalicylate Sodium, 4-Aminosalicylic Acid, Para-Aminosalicylate Sodium, PAS, Paser, Sodium PAS

About Aminosalicylic Acid

Aminosalicylic acid was once a first-choice drug for the treatment of tuberculosis (TB), but its glory days are long past. While it never actually killed the bacteria that cause TB (*Mycobacterium tuberculosis*), it did interfere with the mechanisms that governed their reproduction, so new generations couldn't replace the old ones when they died.

Unfortunately, the wily *M. tuberculosis* has become fairly resistant to aminosalicylic acid, and newer TB drugs have been developed that are not only more effective but also produce fewer side effects. Today, aminosalicylic acid is only used in combination with other drugs to fight TB. It's useful in that role, inhibiting the appearance of bacterial resistance to other anti-TB drugs called streptomycin and isoniazid.

Possible Side Effects

The drug's side effects include fever, anemia, low blood sugar, stomach upset, hepatitis, and jaundice.

Which Nutrients Are Robbed

Taking this medicine may deplete your supply of, increase your need for, or interfere with the activity of:

- Folic acid
- Vitamin B_{12}

Additional Ways This Drug May Upset Your Nutritional Balance

Aminosalicylic acid can cause abdominal pain, low blood sugar (hypoglycemia), nausea, and vomiting, all of which can upset your eating habits and possibly interfere with good nutrition. It can also cause diarrhea, which can hamper nutrient absorption.

Restoring Your Nutritional Balance

To compensate for the nutrient loss caused by this drug, speak to your physician about taking 400–800 mcg folic acid and 500–1,000 mcg vitamin B_{12} per day.

You can also eat foods that contain the depleted nutrients:

- Folic acid: beef liver, fortified breakfast cereals, spinach, great northern beans, asparagus
- Vitamin B_{12}: beef liver, rainbow trout, sockeye salmon, beef, haddock

Consult with your physician before making any changes to your diet or supplemental regimen.

AMITRIPTYLINE (a-mee-TRIP-ti-leen)

Brand Names: Apo-Amitriptyline, Elavil, Endep, Levak, Vanatrip

About Amitriptyline

More than 25 million Americans suffer from migraines, those very intense headaches that can cause nausea, double vision, intolerance of sound and light, bright spots before the eyes, numbness and tingling of the face, slurred speech, confusion, profuse sweating, chills, and diarrhea.

Although there are many theories, we can't say for certain what causes migraines. The vascular theory holds that migraines strike when blood vessels in the brain contract and expand inappropriately, interfering with the flow of blood. The serotonin theory argues that the root problem lies in changes in the amount of the brain's "feel-good" neurotransmitter, serotonin, which causes the inappropriate contraction and expansion of the blood vessels. Then there's the neural theory, which suggests that irritation of certain nerves or a part of the brain stem causes the release of various chemicals that trigger inflammation in the brain. In a small percentage of migraine sufferers, a genetic defect may be responsible for the problem. Whatever the cause of migraines, the result is pain and disability that can last for hours or even days.

There is no cure for migraines. Instead, there are many treatments, including amitriptyline. We're not exactly sure why amitriptyline helps. It may be because the drug prevents the reabsorption of serotonin, correcting serotonin imbalances and allowing more of this neurotransmitter to send its "feel-good" messages throughout the nervous system.

In addition to migraines, amitriptyline is used in treating certain chronic pain conditions and depression in children.

Possible Side Effects

The drug's side effects can include changes in the heart rhythm, restlessness, sedation, constipation, allergic rash, and weight gain.

Which Nutrients Are Robbed

Taking this medicine may deplete your supply of, increase your need for, or interfere with the activity of:

- Riboflavin
- Coenzyme Q_{10}
- Sodium

Restoring Your Nutritional Balance

To compensate for the nutrient loss caused by this drug, speak to your physician about taking 25–100 mg riboflavin and 30–100 mg coenzyme Q_{10} per day. And ask your physician to consider the potential effects of sodium depletion.

You can also eat foods that contain the depleted nutrients:

- Riboflavin: dried sunflower seeds, orange juice, bulgur, spinach noodles, pine nuts
- Coenzyme Q_{10}: beef, chicken, trout, salmon, oranges, broccoli

Consult with your physician before making any changes to your diet or supplemental regimen.

AMMONIUM CHLORIDE (uh-MOE-nee-um KLOR-ide)

About Ammonium Chloride

The mineral chloride is often overlooked and undervalued, but it's vital to good health—indeed, to life itself. Chloride works with potassium and sodium to maintain the proper amount of body fluid and the correct acid-base balance. It's also an effective antibacterial agent and an important ingredient in stomach acid.

If the levels of chloride in the blood fall too far (a condition known as hypochloremia), you may suffer from muscle cramps, loss of appetite, listlessness, shallow breathing, and even coma. Hypochloremia may arise due to prolonged diarrhea or vomiting, to a very strict low-salt vegetarian diet, or to the overuse of diuretics.

Ammonium chloride is used to replenish chloride when you've run short.

Possible Side Effects

The drug's side effects include confusion, rash, headache, stomach upset, low blood levels of potassium, and coma.

Which Nutrients Are Robbed

Taking this medicine may deplete your supply of, increase your need for, or interfere with the activity of:

- Potassium
- Sodium

Additional Ways This Drug May Upset Your Nutritional Balance

Ammonium chloride can cause gastric irritation, nausea, and vomiting, all of which can upset your eating habits and possibly interfere with good nutrition.

Restoring Your Nutritional Balance

To compensate for the nutrient loss caused by this drug, speak to your physician about taking 100–300 mg potassium per day. And ask your physician to consider the potential effects of sodium depletion.

You can also eat foods that contain the depleted nutrient:

- Potassium: dried figs, California avocado, papaya, banana, dates

Consult with your physician before making any changes to your diet or supplemental regimen.

AMOXAPINE (uh-MOKS-uh-peen)

Brand Name: Asendin

About Amoxapine

Depression can be extremely debilitating, striking rich and poor, young and old, and people of all races and cultures. However, the disease does play favorites when it comes to gender: Women are twice as likely as men to become depressed.

Typically, depression settles in over the course of a few days or weeks, and its symptoms vary. For example, depression is said to be "vegetative" if you generally withdraw from others and you eat, speak, and sleep little. It's said to be "atypical" if you eat more, gain weight, feel anxious, and sleep more than usual. Depression may be relatively mild, clear up on its own, and not bother you for months on end. Or it may last for long periods of time or be so intense that you feel there's no reason to keep on living.

Physicians use a variety of drugs to relieve depression. Amoxapine is one of the second-generation antidepressants developed in the 1980s and 1990s. That sounds pretty impressive, but in general the second-generation drugs aren't any stronger than those they were designed to supersede. In fact, amoxapine and many other antidepressants are slowly being pushed aside by a new class of drugs, the selective serotonin reuptake inhibitors (SSRIs).

Still, amoxapine has its uses, and your doctor may prescribe it because of your individual needs or the drug's specific properties, side effects, length of action, and so on.

Possible Side Effects

The drug's more common side effects include drowsiness, blurred vision, constipation, and dry mouth.

Which Nutrients Are Robbed

Taking this medicine may deplete your supply of, increase your need for, or interfere with the activity of:

- Riboflavin
- Coenzyme Q_{10}

Additional Ways This Drug May Upset Your Nutritional Balance

Amoxapine can cause nausea, which can upset your eating habits and interfere with good nutrition.

Restoring Your Nutritional Balance

To compensate for the nutrient loss caused by this drug, speak to your physician about taking 25–100 mg riboflavin and 30–100 mg coenzyme Q_{10} per day.

You can also eat foods that contain the depleted nutrients:

- Riboflavin: dried sunflower seeds, orange juice, bulgur, spinach noodles, pine nuts
- Coenzyme Q_{10}: beef, chicken, trout, salmon, oranges, broccoli

Consult with your physician before making any changes to your diet or supplemental regimen.

AMOXICILLIN (uh-moks-i-SIL-in)

Brand Names: Amoxil, Apo-Amoxi, Moxilin, Novamoxin, Nu-Amoxi, Polymox, Scheinpharm Amoxicillin, Trimox

About Amoxicillin

It's not uncommon for children to develop otitis media, which is doctor-speak for an infection of the middle ear. Chronic otitis media can be caused by an unusual pooling of fluid in the middle ear, a permanent hole in the eardrum, or a noncancerous growth of skinlike material inside the ear.

More commonly, a child's middle ear infection is caused by bacteria or a virus. When the germs take up residence inside the ear, infection sets in and the eardrum becomes red and distended, causing pain.

Amoxicillin, which is related to penicillin, is one of the antibiotics doctors prescribe for middle ear infections caused by bacteria. It destroys bacteria by binding to them and preventing them from building their cellular walls, which results in their death.

Amoxicillin may also be used to treat infections of the skin and the genitourinary and respiratory tracts and to prevent bacterial infections in susceptible people undergoing dental procedures or surgery.

Possible Side Effects

The drug's side effects include diarrhea, vomiting, anxiety, dizziness, confusion, and anemia.

Which Nutrients Are Robbed

Taking this medicine may deplete your supply of, increase your need for, or interfere with the activity of:

- Biotin
- Inositol
- Thiamin
- Riboflavin
- Niacin
- Vitamin B_6
- Vitamin B_{12}
- Vitamin K
- Potassium
- *Bifidobacterium bifidum*
- *Lactobacillus acidophilus*

Additional Ways This Drug May Upset Your Nutritional Balance

Amoxicillin can cause nausea and vomiting, which can upset your eating habits and possibly interfere with good nutrition. It may also trigger diarrhea, which can hamper nutrient absorption.

Restoring Your Nutritional Balance

To compensate for the nutrient loss caused by this drug, speak to your physician about taking 500–1,000 mcg biotin, 250–1,000 mg inositol, 25–100 mg thiamin, 25–100 mg riboflavin, 50–100 mg niacin, 50–100 mg vitamin B_6, 500–1,000 mcg vitamin B_{12}, 60–80 mcg vitamin K, 100–300 mg potassium, 15 billion live *Bifidobacterium bifidum* organisms, and 15 billion live *Lactobacillus acidophilus* organisms per day.

You can also eat foods that contain the depleted nutrients:

- Biotin: beef liver, soybeans, rice bran, peanut butter, barley
- Inositol: cantaloupe, oranges, green beans, grapefruit juice, limes
- Thiamin: braised liver, turkey heart, roasted chicken, gefilte fish, sardines
- Riboflavin: dried sunflower seeds, orange juice, bulgur, spinach noodles, pine nuts
- Niacin: chicken breast, beef liver, mackerel, barley, bulgur
- Vitamin B_6: potato, banana, garbanzo beans, chicken breast, fortified oatmeal
- Vitamin B_{12}: beef liver, rainbow trout, sockeye salmon, beef, haddock
- Vitamin K: kale, broccoli, parsley, Swiss chard, spinach
- Potassium: dried figs, California avocado, papaya, banana, dates

- *Bifidobacterium bifidum*: Jerusalem artichokes, asparagus, garlic, and onions may stimulate the growth or activity of this probiotic
- *Lactobacillus acidophilus*: yogurt containing live lactobacillus cultures, kefir, acidophilus milk

Consult with your physician before making any changes to your diet or supplemental regimen.

AMPHOTERICIN B Amphotericin B Cholesteryl Sulfate Complex, Amphotericin B Conventional, Amphotericin B Liquid Complex, Amphotericin B Liposomal (am-foe-TER-i-sin bee kole-LESS-te-ril SUL-fate KOM-pleks, lye-poe-SOE-mal)

Brand Names: Abelcet, AmBisome, Amphocin, Amphotec, Fungizone

About Amphotericin B

Amphotericin B combats fungi such as *Candida albicans*, one of the organisms most likely to be lurking in the blood.

The drug works by making the fungal cells "bleed" to death. They don't bleed blood, of course. They bleed tiny molecules and other substances that they need to remain alive. When they've lost enough of these vital substances, they die.

Amphotericin B works by targeting certain parts of the fungal cell wall—specifically, it looks for the ergosterol in the cell walls. When it binds to the ergosterol, it changes the permeability of the fungal cell wall, which is something like changing a window into a screen. Turning the ergosterol "windows" into "screens" allows parts of the fungal cell to leak out, and the cell dies.

Unfortunately, amphotericin B can also make certain body cells more permeable and may cause significant damage to the kidneys—sometimes serious enough to require dialysis.

Despite this drawback, amphotericin B is used to rid the body of numerous types of fungi, and some doctors even consider it the drug of choice for many life-threatening fungal infections.

Possible Side Effects

Depending on which form of the drug you use, more common side effects include rapid breathing, low blood pressure, fever, chills, nausea, and generalized pain.

Which Nutrients Are Robbed

Taking this medicine may deplete your supply of, increase your need for, or interfere with the activity of:

- Calcium
- Magnesium
- Potassium
- Sodium

Additional Ways This Drug May Upset Your Nutritional Balance

The various forms of amphotericin can cause abdominal pain, loss of appetite, heartburn, nausea, and vomiting, all of which can upset your eating habits and possibly interfere with good nutrition. It can also cause diarrhea, which can hamper nutrient absorption.

Restoring Your Nutritional Balance

To compensate for the nutrient loss caused by this drug, speak to your physician about taking 1,200 mg calcium, 500–1,000 mg magnesium, and 100–300 mg potassium per day. And ask your physician to consider the potential effects of sodium depletion.

You can also eat foods that contain the depleted nutrients:

- Calcium: milk, dried figs, Swiss cheese, yogurt, tofu
- Magnesium: Florida avocado, toasted wheat germ, almonds, shredded wheat cereal, pumpkin seeds
- Potassium: dried figs, California avocado, papaya, banana, dates

Consult with your physician before making any changes to your diet or supplemental regimen.

AMPICILLIN (am-pi-SIL-in)

Brand Names: Ampicin, Apo-Ampi, Nu-Ampi, Omnipen, Polycillin, Totacillin

About Ampicillin

The bronchi are tubes that carry air in and out of the lungs. The walls of these vital air tubes are elastic so they can expand or relax as necessary to keep the right amount of air flowing through.

In a disease called bronchiectasis, sections of the walls of the air tubes are destroyed. The damaged areas become chronically inflamed, the airways widen and get flabby, and mucus builds up. Bacteria can accumulate, leading to infections, blockage of the airways, and further damage to the bronchial walls.

One of the first symptoms of bronchiectasis can be terribly frightening: coughing up mucus that contains blood. There may also be shortness of breath, chronic coughing, chest pain, fever, and pneumonia.

Several things can cause bronchiectasis, including bacterial infections, and the disease itself can trigger more infections. That's why medicines such as ampicillin may be prescribed. Ampicillin, a penicillin antibiotic, prevents bacteria from building their cell walls. This keeps the bacterial colony from growing and the infection from spreading.

In addition to bronchiectasis, ampicillin may be prescribed for certain skin, sinus, respiratory, genitourinary, or other infections caused by streptococci, pneumococci, staphylococci, and other bacteria.

Possible Side Effects

Depending on the method of administration, ampicillin's side effects include pain at the injection site, rash, allergic reactions, oral candidiasis (yeast infections), and seizures.

Which Nutrients Are Robbed

Taking this medicine may deplete your supply of, increase your need for, or interfere with the activity of:

- Biotin
- Inositol
- Thiamin
- Riboflavin
- Niacin
- Vitamin B_6
- Vitamin B_{12}
- Vitamin K
- Potassium
- *Bifidobacterium bifidum*
- *Lactobacillus acidophilus*

Additional Ways This Drug May Upset Your Nutritional Balance

Ampicillin can cause abdominal cramps and vomiting, which can upset your eating habits and possibly interfere with good nutrition. It may also trigger diarrhea, which can hamper nutrient absorption.

Restoring Your Nutritional Balance

To compensate for the nutrient loss caused by this drug, speak to your physician about taking 500–1,000 mcg biotin, 250–1,000 mg inositol, 25–100 mg thiamin, 25–100 mg riboflavin, 50–100 mg niacin, 50–100 mg vitamin B_6, 500–1,000 mcg vitamin B_{12}, 60–80 mcg vitamin K, 100–300 mg potassium,

15 billion live *Bifidobacterium bifidum* organisms, and 15 billion live *Lactobacillus acidophilus* organisms per day.

You can also eat foods that contain the depleted nutrients:

- Biotin: beef liver, soybeans, rice bran, peanut butter, barley
- Inositol: cantaloupe, oranges, green beans, grapefruit juice, limes
- Thiamin: braised liver, turkey heart, roasted chicken, gefilte fish, sardines
- Riboflavin: dried sunflower seeds, orange juice, bulgur, spinach noodles, pine nuts
- Niacin: chicken breast, beef liver, mackerel, barley, bulgur
- Vitamin B_6: potato, banana, garbanzo beans, chicken breast, fortified oatmeal
- Vitamin B_{12}: beef liver, rainbow trout, sockeye salmon, beef, haddock
- Vitamin K: kale, broccoli, parsley, Swiss chard, spinach
- Potassium: dried figs, California avocado, papaya, banana, dates
- *Bifidobacterium bifidum*: Jerusalem artichokes, asparagus, garlic, and onions may stimulate the growth or activity of this probiotic
- *Lactobacillus acidophilus*: yogurt containing live lactobacillus cultures, kefir, acidophilus milk

Consult with your physician before making any changes to your diet or supplemental regimen.

ARSENIC TRIOXIDE (AR-se-nik trye-OKS-ide)

Brand Name: Trisenox

About Arsenic Trioxide

Cancer brings to mind images of large masses growing in or pressing down on organs. But sometimes the cancer is small enough to fit inside very tiny cells, such as the blood cells.

Leukemia is one of those cancers, so named because it strikes the leukocytes, or white blood cells, which are an important part of the body's immune system. Cancerous white blood cells reproduce rapidly, too rapidly. They take over the bone marrow, where blood cells are born, interfering with the development of other blood cells. They may also invade the brain, liver, spleen, or other organs.

In adults, the most common form of leukemia is called acute myelocytic leukemia. This disease causes the rapidly reproducing, immature white blood cells to destroy other developing blood cells in the bone marrow. Then they dive into the bloodstream and travel to various organs, where they continue multiplying. These cells may cause infection, sweats, fever, fatigue, and other symptoms linked to a malfunctioning immune system. If the errant white blood cells congregate in the brain, they can trigger inflammation of the brain lining, headaches, vomiting, and mood changes. If they settle in the skeletal system, they can cause bone pain.

Arsenic trioxide is used to treat a subtype of acute myelocytic leukemia called acute promyelocytic leukemia. We don't know exactly how it works, but it does bring about remission in some 70 percent of those with severe cases or in those who have already suffered a relapse.

Possible Side Effects

The drug's more common side effects include rapid heartbeat, fatigue, diarrhea, fever, headache, nausea, and cough.

Which Nutrients Are Robbed

Taking this medicine may deplete your supply of, increase your need for, or interfere with the activity of:

- Calcium
- Magnesium
- Potassium

Additional Ways This Drug May Upset Your Nutritional Balance

Arsenic trioxide can cause nausea, abdominal pain, hypoglycemia, vomiting, and loss of appetite, all of which can upset your eating habits and possibly interfere with good nutrition. It can also cause diarrhea, which can hamper nutrient absorption.

This drug can also trigger hyperkalemia, or too much potassium in the blood.

Restoring Your Nutritional Balance

To compensate for the nutrient loss caused by this drug, speak to your physician about taking 1,200 mg calcium and 500–1,000 mg magnesium per day. And ask your physician to monitor your potassium status.

You can also eat foods that contain the depleted nutrients:

- Calcium: milk, dried figs, Swiss cheese, yogurt, tofu
- Magnesium: Florida avocado, toasted wheat germ, almonds, shredded wheat cereal, pumpkin seeds

Consult with your physician before making any changes to your diet or supplemental regimen.

ASPIRIN, ASPIRIN PLUS EXTENDED-RELEASE DIPYRIDAMOLE (ASS-pir-in, dye-peer-ID-uh-mole)

Brand Names: Aspirin: Anacin, Apo-ASA, A.S.A., Asaphen, Ascriptin, Aspergum, Asprimox, Bayer (Aspirin, Buffered Aspirin, Extra Strength, Extra Strength Plus, Low Adult Strength), Bufferin, Buffex, Carma Arthritis Pain Reliever, Easprin, Ecotrin, Ecotrin Low Adult Strength, Empirin, Entrophen, Extra Strength Adprin-B, Enteric 500 Aspirin, MSD Enteric Coated ASA, St. Joseph Adult Chewable Aspirin, Novasen, ZORprin
Aspirin plus dipyridamole: Aggrenox

About Aspirin, Aspirin plus Dipyridamole

It's the oldest and least expensive of the painkillers: aspirin, known more technically as acetylsalicylic acid (ASA). Humans began using aspirin, or something close to it, long before they had any idea what it was or how it worked. Ancient Romans used the extract of willow bark, which contains a chemical "ancestor" of aspirin, to cool off fevers. Aspirin itself was formulated in the 1800s and became very popular as the nineteenth century made way for the twentieth and the drug's anti-inflammatory properties were recognized.

Aspirin has many actions. It helps reduce:

- *Fever,* by hindering the release of substances in the body that raise the temperature.
- *Inflammation,* by interfering with the action of the COX enzymes which produce the prostaglandins that spur the inflammation response when body tissue is injured or invaded. It also hampers other inflammation responses in the body. This anti-inflammatory action makes aspirin very useful for treating rheumatoid arthritis and other problems that cause inflamed joints.
- *Pain,* by reducing inflammation and inhibiting pain signals in the nervous system.
- *The risk of a heart attack or stroke* and related problems, by "thinning" the blood and making it less likely to clot.

Aspirin would seem to be the ideal medicine for pain and inflammation—indeed, for years it was the "gold standard" against which all other anti-inflammatory medicines were measured. And you can buy over 200 aspirin and aspirin-based products without a prescription. Unfortunately, it can severely irritate the lining of the stomach and it increases the risk of bleeding in various parts of the body. Ibuprofen and naproxen, two popular anti-inflammatories that don't contain aspirin, are easier on the stomach, so the use of aspirin has declined in recent years.

However, taking aspirin is still considered a good way to reduce the risk of transient ischemic attacks (TIAs, or "baby strokes"), as well as full-fledged strokes and heart attacks in people at risk for these ailments. It does this by reducing the tendency of platelets to clump together, "crowd around" plaque in your arteries, and release substances that can encourage a heart attack or stroke. Dipyridamole also thins the blood, which is why it may be combined with aspirin to prevent heart attacks or strokes in at-risk patients.

Possible Side Effects

Aspirin's side effects include anemia, insomnia, rapid heartbeat, stomach ulcers, and liver damage. The more common side effects seen with aspirin plus dipyridamole include headache, stomach upset, and abdominal pain.

Which Nutrients Are Robbed

Taking this medicine may deplete your supply of, increase your need for, or interfere with the activity of:

- Folic acid
- Vitamin C
- Iron
- Potassium
- Sodium
- Zinc

Additional Ways This Drug May Upset Your Nutritional Balance

Aspirin can cause heartburn, stomach pain, nausea, and vomiting. Aspirin plus dipyridamole can cause loss of appetite and vomiting. These side effects can upset your eating habits and possibly interfere with good nutrition. Aspirin plus dipyridamole may also trigger diarrhea, which can hamper nutrient absorption.

Aspirin can also trigger hyperkalemia, or too much potassium in the blood. Buffered aspirin and sodium salicylate, which contain large amounts of sodium, may cause hypernatremia, or too much sodium in the blood.

Restoring Your Nutritional Balance

To compensate for the nutrient loss caused by this drug, speak to your physician about taking 400–800 mcg folic acid, 250–1,500 mg vitamin C, and 50–200 mg zinc per day. And ask your physician to consider the potential effects of iron and sodium depletion and to monitor your potassium status.

You can also eat foods that contain the depleted nutrients:

- Folic acid: beef liver, fortified breakfast cereals, spinach, great northern beans, asparagus
- Vitamin C: papaya, guava, red pepper, cantaloupe, black currants
- Zinc: oysters, beef shank, chicken, pork tenderloin, plain yogurt

Consult with your physician before making any changes to your diet or supplemental regimen.

ATENOLOL (uh-TEN-oh-lole)

Brand Names: Apo-Atenol, Novo-Atenol, PMS-Atenolol, Rhoxal-atenolol, Tenolin, Tenormin

About Atenolol

You wouldn't think that fixing a heart problem could cause an equally dangerous breathing problem. But it can happen when drugs called beta-blockers are used to treat elevated blood pressure, angina, and certain other ailments.

Beta-blockers work by "blockading" specialized areas in the heart and elsewhere called beta-receptors. That is, they insert themselves into these beta-receptors and interfere with chemical messengers that would otherwise plug in and force the heart to work harder. With these "work-hard" messages blocked out, the heart can relax a bit, allowing blood pressure to fall.

That's fine, except that beta-receptors are also found in the respiratory system. And when those beta-receptors are blocked, the airways may constrict and breathing can become very difficult. This is especially troublesome for people who already have certain breathing difficulties.

The solution is to block the beta-receptors of the heart (called the Beta$_1$-receptors), while generally staying away from the beta-receptors of the airways (the Beta$_2$-receptors). Certain beta-blockers, including atenolol, do just that. Called selective beta-blockers, they "prefer" the

Beta$_1$-receptors of the heart. Although they don't completely avoid the Beta$_2$-receptors in the airways, they're much more likely to interact with the Beta$_1$-receptors.

Atenolol is used to treat elevated blood pressure, especially when it's associated with certain diseases of the airways. It's also used for angina, to prevent migraines, and to reduce the odds of further problems in those who have had a heart attack.

Possible Side Effects

The drug's more common side effects include slow heartbeat, low blood pressure, lethargy, nightmares, impotence, and depression.

Which Nutrients Are Robbed

Taking this medicine may deplete your supply of, increase your need for, or interfere with the activity of:

- Coenzyme Q$_{10}$ • Melatonin

Additional Ways This Drug May Upset Your Nutritional Balance

Atenolol can cause hypoglycemia and nausea, which can upset your eating habits and possibly interfere with good nutrition. It may also trigger diarrhea, which can hamper nutrient absorption.

Restoring Your Nutritional Balance

To compensate for the nutrient loss caused by this drug, speak to your physician about taking 30–100 mg coenzyme Q$_{10}$ and 1–3 mg melatonin per day.

You can also eat foods that contain the depleted nutrient:

- Coenzyme Q$_{10}$: beef, chicken, trout, salmon, oranges, broccoli

Consult with your physician before making any changes to your diet or supplemental regimen.

ATENOLOL PLUS CHLORTHALIDONE (uh-TEN-oh-lole, klor-THAL-i-dohn)

Brand Name: Tenoretic

About Atenolol plus Chlorthalidone

Everybody on a football team has a specialty. The center hikes the ball to the quarterback. The quarterback throws the ball, runs with it, or hands it off to a running back. The running back tries to run the ball down to the end zone. And they're all protected by the linesmen, who block the other team and prevent them from tackling "our guys."

Atenolol is like a football lineman. Its job is to block chemical messengers that try to get into the tiny beta-receptors in the heart. If these messengers do get into the beta-receptors, they can force the heart to work harder. But when atenolol blocks them, the heart can relax a bit, which can help reduce elevated blood pressure, ease angina, and protect the hearts of people who have had heart attacks.

When treating elevated blood pressure, physicians often combine two drugs to take advantage of their different actions. It's like sending two football players, each with a different talent, into the game. If one doesn't knock the opponent flat, perhaps the other one will. Or maybe the combination of the two will do the trick.

Such is the case with the combination of atenolol plus chlorthalidone, both of which are designed to treat hypertension by taking a load off the heart. Atenolol helps the heart relax, and chlorthalidone stimulates the kidneys to excrete larger amounts of fluid, which reduces the blood volume. Both make it possible for the heart to relax a little more.

Possible Side Effects

Atenolol's more common side effects include slow heartbeat, low blood pressure, lethargy, nightmares, impotence, and depression. Chlorthalidone's side effects include dizziness, drowsiness, and weakness.

Which Nutrients Are Robbed

Taking this medicine may deplete your supply of, increase your need for, or interfere with the activity of:

- Magnesium
- Phosphorus
- Potassium
- Sodium
- Zinc
- Coenzyme Q_{10}

Additional Ways This Drug May Upset Your Nutritional Balance

Atenolol can cause hypoglycemia and nausea, which can upset your eating habits and possibly interfere with good nutrition. It may also trigger diarrhea, which can hamper nutrient absorption. Chlorthalidone may cause nausea and vomiting.

Restoring Your Nutritional Balance

To compensate for the nutrient loss caused by this drug, speak to your physician about taking 500–1,000 mg magnesium, 700 mg phosphorus, 50–200 mg zinc, and 30–100 mg coenzyme Q_{10} per day. And ask your physician to consider the potential effects of sodium depletion.

A Note on Potassium: "Regular" diuretics lower potassium levels, while potassium-sparing diuretics do not—they may increase levels instead. It is not uncommon for doctors to prescribe two different diuretics. That's why you should speak to your physician about your potassium levels, and whether it is appropriate for you to take supplements or eat potassium-rich foods.

You can also eat foods that contain the depleted nutrients:

- Magnesium: Florida avocado, toasted wheat germ, almonds, shredded wheat cereal, pumpkin seeds
- Phosphorus: plain nonfat yogurt, lentils, salmon, milk, halibut
- Zinc: oysters, beef shank, chicken, pork tenderloin, plain yogurt
- Coenzyme Q_{10}: beef, chicken, trout, salmon, oranges, broccoli

Consult with your physician before making any changes to your diet or supplemental regimen.

ATORVASTATIN (uh-TORE-vuh-stat-in)

Brand Name: Lipitor

About Atorvastatin

The famous Framingham Heart Study, which was launched in 1948, was the first major study to link elevated cholesterol levels to heart attacks. Although it didn't prove that elevated cholesterol *caused* heart attacks, it did show that the two were associated, and that was good enough to convince physicians that everyone should keep their cholesterol levels under certain limits. But how do you do that?

Cholesterol doesn't just spring to life in the body. It's produced, one step at a time, by the body's biochemical machinery. One of the strategies for lowering cholesterol levels is to throw a monkey wrench into the biochemical machinery. And that's exactly what atorvastatin does.

A substance known as HMG-CoA reductase plays a key role at an early point in the cholesterol manufacturing process. Atorvastatin interferes with the activity of HMG-CoA reductase, which is why it's called a HMG-CoA reductase *inhibitor*. In essence, atorvastatin "disengages" part of the body's cholesterol-making machinery, so cholesterol levels fall. Unfortunately, part of that same biochemical machinery is used to synthesize coenzyme Q_{10}, which is indispensable for good heart health.

Belonging to the popular group of drugs known as the statins, atorvastatin is used to reduce blood levels of cholesterol and fat.

Possible Side Effects

The drug's more common side effects include headache, chest pain, rash, stomach upset, urinary tract infection, and pain in the joints and muscles.

Which Nutrients Are Robbed

Taking this medicine may deplete your supply of, increase your need for, or interfere with the activity of:

- Coenzyme Q_{10}

Additional Ways This Drug May Upset Your Nutritional Balance

Atorvastatin can cause abdominal pain, dyspepsia, and nausea, all of which can upset your eating habits and possibly interfere with good nutrition. It may also trigger diarrhea, which can hamper nutrient absorption.

The drug may cause blood levels of vitamin A to rise.

Restoring Your Nutritional Balance

To compensate for the nutrient loss caused by this drug, speak to your physician about taking 30–100 mg coenzyme Q_{10} per day.

You can also eat foods that contain the depleted nutrient:

- Coenzyme Q_{10}: beef, chicken, trout, salmon, oranges, broccoli

Consult with your physician before making any changes to your diet or supplemental regimen.

AZITHROMYCIN (az-ith-roe-MYE-sin)

Brand Name: Zithromax

About Azithromycin

Because there are thousands of kinds of bacteria, we've had to develop a whole arsenal of antibiotics that can attack the "enemy" in different ways. They may prevent the germs from building their cells walls, interfere as they attempt to make new DNA, specialize in tracking them down in a particular kind of body tissue, and so on.

Azithromycin is an antibiotic that's particularly good at working its way into organs, tissues, and even certain white blood cells, which means that bacteria have a hard time hiding from it. It also has a very long half-life, which means it continues working long after other drugs have been broken down and deactivated.

These and other properties make it useful for treating a variety of bacterial infections, including infection of the urethra (urethritis), which attacks the tube that carries urine from the bladder to the outside of the body. A variety of organisms—bacteria, viruses and fungi—can infect the urethra, causing discharge and painful urination. Urethritis caused by bacteria can be treated with azithromycin, a single dose of which is believed to be as good as a week-long course of doxycycline.

In addition to urethritis, azithromycin is used to treat upper and lower respiratory tract infections, infections of the skin and skin structure, community-acquired pneumonia, and other ailments.

Possible Side Effects

The drug's more common side effects include nausea, vomiting, diarrhea, abdominal pain, and irregular heartbeat (especially when a single high dose is taken).

Which Nutrients Are Robbed

Taking this medicine may deplete your supply of, increase your need for, or interfere with the activity of:

- Biotin
- Inositol
- Thiamin
- Vitamin B_6
- Vitamin B_{12}
- Vitamin K

- Riboflavin
- Niacin
- *Bifidobacterium bifidum*
- *Lactobacillus acidophilus*

Additional Ways This Drug May Upset Your Nutritional Balance

Azithromycin can cause nausea, vomiting, and abdominal pain, all of which can upset your eating habits and possibly interfere with good nutrition. It may also trigger diarrhea, which can hamper nutrient absorption.

This drug can also cause hyperkalemia, or too much potassium in the blood.

Restoring Your Nutritional Balance

To compensate for the nutrient loss caused by this drug, speak to your physician about taking 500–1,000 mcg biotin, 250–1,000 mg inositol, 25–100 mg thiamin, 25–100 mg riboflavin, 50–100 mg niacin, 50–100 mg vitamin B_6, 500–1,000 mcg vitamin B_{12}, 60–80 mcg vitamin K, 15 billion live *Bifidobacterium bifidum* organisms, and 15 billion live *Lactobacillus acidophilus* organisms per day.

You can also eat foods that contain the depleted nutrients:

- Biotin: beef liver, soybeans, rice bran, peanut butter, barley
- Inositol: cantaloupe, oranges, green beans, grapefruit juice, limes
- Thiamin: braised liver, turkey heart, roasted chicken, gefilte fish, sardines
- Riboflavin: dried sunflower seeds, orange juice, bulgur, spinach noodles, pine nuts
- Niacin: chicken breast, beef liver, mackerel, barley, bulgur
- Vitamin B_6: potato, banana, garbanzo beans, chicken breast, fortified oatmeal
- Vitamin B_{12}: beef liver, rainbow trout, sockeye salmon, beef, haddock
- Vitamin K: kale, broccoli, parsley, Swiss chard, spinach
- *Bifidobacterium bifidum*: Jerusalem artichokes, asparagus, garlic, and onions may stimulate the growth or activity of this probiotic
- *Lactobacillus acidophilus*: yogurt containing live lactobacillus cultures, kefir, acidophilus milk

Consult with your physician before making any changes to your diet or supplemental regimen.

BALSALAZIDE (bal-SAL-uh-zide)

Brand Name: Colazal

About Balsalazide

The large intestine (also known as the colon) is the final processing station for the food you eat. There, fluid is taken out of the food and absorbed by the body; bacteria break down the remaining food remnants, creating gas and vitamin K; and waste products are converted into stool.

Ulcerative colitis is a disease in which the colon becomes inflamed and pitted with erosions. The problem tends to wax and wane, and during flare-ups you may be hit with abdominal cramps, fever, and bloody diarrhea. Although ulcerative colitis can strike at any age, people between the ages of 15 and 30 are the most frequent targets.

Balsalazide helps combat ulcerative colitis by dampening inflammation. It doesn't do this directly: instead, balsalazide is converted in the body to 5-amino-salicylic acid, among other things. It's the 5-amino-salicylic acid that's believed to interfere with the production of substances that cause inflammation in the lining of the colon.

Possible Side Effects

The drug's more common side effects include headache, abdominal pain, diarrhea, joint pain, and respiratory infection.

Which Nutrients Are Robbed

Taking this medicine may deplete your supply of, increase your need for, or interfere with the activity of:

- Folic acid

Other Ways This Drug May Upset Your Nutritional Balance

Balsalazide can cause abdominal pain, nausea, vomiting, loss of appetite, cramps, and dry mouth, all of which can upset your eating habits and possibly interfere with good nutrition. It may also trigger diarrhea, which can hamper nutrient absorption.

Restoring Your Nutritional Balance

To compensate for the nutrient loss caused by this drug, speak to your physician about taking 400–800 mcg folic acid per day.

You can also eat foods that contain the depleted nutrient:

- Folic acid: beef liver, fortified breakfast cereals, spinach, great northern beans, asparagus

Consult with your physician before making any changes to your diet or supplemental regimen.

BASILIXIMAB (bay-si-LIKS-i-mab)

Brand Name: Simulect

About Basiliximab

An antibody is a weapon designed by the immune system to destroy one specific antigen, that is, one thing that the immune system considers harmful. After destroying the immediate problem (such as the germ that causes measles), some antibodies will continue to protect you against that problem for the rest of your life.

Sometimes it's extremely helpful to have large quantities of specific antibodies on hand to fight a certain disease right now. Rather than wait for these antibodies to be produced by your body—or by some poor lab animal pressed into service on your behalf—lab technicians can whip up a batch using monoclonal antibody technology. When a cell that produces a particular antibody is fused with a cell that keeps replicating, the combination cell can churn out copies of the needed antibody in large amounts.

Basiliximab is a monoclonal antibody with a very specific purpose. It doesn't destroy a particular germ. Instead, it helps prevent transplanted tissue—like a kidney—from being rejected. It does this by binding to and interfering with certain T-cells that would otherwise destroy the foreign tissue. Attacking your own T-cells may not seem like a good idea, but in this case you don't want the T-cells to do their duty.

Basiliximab is used in conjunction with other medicines to prevent the body from rejecting kidney transplants. Because the drug is made up of two things that do not combine on their own, it's called a chimeric monoclonal antibody. (In Greek mythology, a chimera is a monster with the head of a lion, the body of a goat, and the tail of a serpent.)

Possible Side Effects

The drug's more common side effects include irregular heartbeat, high blood pressure, difficulty breathing, stomach upset, fever, insomnia, and acne.

Which Nutrients Are Robbed

Taking this medicine may deplete your supply of, increase your need for, or interfere with the activity of:

- Calcium
- Phosphorus
- Potassium

Other Ways This Drug May Upset Your Nutritional Balance

Basiliximab can cause nausea, vomiting, and abdominal pain, all of which can upset your eating habits and possibly interfere with good nutrition. It may also trigger diarrhea, which can hamper nutrient absorption.

The drug can also cause hyperkalemia, or too much potassium in the blood, and hypercalcemia, or too much calcium in the blood.

Restoring Your Nutritional Balance

To compensate for the nutrient loss caused by this drug, speak to your physician about taking 1,200 mg calcium, 100–300 mg potassium, and 700 mg phosphorus per day.

You can also eat foods that contain the depleted nutrients:

- Calcium: milk, dried figs, Swiss cheese, yogurt, tofu
- Potassium: dried figs, California avocado, papaya, banana, dates
- Phosphorus: plain nonfat yogurt, lentils, salmon, milk, halibut

Consult with your physician before making any changes to your diet or supplemental regimen.

BECLOMETHASONE (be-kloe-METH-uh-sohn)

Brand Names: Alti-Beclomethasone, Apo-Beclomethasone, Beconase, Propaderm, QVAR, Vancenase, Vancenase Pockethaler, Vanceril

About Beclomethasone

The eardrum is a thin membrane (technically, the tympanic membrane) that separates the ear canal and the middle ear, and that transmits sound vibrations to the inner ear. The eardrum is exposed to air and air pressure from the outside world, as you well know if anyone has ever blown into your ear.

To balance the air pressure from the outside, the Eustachian tube connects the middle ear to the back of the nose. This tube opens and closes when you swallow or yawn, allowing air to flow in and out and balance the pressure exerted on the eardrum. It also allows fluid to drain out of the middle ear.

If you have an upper respiratory tract infection, an allergy, or some other ailment that interferes with the Eustachian tube, the air in your middle ear can be absorbed, creating negative pressure, or a "pull," on the eardrum. This can interfere with hearing and give you a feeling of fullness in your ear.

The problem may go away on its own when the underlying condition clears up, or it may require a medical assist. Beclomethasone, a corticosteroid, is sprayed into the nostrils to help control the inflammation that contributes to fullness in the ear. It's also used to treat asthma and nasal polyps.

Possible Side Effects

The drug's side effects include agitation, dizziness, rash, nosebleeds, and dryness and irritation of the nose, mouth, and throat.

Which Nutrients Are Robbed

Taking this medicine may deplete your supply of, increase your need for, or interfere with the activity of:

- Vitamin A
- Vitamin B_6
- Vitamin C
- Vitamin D
- Vitamin K
- Calcium
- Magnesium
- Potassium
- Zinc
- Melatonin

Additional Ways This Drug May Upset Your Nutritional Balance

Beclomethasone can cause nausea, vomiting, and changes in taste, all of which can upset your eating habits and possibly interefere with good nutrition.

Restoring Your Nutritional Balance

To compensate for the nutrient loss caused by this drug, speak to your physician about taking 5,000 IU vitamin A, 50–100 mg vitamin B_6, 250–1,500 mg vitamin C, 400 IU vitamin D, 60–80 mcg vitamin K, 1,200 mg calcium,

500–1,000 mg magnesium, 100–300 mg potassium, 50–200 mg zinc, and 1–3 mg melatonin per day.

You can also eat foods that contain the depleted nutrients:

- Vitamin A: beef liver, chicken liver, cheese pizza, whole milk, cheddar cheese
- Vitamin B_6: potato, banana, garbanzo beans, chicken breast, fortified oatmeal
- Vitamin C: papaya, guava, red pepper, cantaloupe, black currants
- Vitamin D: salmon, mackerel, sardines, eel, fortified milk
- Vitamin K: kale, broccoli, parsley, Swiss chard, spinach
- Calcium: milk, dried figs, Swiss cheese, yogurt, tofu
- Magnesium: Florida avocado, toasted wheat germ, almonds, shredded wheat cereal, pumpkin seeds
- Potassium: dried figs, California avocado, papaya, banana, dates
- Zinc: oysters, beef shank, chicken, pork tenderloin, plain yogurt

Consult with your physician before making any changes to your diet or supplemental regimen.

BENAZEPRIL (ben-AY-ze-pril)

Brand Name: Lotensin

About Benazepril

Hypertension (elevated blood pressure) is usually brought about by a complex series of biochemical events. But many times, doctors have no idea what triggered the cascade. When that's the case, they label it primary or essential hypertension. (Used this way, "essential" doesn't mean "really important," because you don't need permanently elevated blood pressure. It's doctor-speak for "I have no idea what caused it.")

There are many treatments for elevated blood pressure, including benazepril, which belongs to a group of medications known as ACE inhibitors.

ACE stands for angiotensin converting enzyme, one of many factors in the blood pressure equation. ACE helps push blood pressure up. As an ACE inhibitor, benazepril helps to keep the pressure down. (By the way,

ACE is not bad, because blood pressure that's too low can be just as dangerous as pressure that's too high. We need mechanisms that can push the blood pressure up quickly and reliably, just as we need those that can bring it back down when necessary. Problems arise only when there's too much of a push, one way or the other.)

Benazepril is used, either by itself or with other medications, to treat hypertension. It's also used to treat problems with the heart following a heart attack.

Possible Side Effects

The drug's more common side effects include headache, dizziness, cough, and fatigue.

Which Nutrients Are Robbed

Taking this medicine may deplete your supply of, increase your need for, or interfere with the activity of:

• Zinc

Other Ways This Drug May Upset Your Nutritional Balance

Benazepril can cause nausea, which can upset your eating habits and possibly interfere with good nutrition.

The drug can also cause hyperkalemia, or too much potassium in the blood.

Restoring Your Nutritional Balance

To compensate for the nutrient loss caused by this drug, speak to your physician about taking 50–200 mg zinc per day.

You can also eat foods that contain the depleted nutrient:

• Zinc: oysters, beef shank, chicken, pork tenderloin, plain yogurt

Consult with your physician before making any changes to your diet or supplemental regimen.

BETAMETHASONE (bay-tuh-METH-uh-sohn)

Brand Names: Alphatrex, Betaderm, Betatrex, Beta-Val, Celestoderm-EV/2, Diprolene, Luxiq, Maxivate, Topisone

About Betamethasone

Seborrheic dermatitis causes "dandruff of the skin" and other symptoms, and usually occurs either in infants or in adults between the ages of 30 and 70. No one fully understands what brings on seborrheic dermatitis, or why it tends to skip children, teens, young adults, and the elderly in favor of infants and the 30-to-70 crowd.

What we do know is that the disease triggers chronic inflammation and the formation of scales on the face, scalp, and sometimes the body. The first symptom is generally dandruff, or the appearance of scaly skin on the head. There may also be reddish or yellowish pimples on the head, face, chest, and upper back. In newborns, the disease may produce cradle cap: a yellowish, crusty rash on the scalp, and maybe facial pimples and scaling of the skin behind the ears.

Betamethasone is a steroid that reduces the inflammation seen with seborrheic dermatitis. It's also used to treat atopic dermatitis, neurodermatitis, psoriasis, and inflammatory diseases.

Possible Side Effects

The drug's more common side effects include insomnia, nervousness, increased appetite, and indigestion.

Which Nutrients Are Robbed

Taking this medicine may deplete your supply of, increase your need for, or interfere with the activity of:

- Vitamin A
- Folic acid
- Vitamin B_6
- Vitamin C
- Vitamin D
- Vitamin K
- Calcium
- Magnesium
- Phosphorus
- Potassium
- Selenium
- Zinc

Other Ways This Drug May Upset Your Nutritional Balance

Betamethasone can cause an increase in appetite and indigestion, which may upset your eating habits and possibly interfere with good nutrition.

Restoring Your Nutritional Balance

To compensate for the nutrient loss caused by this drug, speak to your physician about taking 5,000 IU vitamin A, 400–800 mcg folic acid, 50–100 mg vitamin B_6, 250–1,500 mg vitamin C, 400 IU vitamin D, 60–80 mcg vitamin K, 1,200 mg calcium, 500–1,000 mg magnesium, 700 mg phosphorus, 100–300 mg potassium, 20–100 mcg selenium, and 50–200 mg zinc per day.

You can also eat foods that contain the depleted nutrients:

- Vitamin A: beef liver, chicken liver, cheese pizza, whole milk, cheddar cheese
- Folic acid: beef liver, fortified breakfast cereals, spinach, great northern beans, asparagus
- Vitamin B$_6$: potato, banana, garbanzo beans, chicken breast, fortified oatmeal
- Vitamin C: papaya, guava, red pepper, cantaloupe, black currants
- Vitamin D: salmon, mackerel, sardines, eel, fortified milk
- Vitamin K: kale, broccoli, parsley, Swiss chard, spinach
- Calcium: milk, dried figs, Swiss cheese, yogurt, tofu
- Magnesium: Florida avocado, toasted wheat germ, almonds, shredded wheat cereal, pumpkin seeds
- Phosphorus: plain nonfat yogurt, lentils, salmon, milk, halibut
- Potassium: dried figs, California avocado, papaya, banana, dates
- Selenium: Brazil nuts, tuna, beef liver, turkey breast, spaghetti with meat sauce
- Zinc: oysters, beef shank, chicken, pork tenderloin, plain yogurt

Consult with your physician before making any changes to your diet or supplemental regimen.

BETAXOLOL, BISOPROLOL, NADOLOL (bay-TAKS-oh-lol, bis-OH-proe-lol, nay-DOE-lole)

Brand Names: Betaxolol: Betoptic S, Kerlone
Bisoprolol: Monocor, Zebeta
Nadolol: Alti-Nadolol, Apo-Nadol, Corgard, Novo-Nadolol

About Betaxolol, Bisoprolol, and Nadolol

Among the beta-blockers used to treat hypertension and glaucoma (increased pressure within the eyeball), these three—betaxolol, bisoprolol, and nadolol—stand out because of their long half-lives.

A half-life is the amount of time it takes for half the amount of a drug you've taken to be "deactivated" by your liver or other bodily processes. The longer the half-life, the longer the drug keeps working. A longer half-life can be good and bad: good because you have to take the drug less often than one with a shorter half-life, or bad because the drug can continue to circulate throughout your body after you no longer need it.

Nadolol has a half-life of 14 to 24 hours; betaxolol, 14 to 22 hours; and bisoprolol 9 to 12 hours. Because some of the other beta-blockers don't last nearly as long, they must be taken more often.

Betaxolol is used to treat glaucoma and elevated blood pressure. Bisoprolol is used to treat elevated blood pressure, certain kinds of irregular heartbeat, and angina. Nadolol is used to prevent migraine headaches, although no one knows exactly how it does so. It's also used to treat elevated blood pressure and angina.

Possible Side Effects

When used to treat glaucoma, betaxolol's more common side effects include enlargement of the blood vessels in the conjunctiva (the membrane covering the inside of the eyelids and part of the eyeball), vision disturbances, and eye pain. When it's used to treat elevated blood pressure, more common side effects include drowsiness, insomnia, spasms in the breathing tubes, and heart palpitations.

More common side effects of bisoprolol and nadolol include drowsiness, insomnia, and decreased sexual ability.

Which Nutrients Are Robbed

Taking these medicines may deplete your supply of, increase your need for, or interfere with the activity of:

- Coenzyme Q_{10}
- Melatonin

Other Ways These Drugs May Upset Your Nutritional Balance

Betaxolol can cause hypoglycemia, nausea, vomiting, and stomach discomfort, all of which can upset your eating habits and possibly interfere with good nutrition. It may also trigger diarrhea, which can hamper nutrient absorption.

Bisoprolol can cause stomach discomfort, nausea, and vomiting, all of which can upset your eating habits and possibly interfere with good nutrition. It can also cause diarrhea, which can hamper nutrient absorption.

Nadolol can cause stomach discomfort, nausea, and vomiting, all of which can upset your eating habits and possibly interfere with good nutrition. It can also cause diarrhea, which can hamper nutrient absorption.

Restoring Your Nutritional Balance

To compensate for the nutrient loss caused by these drugs, speak to your physician about taking 30–100 mg coenzyme Q_{10} and 1–3 mg melatonin per day.

You can also eat foods that contain the depleted nutrient:

- Coenzyme Q_{10}: beef, chicken, trout, salmon, oranges, broccoli

Consult with your physician before making any changes to your diet or supplemental regimen.

BISACODYL (bis-uh-KOE-dil)

Brand Names: Bisaco-Lax, Carter's Little Pills, Correctol, Dacodyl, Dulcolax, Feen-a-Mint, Femilax, PMS-Bisacodyl

About Bisacodyl

Constipation (infrequent or difficult bowel movements) can be triggered by many things, including certain drugs, a lack of physical activity, hypothyroidism, excessive levels of calcium in the blood, and lack of dietary fiber.

"The slows" may also be to blame. When the transit time of ingested food lengthens, the stool remains in the intestine longer, allowing the body to reabsorb more of its water. What remains becomes dry, hard, and difficult to pass.

Dehydration can also cause constipation. A less-than-adequate intake of fluid can prompt the body to pull additional water out of the stool, so even if food moves through the intestines at a normal pace, the stool can become hard and dry. A lack of fiber in the diet can cause similar results, as fiber helps hold water in the stool.

Cancerous growths, fibrous tissues (adhesions) from abdominal surgery, and foreign objects can obstruct the flow of stool and cause constipation, a condition that can be encouraged by chronic pain, both physical and psychological.

Whatever the cause, constipation can be uncomfortable, at best, and dangerous, at worst. It may lead to diverticular disease, in which little pouches form in the wall of the intestines and can trap undigested food, causing inflammation and infection. There may be fecal impaction, in which hard stool becomes lodged in the colon or rectum and refuses to move.

There are several approaches to treating constipation. One is to use stimulant laxatives like bisacodyl to encourage muscle contraction in the bowel (a process called peristalsis) to push the stool through.

Bisacodyl is a strong peristalsis stimulant that is used to treat constipation and to clear out the bowels before surgery or bowel X-rays.

Possible Side Effects

The drug's side effects include abdominal cramps, rectal burning, and, when used over time, muscle weakness.

Which Nutrients Are Robbed

Taking this medicine may deplete your supply of, increase your need for, or interfere with the activity of:

- Calcium
- Sodium
- Potassium

Other Ways This Drug May Upset Your Nutritional Balance

Bisacodyl can cause nausea, which can upset your eating habits and possibly interfere with good nutrition. It may also trigger diarrhea, which can hamper nutrient absorption.

Restoring Your Nutritional Balance

To compensate for the nutrient loss caused by this drug, speak to your physician about taking 1,200 mg calcium and 100–300 mg potassium per day. And ask your physician to consider the potential effects of sodium depletion.

You can also eat foods that contain the depleted nutrients:

- Calcium: milk, dried figs, Swiss cheese, yogurt, tofu
- Potassium: dried figs, California avocado, papaya, banana, dates

Consult with your physician before making any changes to your diet or supplemental regimen.

BUDESONIDE (byoo-DESS-oh-nide)

Brand Names: Entocort, Gen-Budesonide AQ, Pulmicort, Pulmicort Turbuhaler, Rhinocort, Rhinocort Aqua

About Budesonide

Crohn's disease, a chronic inflammatory disease, can turn the intenstines into a patchwork of healthy and diseased tissue. The symptoms often appear gradually and usually include abdominal pain, diarrhea, fever, fatigue, and weight loss. Inside the body, portions of the intestines may be severely inflamed, narrowing the passageway and creating abnormal openings in the intestines called fistulas. Crohn's disease can be mild or severe, and tends to flare up and then recede. It appears to be more common in Jewish people of Ashkenazi background and less common in African Americans.

We don't know what causes Crohn's disease, but suspects include genetics, allergies, and immune disorders. Although it is incurable, it can usually be managed medically, keeping the symptoms to a minimum.

The treatments for Crohn's disease include surgery, lifestyle changes, and medicines that suppress the immune system, reduce inflammation, and control diarrhea.

Budesonide is a corticosteroid used to suppress the inflammation seen in Crohn's disease, thereby reducing the symptoms. Use of this drug leads to remission in at least half of those with mild to moderate Crohn's disease located in certain areas of the intestines.

Possible Side Effects

The drug's more common side effects include headache, nausea, and respiratory infection.

Which Nutrients Are Robbed

Taking this medicine may deplete your supply of, increase your need for, or interfere with the activity of:

- Vitamin A
- Calcium
- Vitamin B_6
- Magnesium
- Folic acid
- Potassium
- Vitamin C
- Selenium
- Vitamin D
- Zinc
- Vitamin K
- Melatonin

Other Ways This Drug May Upset Your Nutritional Balance

Budesonide can cause nausea, changes in taste, abdominal pain, loss of appetite, and vomiting, all of which can upset your eating habits and possibly interfere with good nutrition.

Restoring Your Nutritional Balance

To compensate for the nutrient loss caused by this drug, speak to your physician about taking 5,000 IU vitamin A, 50–100 mg vitamin B_6,

400–800 mcg folic acid, 250–1,500 mg vitamin C, 400 IU vitamin D, 60–80 mcg vitamin K, 1,200 mg calcium, 500–1,000 mg magnesium, 100–300 mg potassium, 20–100 mcg selenium, 50–200 mg zinc, and 1–3 mg melatonin per day.

You can also eat foods that contain the depleted nutrients:

- Vitamin A: beef liver, chicken liver, cheese pizza, whole milk, cheddar cheese
- Vitamin B$_6$: potato, banana, garbanzo beans, chicken breast, fortified oatmeal
- Folic acid: beef liver, fortified breakfast cereals, spinach, great northern beans, asparagus
- Vitamin C: papaya, guava, red pepper, cantaloupe, black currants
- Vitamin D: salmon, mackerel, sardines, eel, fortified milk
- Vitamin K: kale, broccoli, parsley, Swiss chard, spinach
- Calcium: milk, dried figs, Swiss cheese, yogurt, tofu
- Magnesium: Florida avocado, toasted wheat germ, almonds, shredded wheat cereal, pumpkin seeds
- Potassium: dried figs, California avocado, papaya, banana, dates
- Selenium: Brazil nuts, tuna, beef liver, turkey breast, spaghetti with meat sauce
- Zinc—oysters, beef shank, chicken, pork tenderloin, plain yogurt

Consult with your physician before making any changes to your diet or supplemental regimen.

BUMETANIDE (byoo-MET-uh-nide)

Brand Names: Bumex, Burinex

About Bumetanide

The healthy heart can pump tirelessly for seven, eight, or even more decades, rarely missing a beat. But in about 1 percent of Americans, it fails. Although it doesn't actually stop beating, it simply can't do its job well anymore. Obviously this is a problem because the heart is responsible for delivering oxygen and nutrients to every cell in the body via the blood.

One of the dangerous symptoms of heart failure is the buildup of fluid in various parts of the body. Where that fluid accumulates depends on which side of the heart is failing.

The right side of the heart collects used blood from all over the body and sends it to the lungs to be refreshed with new oxygen. If the right side of the heart fails, the excess fluid pools in the legs, ankles, feet, and abdomen. And that fluid may move around as you do. For example, when you lie down, it may pool in your lower back.

The left side of your heart receives refreshed blood from the lungs, then pumps it to all parts of the body. If this side of your heart fails, the fluid gathers in your lungs and can literally take your breath away.

Besides treating the underlying cause of your heart failure, your physician may also prescribe diuretics such as bumetanide to force excess fluid out of your body via the urine. Bumetanide works by slowing the reabsorption of sodium and chloride in the kidneys, which forces you to expel more water in order to carry out the sodium and chloride that isn't returned to the circulation.

In addition to water retention, bumetanide may be used to treat elevated blood pressure.

Possible Side Effects

The drug's most common side effects include muscle cramps and dizziness; high blood levels of uric acid, nitrogen-type wastes, and glucose; and low blood levels of sodium, chloride, and potassium.

Which Nutrients Are Robbed

Taking this medicine may deplete your supply of, increase your need for, or interfere with the activity of:

- Thiamin
- Vitamin B_6
- Vitamin C
- Calcium
- Chloride
- Magnesium
- Potassium
- Sodium
- Zinc

Restoring Your Nutritional Balance

To compensate for the nutrient loss caused by this drug, speak to your physician about taking 25–100 mg thiamin, 50–100 mg vitamin B_6, 250–1,500 mg vitamin C, 1,200 mg calcium, 500–1,000 mg magnesium, and 50–200 mg zinc per day. And ask your physician to consider the potential effects of sodium and chloride depletion.

A Note on Potassium: "Regular" diuretics lower potassium levels, while potassium-sparing diuretics do not—they may increase levels instead. It is not uncommon for doctors to prescribe two different diuretics. That's why you should speak to your physician about your potassium levels, and whether it is appropriate for you to take supplements or eat potassium-rich foods.

You can also eat foods that contain the depleted nutrients:

- Thiamin: braised liver, turkey heart, roasted chicken, gefilte fish, sardines
- Vitamin B₆: potato, banana, garbanzo beans, chicken breast, fortified oatmeal
- Vitamin C: papaya, guava, red pepper, cantaloupe, black currants
- Calcium: milk, dried figs, Swiss cheese, yogurt, tofu
- Magnesium: Florida avocado, toasted wheat germ, almonds, shredded wheat cereal, pumpkin seeds
- Zinc: oysters, beef shank, chicken, pork tenderloin, plain yogurt

Consult with your physician before making any changes to your diet or supplemental regimen.

BUSULFAN (byoo-SUL-fan)

Brand Names: Busulfex, Myleran

About Busulfan

Normally, cells called neutrophils, basophils, eosinophils, and monocytes protect the body from bacteria, viruses, and other invaders. These cells are born in the bone marrow, where they receive their "training" before being released into circulation. But with chronic myelogenous leukemia (CML), something goes wrong in the marrow, and the immature cells that were meant to become these body protectors become cancerous instead.

CML can strike at any age, but it typically targets middle-age men and women. The first symptoms are often fatigue, weakness, loss of appetite and weight, fever, and night sweats. As the disease progresses, the cancerous cells crowd out the red blood cells, causing anemia. They can also squeeze out the platelets, making bruising and bleeding more likely because the blood can't clot properly.

Busulfan may be used in combination with other drugs to send CML into remission. It works by interfering with the ability of the cancer cells to manufacture DNA. In younger people who are in remission, physicians may attempt bone marrow transplants in the hopes that the new marrow will produce healthy neutrophils, basophils, eosinophils, and monocytes.

In addition to chronic myelogenous leukemia, busulfan may be used to treat other disorders of the bone marrow.

Possible Side Effects

The drug's more common side effects include fever, headache, bone marrow suppression, severe anemia, and a decrease in the number of all types of blood cells.

Which Nutrients Are Robbed

Taking this medicine may deplete your supply of, increase your need for, or interfere with the activity of:

- Magnesium   • Phosphorus
- Potassium

Other Ways This Drug May Upset Your Nutritional Balance

Busulfan can cause nausea, loss of appetite, and vomiting, all of which can upset your eating habits and possibly interfere with good nutrition. It may also trigger diarrhea, which can hamper nutrient absorption.

Restoring Your Nutritional Balance

To compensate for the nutrient loss caused by this drug, speak to your physician about taking 500–1,000 mg magnesium, 100–300 mg potassium, and 700 mg phosphorus per day.

You can also eat foods that contain the depleted nutrients:

- Magnesium: Florida avocado, toasted wheat germ, almonds, shredded wheat cereal, pumpkin seeds
- Potassium: dried figs, California avocado, papaya, banana, dates
- Phosphorus: plain nonfat yogurt, lentils, salmon, milk, halibut

Consult with your physician before making any changes to your diet or supplemental regimen.

BUTABARBITAL (byoo-tuh-BAR-bi-tall)

Brand Names: Busodium, Butalan, Butisol

About Butabarbital

Butabarbital is a barbiturate, or a sedative-hypnotic drug. A sedative calms and reduces anxiety, while a hypnotic makes it easier to fall asleep and stay asleep. The barbiturates were once very popular remedies for sleep problems. First made available about 100 years ago, they were widely used—and abused. But over the past several decades, they've been pushed to the back of the doctor's little black bag by newer drugs.

Butabarbital and other barbiturates work by depressing the central nervous system, thus lowering the temperature, blood pressure, and respiratory rate. It may be used as a sedative or a sleep aid.

Possible Side Effects

The drug's more common side effects include dizziness, light-headedness, and drowsiness.

Which Nutrients Are Robbed

Taking this medicine may deplete your supply of, increase your need for, or interfere with the activity of:

- Biotin
- Folic acid
- Vitamin D
- Vitamin K
- Calcium

Other Ways This Drug May Upset Your Nutritional Balance

Butabarbital can cause nausea and vomiting, which can upset your eating habits and possibly interfere with good nutrition.

Restoring Your Nutritional Balance

To compensate for the nutrient loss caused by this drug, speak to your physician about taking 500–1,000 mcg biotin, 400–800 mcg folic acid, 400 IU vitamin D, 60–80 mcg vitamin K, and 1,200 mg calcium per day.

You can also eat foods that contain the depleted nutrients:

- Biotin: beef liver, soybeans, rice bran, peanut butter, barley

- Folic acid: beef liver, fortified breakfast cereals, spinach, great northern beans, asparagus
- Vitamin D: salmon, mackerel, sardines, eel, fortified milk
- Vitamin K: kale, broccoli, parsley, Swiss chard, spinach
- Calcium: milk, dried figs, Swiss cheese, yogurt, tofu

Consult with your physician before making any changes to your diet or supplemental regimen.

BUTALBITAL PLUS ACETAMINOPHEN PLUS CAFFEINE
(byoo-TAL-bi-tall, uh-seet-uh-MIN-oh-fen, kaf-EEN)

Brand Names: Amaphen, Esgic, Esgic-Plus, Fioricet, Repan

About Butalbital plus Acetaminophen plus Caffeine
We all get them, those tension headaches that sneak up on us when we're rushing to get somewhere important, before a big test or presentation, at the end of a long day, or when we're just plain stressed.

Tension headaches are quite common, typically producing mild to moderate pain. Unlike migraine headaches, tension headaches have no aura, nausea, or "after fatigue" to worry about. Neither do they strike in groups, like cluster headaches. Tension headaches may hurt, but they're rarely a cause for worry because they're likely to disappear without leaving any damage behind.

Luckily, tension headaches are usually easy to treat with over-the-counter medicines. Acetaminophen is a popular remedy, and sometimes caffeine is added to the drug to make it even more effective. But when a tension headache is more intense than usual, you may need a prescription medicine. The trio of butalbital (a barbiturate with sedative effects on the body) combined with acetaminophen and caffeine is sometimes prescribed for these headaches.

Possible Side Effects
The side effects of butalbital plus acetaminophen include bleeding sores on the lips, fever, muscle cramps, and scaly skin. Overuse of caffeine can contribute to chronic daily headaches, especially on withdrawal.

Which Nutrients Are Robbed

Taking this medicine may deplete your supply of, increase your need for, or interfere with the activity of:

- Biotin
- Folic acid
- Vitamin D
- Vitamin K
- Calcium
- Glutathione

Restoring Your Nutritional Balance

To compensate for the nutrient loss caused by this drug, speak to your physician about taking 500–1,000 mcg biotin, 400–800 mcg folic acid, 400 IU vitamin D, 60–80 mcg vitamin K, 1,200 mg calcium, and 800–2,000 mg n-acetyl cysteine (a precursor to glutathione) per day.

You can also eat foods that contain the depleted nutrients:

- Biotin: beef liver, soybeans, rice bran, peanut butter, barley
- Folic acid: beef liver, fortified breakfast cereals, spinach, great northern beans, asparagus
- Vitamin D: salmon, mackerel, sardines, eel, fortified milk
- Vitamin K: kale, broccoli, parsley, Swiss chard, spinach
- Calcium: milk, dried figs, Swiss cheese, yogurt, tofu

Consult with your physician before making any changes to your diet or supplemental regimen.

BUTALBITAL PLUS ASPIRIN PLUS CAFFEINE (byoo-TAL-bi-tall, ASS-pir-in, kaf-EEN)

Brand Names: Axotal, B-A-C, Butalbital Compound, Fiorinal, Lanorinal, Marnal

About Butalbital plus Aspirin plus Caffeine

Muscle tension headaches are often brought on by stress or "mechanical irritation" of the muscles or supporting tissues, making your head feel like it's caught in a vise. And sometimes it's not just the head; the pain may spread to your neck and shoulders. Fortunately, pain is the only symptom of tension headaches, because they don't cause the vomiting, sensitivity to light, and other symptoms seen with migraine headaches. People of all ages can be struck by muscle tension headaches, which can last anywhere from 30 minutes to a couple of days.

The best way to deal with tension headaches is to figure out what's causing the tension, then learn to avoid it or handle it in a more positive way. Stress reduction techniques can be a big help, as can painkillers and caffeine (which constricts throbbing blood vessels). If more powerful pain relief is needed, your doctor may prescribe the combination of butalbital (a barbiturate with sedative effects on the body) plus aspirin and caffeine.

Possible Side Effects

The side effects of butalbital plus aspirin plus caffeine include drowsiness, light-headedness, and confusion. Aspirin's side effects include anemia, insomnia, rapid heartbeat, stomach ulcers, and liver damage.

Which Nutrients Are Robbed

Taking this medicine may deplete your supply of, increase your need for, or interfere with the activity of:

- Biotin
- Calcium
- Folic acid
- Iron
- Vitamin C
- Potassium
- Vitamin D
- Sodium
- Vitamin K

Other Ways This Drug May Upset Your Nutritional Balance

Butalbital plus aspirin plus caffeine can cause heartburn, nausea, and vomiting, which can upset your eating habits and possibly interfere with good nutrition. It may also trigger diarrhea, which can hamper nutrient absorption.

Aspirin can also trigger hyperkalemia, or too much potassium in the blood.

Restoring Your Nutritional Balance

To compensate for the nutrient loss caused by this drug, speak to your physician about taking 500–1,000 mcg biotin, 400–800 mcg folic acid, 250–1,500 mg vitamin C, 400 IU vitamin D, 60–80 mcg vitamin K, and 1,200 mg calcium per day. And ask your physician to consider the potential effects of iron and sodium depletion and to monitor your potassium status.

You can also eat foods that contain the depleted nutrients:

- Biotin: beef liver, soybeans, rice bran, peanut butter, barley
- Folic acid: beef liver, fortified breakfast cereals, spinach, great northern beans, asparagus
- Vitamin C: papaya, guava, red pepper, cantaloupe, black currants
- Vitamin D: salmon, mackerel, sardines, eel, fortified milk
- Vitamin K: kale, broccoli, parsley, Swiss chard, spinach
- Calcium: milk, dried figs, Swiss cheese, yogurt, tofu

Consult with your physician before making any changes to your diet or supplemental regimen.

CALCIUM CARBONATE (KAL-see-um KAR-buh-nate)

Brand Names: Alka-Mints, Alkets, Apo-Cal, Calci-Chew, Calcite-500, Caltrate, Os-Cal, Rolaids Calcium Rich, Tums

About Calcium Carbonate

The mineral calcium comes in many different forms, including calcium gluconate, calcium phosphate, calcium lactate, calcium citrate, and calcium carbonate.

The various forms are not pure calcium; each contains a different amount of the mineral. For example, calcium carbonate is 40 percent elemental calcium, calcium phosphate is 25 percent elemental calcium, and calcium lactate is 13 percent elemental calcium. Due to their varying amounts of calcium and different chemical properties, each form is useful for treating different ailments.

Calcium carbonate (think Tums) is commonly used as an antacid. It's also put to work to counteract low blood levels of calcium (hypocalcemia) or high blood levels of phosphate (hyperphosphatemia). These problems occur in those suffering from osteoporosis, mild kidney insufficiency, rickets, and related ailments.

Possible Side Effects

The drug's side effects include headache and constipation.

Which Nutrients Are Robbed

Taking this medicine may deplete your supply of, increase your need for, or interfere with the activity of:

- Chromium
- Iron
- Manganese
- Phosphorus

Other Ways This Drug May Upset Your Nutritional Balance

Although calcium carbonate is usually well tolerated, it can cause nausea, vomiting, loss of appetite, and abdominal pain, all of which can upset your eating habits and possibly interfere with good nutrition.

This drug can also cause hypercalcemia, or too much calcium in the blood.

Restoring Your Nutritional Balance

To compensate for the nutrient loss caused by this drug, speak to your physician about taking 1,000 mcg chromium and 50–100 mg manganese per day. Ask your physician to consider the potential effects of iron and phosphorus depletion. (If you're using calcium carbonate as a phosphate binder, you may want to have less phosphate in your diet.)

You can also eat foods that contain the depleted nutrients:

- Chromium: broccoli, green beans, potatoes, grape juice, orange juice
- Manganese: oat bran, brown rice, almonds, hazel nuts, peanuts

Consult with your physician before making any changes to your diet or supplemental regimen.

CALCIUM CHLORIDE (KAL-see-um KLOR-ide)

Brand Name: Calciject

About Calcium Chloride

Hypermagnesemia is doctor-speak for the presence of too much magnesium in the blood. It's most likely to appear in those whose weakened kidneys can't filter out excessive amounts of magnesium, whether it stems from food sources or magnesium-containing drugs such as certain laxatives and antacids.

If your blood levels of magnesium rise too high, you may develop symptoms such as confusion, muscle weakness, low blood pressure, and trouble breathing. If the problem is severe enough, your heart may stop beating, or the muscles that allow you to breathe may stop working.

Calcium balances magnesium in several body functions, so those with hypermagnesemia may be given calcium chloride intravenously to balance their high magnesium levels.

Possible Side Effects

The drug's side effects include slow heartbeat, irregular heartbeat, and high blood levels of calcium.

Which Nutrients Are Robbed

Taking this medicine may deplete your supply of, increase your need for, or interfere with the activity of:

• Magnesium

Additional Ways This Drug May Upset Your Nutritional Balance

Calcium chloride can trigger hypercalcemia, or too much calcium in the blood.

Restoring Your Nutritional Balance

Ask your physician to monitor your magnesium status.

Consult with your physician before making any changes to your diet or supplemental regimen.

CAPTOPRIL (KAP-toe-pril)

Brand Names: Alti-Captopril, Apo-Capto, Capoten, Novo-Captopril, Nu-Capto, PMS-Captopril

About Captopril

If you're reading about this drug, you've probably already had a sit-down with your physician and heard about the benefits of suppressing the renin-aldosterone system and the conversion of angiotensin I to angiotensin II.

Your physician was describing one of the ways the body keeps blood pressure "in the zone"—not too high, not too low. It's a complex system, a key part of which is the angiotensin conversion process.

Here's the crux of the matter: Angiotensin I is a relatively inactive substance manufactured by the body that primarily waits around to be converted into angiotensin II. Once in the form of angiotensin II, it becomes capable of, among other things, constricting blood vessels and encouraging the body to retain more water. Both of these actions can raise blood pressure.

It's good that angiotensin II can raise blood pressure and keep it in the zone—most of the time. Unfortunately, millions of Americans have blood pressure that is already way too high. They need to reduce the pressure, and one way to do that is to prevent the weak, inactive angiotensin I from being converted into the powerful angiotensin II.

Fortunately, captopril does just that, by blocking the action of an enzyme called ACE (angiotensin converting enzyme) that turns angiotensin I into angiotensin II. Captopril is an ACE inhibitor; it prevents ACE from doing its job, so blood pressure doesn't rise.

Captopril is used to treat elevated blood pressure, as well as congestive heart failure, and other ailments.

Possible Side Effects

The drug's more common side effects include rash, fever, joint pain, and eosinophillia (accumulation of an abnormally large amount of white blood cells).

Which Nutrients Are Robbed

Taking this medicine may deplete your supply of, increase your need for, or interfere with the activity of:

- Sodium
- Zinc

Additional Ways This Drug May Upset Your Nutritional Balance

Captopril can trigger hyperkalemia, or too much potassium in the blood.

Restoring Your Nutritional Balance

To compensate for the nutrient loss caused by this drug, speak to your physician about taking 50–200 mg zinc per day. And ask your physician to consider the potential effects of sodium depletion.

You can also eat foods that contain the depleted nutrient:

- Zinc: oysters, beef shank, chicken, pork tenderloin, plain yogurt

Consult with your physician before making any changes to your diet or supplemental regimen.

CARBAMAZEPINE (kar-buh-MAZ-e-peen)

Brand Names: Atretol, Carbatrol, Epitol, Novo-Carbamaz, Nu-Carbamazepine, Tegretol

About Carbamazepine

To laypeople, a seizure is uncontrolled muscle spasms, perhaps a loss of consciousness, and other symptoms caused by an unexpected flurry of electrical firing in the brain.

To doctors, however, there are different types of seizures, each with its own distinct pattern and symptoms. For example, there are partial seizures that strike on only one side of the brain and generalized seizures that attack large portions of both sides of the brain. If you're fully conscious during your seizure it's dubbed a simple seizure, but if your consciousness is impaired it's called a complex seizure. There are grand mal seizures, petit mal seizures, and more.

All of this terminology is more than medical hairsplitting, for different types of seizures are best treated by different drugs.

Carbamazepine is looked on as a drug of choice for partial seizures. A relative of certain antidepressants, it is also used for bipolar depression, as well as mania. In fact, it is sometimes used in place of lithium when that drug is not working well enough. It may also be used to treat those suffering from certain types of pain.

Carbamazepine works by reducing synaptic activity in the central nervous system.

Possible Side Effects

The drug's side effects include uncoordinated movements (ataxia), drowsiness, chills, fever, blurred vision, rashes, fainting, and blood pressure that is too high or too low.

Which Nutrients Are Robbed

Taking this medicine may deplete your supply of, increase your need for, or interfere with the activity of:

- Biotin
- Folic acid
- Vitamin D
- Calcium
- Sodium
- Carnitine

Additional Ways This Drug May Upset Your Nutritional Balance

Carbamazepine can cause nausea, vomiting, gastric distress, abdominal pain, and loss of appetite, all of which can upset your eating habits and possibly interfere with good nutrition. It can also cause diarrhea, which can hamper nutrient absorption.

Restoring Your Nutritional Balance

To compensate for the nutrient loss caused by this drug, speak to your physician about taking 500–1,000 mcg biotin, 400 IU vitamin D, 1,200 mg calcium, and 250–1,000 mg carnitine per day. And ask your physician to consider the potential effects of sodium depletion. Taking folic acid may increase the risk of seizures in some people, so discuss the use of this nutrient with your physician.

You can also eat foods that contain the depleted nutrients:

- Biotin: beef liver, soybeans, rice bran, peanut butter, barley
- Vitamin D: salmon, mackerel, sardines, eel, fortified milk
- Calcium: milk, dried figs, Swiss cheese, yogurt, tofu
- Carnitine: ground beef, pork, Canadian bacon, whole milk, cod

Consult with your physician before making any changes to your diet or supplemental regimen.

CARBENICILLIN (kar-ben-i-SIL-in)

Brand Names: Geocillin, Geopen

About Carbenicillin

The prostate is a small gland that sits just below a man's bladder and wraps itself around the urethra (the tube that carries urine out of the body). In infants the prostate is about the size of a pea, and it grows to the size of a walnut in young men. Its job is to produce fluid that combines with sperm to form semen.

Unfortunately, the prostate can easily become infected, a condition called prostatitis. Bacteria might work its way down from the bladder or up from the entry to the penis, or it might even travel through the bloodstream and take up residence in the prostate, causing pain and swelling.

Symptoms of a prostate infection include pain in the lower back, perineum, penis, and testicles; urinary urgency (the need to urinate *right now!*); frequent need to urinate; pain or burning when urinating; difficulty getting an erection; and painful ejaculation.

Antibiotics such as carbenicillin may be prescribed for prostatitis. This chemical cousin of penicillin works by preventing bacteria from building their cellular walls, killing the bacteria in the making. Carbenicillin is also used to treat urinary tract infections.

Possible Side Effects

The drug's more common side effects include diarrhea, stomach upset, and flatulence.

Which Nutrients Are Robbed

Taking this medicine may deplete your supply of, increase your need for, or interfere with the activity of:

- Biotin
- Inositol
- Thiamin
- Riboflavin
- Niacin
- Vitamin B_6

- Vitamin B_{12}
- Vitamin K
- Potassium
- *Bifidobacterium bifidum*
- *Lactobacillus acidophilus*

Additional Ways This Drug May Upset Your Nutritional Balance

Carbenicillin can cause a bad taste, nausea, and vomiting, all of which can upset your eating habits and possibly interfere with good nutrition. It can also cause diarrhea, which can hamper nutrient absorption.

Restoring Your Nutritional Balance

To compensate for the nutrient loss caused by this drug, speak to your physician about taking 500–1,000 mcg biotin, 250–1,000 mg inositol, 25–100 mg thiamin, 25–100 mg riboflavin, 50–100 mg niacin, 50–100 mg vitamin B_6, 500–1,000 mcg vitamin B_{12}, 60–80 mcg vitamin K, 100–300 mg potassium, 15 billion live *Bifidobacterium bifidum* organisms, and 15 billion live *Lactobacillus acidophilus* organisms per day.

You can also eat foods that contain the depleted nutrients:

- Biotin: beef liver, soybeans, rice bran, peanut butter, barley
- Inositol: cantaloupe, oranges, green beans, grapefruit juice, limes
- Thiamin: braised liver, turkey heart, roasted chicken, gefilte fish, sardines

- Riboflavin: dried sunflower seeds, orange juice, bulgur, spinach noodles, pine nuts
- Niacin: chicken breast, beef liver, mackerel, barley, bulgur
- Vitamin B$_6$: potato, banana, garbanzo beans, chicken breast, fortified oatmeal
- Vitamin B$_{12}$: beef liver, rainbow trout, sockeye salmon, beef, haddock
- Vitamin K: kale, broccoli, parsley, Swiss chard, spinach
- Potassium: dried figs, California avocado, papaya, banana, dates
- *Bifidobacterium bifidum*: Jerusalem artichokes, asparagus, garlic, and onions may stimulate the growth or activity of this probiotic
- *Lactobacillus acidophilus*: yogurt containing live lactobacillus cultures, kefir, acidophilus milk

Consult with your physician before making any changes to your diet or supplemental regimen.

CARBOPLATIN (KAR-boe-plat-in)

Brand Names: Paraplatin, Paraplatin-AQ

About Carboplatin

Carboplatin destroys cancer cells by cross-linking DNA strands. You can imagine the way this works by thinking about what happens when you're trying to comb a head of tangled hair. It's hard to separate the tangled strands and make the hair behave. In a way, carboplatin is a "tangler" that prevents DNA from performing. And because DNA contains all of the instructions a cell needs to live and replicate, if it gets tangled up and can't do its job, the cancer cell is in trouble.

Carboplatin is used to treat ovarian cancer, a disease that can be difficult to detect in its early stages because it often doesn't produce obvious symptoms until it's advanced. A woman's chance of survival depends on how soon her treatment begins. If it starts when the cancer is still at stage I, there's a 70 percent or greater chance of surviving five years after the diagnosis. If treatment isn't begun until the cancer is in stage III or IV, the five-year survival odds drop to 5 to 40 percent.

Carboplatin is officially approved for use in ovarian cancer. But it's also been used or at least studied as a treatment for cancers of the lung, neck, head, esophagus, breast, and other parts of the body.

Possible Side Effects

The drug's more common side effects include low blood levels of calcium, magnesium, sodium, and potassium; nausea, vomiting, weakness, hearing loss; and a decreased number of white blood cells.

Which Nutrients Are Robbed

Taking this medicine may deplete your supply of, increase your need for, or interfere with the activity of:

- Calcium
- Magnesium
- Potassium
- Sodium

Additional Ways This Drug May Upset Your Nutritional Balance

Carboplatin can cause nausea, vomiting, and loss of appetite, all of which can upset your eating habits and possibly interfere with good nutrition. It can also cause diarrhea, which can hamper nutrient absorption.

Restoring Your Nutritional Balance

To compensate for the nutrient loss caused by this drug, speak to your physician about taking 1,200 mg calcium, 500–1,000 mg magnesium, and 100–300 mg potassium per day. And ask your physician to consider the potential effects of sodium depletion.

You can also eat foods that contain the depleted nutrients:

- Calcium: milk, dried figs, Swiss cheese, yogurt, tofu
- Magnesium: Florida avocado, toasted wheat germ, almonds, shredded wheat cereal, pumpkin seeds
- Potassium: dried figs, California avocado, papaya, banana, dates

Consult with your physician before making any changes to your diet or supplemental regimen.

CARISOPRODOL PLUS ASPIRIN, CARISOPRODOL PLUS ASPIRIN PLUS CODEINE (kar-eye-soe-PROE-dole, ASS-pir-in, KOE-deen)

Brand Names: Carisoprodol plus aspirin: Soma Compound
Carisoprodol plus aspirin plus codeine: Soma Compound with Codeine

About Carisoprodol plus Aspirin, Carisoprodol plus Aspirin plus Codeine

Carisoprodol is a spasmolytic. In everyday language, it's a muscle relaxant, but not one that you would use for everyday muscle spasms, the kind that might strike after ballet class or a session at the gym. Instead, carisoprodol and other spasmolytics typically are reserved for the more powerful spasms seen with painful musculoskeletal ailments.

We know that carisoprodol works in the central nervous system, although we don't know exactly what it does there to relax the muscles. Carisoprodol may be combined with aspirin, which reduces pain and inflammation by interfering with the production of prostaglandins. To make the pain-relieving effects even stronger, codeine may be combined with carisoprodol and aspirin.

Possible Side Effects

Carisoprodol's more common side effects include drowsiness, chest tightness, allergic fever, stomach upset, and trembling. Those seen with aspirin use include anemia, insomnia, rapid heartbeat, stomach upset, and liver damage. The side effects of codeine include drowsiness, constipation, dizziness, and low blood pressure.

Which Nutrients Are Robbed

Taking this medicine may deplete your supply of, increase your need for, or interfere with the activity of:

- Folic acid
- Vitamin C
- Iron
- Potassium
- Sodium

Additional Ways This Drug May Upset Your Nutritional Balance

Carisoprodol can cause nausea, vomiting, and stomach cramps, all of which can upset your eating habits and possibly interfere with good nutrition.

Aspirin can cause heartburn, stomach pain, nausea, and vomiting. Aspirin can also trigger hyperkalemia, or too much potassium in the blood.

Codeine can cause dry mouth, loss of appetite, nausea, and vomiting, all of which can upset your eating habits and possibly interfere with good nutrition.

Restoring Your Nutritional Balance

To compensate for the nutrient loss caused by these drugs, speak to your physician about taking 400–800 mcg folic acid and 250–1,500 mg vitamin C per day. And ask your physician to consider the potential effects of iron and sodium depletion and to monitor your potassium status, for too much potassium may be a problem for those taking these combinations of drugs.

You can also eat foods that contain the depleted nutrients:

- Folic acid: beef liver, fortified breakfast cereals, spinach, great northern beans, asparagus
- Vitamin C: papaya, guava, red pepper, cantaloupe, black currants

Consult with your physician before making any changes to your diet or supplemental regimen.

CARTEOLOL (KAR-tee-oh-lole)

Brand Names: Cartrol Oral, Ocupress Ophthalmic

About Carteolol

When you think about carteolol, think about ringing a bell, but gently.

The human heart and other parts of the body are constantly receiving instructions from the brain to "work faster" or "work slower," "produce more" or "produce less." Of course, the brain doesn't actually talk to the heart when it sends these instructions. Instead, it communicates by sending messengers to select parts of the heart called beta-receptors. By plugging into the beta-receptors, these messengers, in effect, "ring a bell" that notifies the heart that it's time to work harder.

The drug carteolol also "rings a bell," but only a little. Just like the messengers, carteolol plugs into the beta-receptors. But while the messengers "ring the bell" loudly, carteolol rings it gently. Instead of bells pealing and the heart scrambling to work harder, with carteolol there are just a few quiet dings. Because carteolol takes up the space that would have been occupied by the messengers, the result is a more relaxed heart and blood pressure that eases back toward normal levels.

Carteolol, the gentle "bell ringer," is used to help reduce elevated blood pressure, as well as to treat glaucoma (the buildup of pressure within the eyeball).

Possible Side Effects

The drug's side effects include heart failure and spasms of the bronchial tubes. When used to treat glaucoma, carteolol's more common side effects include enlargement of the blood vessels in the conjunctiva (the membrane covering the inside of the eyelids and part of the eyeball), eye pain, vision disturbances, and other eye problems. When used to treat high blood pressure, its more common side effects include drowsiness, insomnia, and decreased sexual ability.

Which Nutrients Are Robbed

Taking this medicine may deplete your supply of, increase your need for, or interfere with the activity of:

- Coenzyme Q_{10} • Melatonin

Additional Ways This Drug May Upset Your Nutritional Balance

Carteolol can cause hypoglycemia, nausea, vomiting, and stomach discomfort, all of which can upset your eating habits and possibly interfere with good nutrition. It can also cause diarrhea, which can hamper nutrient absorption.

Restoring Your Nutritional Balance

To compensate for the nutrient loss caused by this drug, speak to your physician about taking 30–100 mg coenzyme Q_{10} and 1–3 mg melatonin per day.

You can also eat foods that contain the depleted nutrient:

- Coenzyme Q_{10} beef, chicken, trout, salmon, oranges, broccoli

Consult with your physician before making any changes to your diet or supplemental regimen.

CARVEDILOL (KAR-ve-dil-ole)

Brand Name: Coreg

About Carvedilol

The heart and blood vessels receive instructions from the sympathetic nervous system that dictate how rapidly and forcefully the blood should be pumped, and how much the blood flow should be resisted. If the heart pumps more rapidly or forcefully, and/or the blood vessels offer more resistance, the blood pressure rises. If the heart pumps more slowly or less forcefully, and/or the vessels decrease resistance by opening wider, the blood pressure falls.

The sympathetic nervous system communicates with the heart and blood vessels via chemical messengers called neurotransmitters. These neurotransmitters travel to certain receptor sites in the heart, including the $Beta_1$-receptor sites, to tell the heart to beat faster. You can think of the neurotransmitters as "delivery boys" carrying orders to "crank up" the heart rate. Unfortunately, cranking up the speed can also make the blood pressure rise. If you can prevent these orders from getting through to the heart, elevated blood pressure can ease back down toward normal.

That's exactly what carvedilol does. It inserts itself into the $Beta_1$-receptor sites on the heart, preventing the delivery boys from dropping off their messages. The heart rate slows, and blood pressure falls. This makes carvedilol useful in treating elevated blood pressure, heart failure, and angina.

Possible Side Effects

The drug's more common side effects include dizziness, fatigue, weakness, diarrhea, elevated blood sugar, infections of the upper respiratory tract, and weight gain.

Which Nutrients Are Robbed

Taking this medicine may deplete your supply of, increase your need for, or interfere with the activity of:

- Coenzyme Q_{10}
- Melatonin

Additional Ways This Drug May Upset Your Nutritional Balance

Carvedilol can cause hypoglycemia, nausea, and vomiting, which can upset your eating habits and possibly interfere with good nutrition. It can also cause diarrhea, which can hamper nutrient absorption.

This drug can also trigger hyperkalemia, or too much potassium in the blood.

Restoring Your Nutritional Balance

To compensate for the nutrient loss caused by this drug, speak to your physician about taking 30–100 mg coenzyme Q_{10} and 1–3 mg melatonin per day.

You can also eat foods that contain the depleted nutrient:

- Coenzyme Q_{10}: beef, chicken, trout, salmon, oranges, broccoli

Consult with your physician before making any changes to your diet or supplemental regimen.

CASCARA (kas-KAR-uh)

Also Known as: Cascara sagrada

About Cascara

Food doesn't just slide through the digestive tract; it's up to the intestines to keep it moving with a series of rhythmic movements called peristalsis. The muscles in the intestinal walls squeeze in a coordinated way that causes ripples through the bowel that push food and liquid on down the line.

You can imagine the action of peristalsis by thinking back to those old Esther Williams movies. A favorite scene was to show 20 or 30 bathing beauties lined up on the edge of a pool. On cue, each bathing beauty dove into the water one at a time, *splash, splash, splash,* right down the line. Mentally picture those diving bathing beauties and you'll get an idea of how the intestinal muscles squeeze, one after another, to move your food along.

Cascara is used to treat constipation by stimulating peristalsis. Although it doesn't cure the underlying cause of constipation, cascara can solve the immediate problem.

Possible Side Effects

The drug's side effects include confusion, irregular heartbeat, and muscle cramps.

Which Nutrients Are Robbed

Taking this medicine may deplete your supply of, increase your need for, or interfere with the activity of:

- Vitamin D
- Calcium
- Potassium
- Sodium

Restoring Your Nutritional Balance

To compensate for the nutrient loss caused by this drug, speak to your physician about taking 400 IU vitamin D, 1,200 mg calcium, and 100–300 mg potassium per day. And ask your physician to consider the effects of sodium depletion.

You can also eat foods that contain the depleted nutrients:

- Vitamin D: salmon, mackerel, sardines, eel, fortified milk
- Calcium: milk, dried figs, Swiss cheese, yogurt, tofu
- Potassium: dried figs, California avocado, papaya, banana, dates

Consult with your physician before making any changes to your diet or supplemental regimen.

CASPOFUNGIN (kas-poe-FUN-jin)

Brand Name: Cancidas

About Caspofungin

Infections caused by a fungus known as *Candida* are fairly common but are usually limited to the skin, mouth, intestines, or vagina, where they are held in check by the immune system.

But if your immune system has been weakened, or if you have diabetes or other conditions that favor the growth of fungi such as *Candida,* there's a greater risk that a fungal infection will spread throughout your body. If it infects the valves of your heart, it can cause a heart murmur. If your retinas are the targets, you may lose your sight. If your blood is infected, you may develop a fever and low blood pressure.

Caspofungin is used to treat infections caused by *Candida, Aspergillus,* and certain other fungi. It works by preventing the fungi from synthesizing essential parts of their cellular walls.

Possible Side Effects

The drug's more common side effects include headache and phlebitis (inflammation of the veins).

Which Nutrients Are Robbed

Taking this medicine may deplete your supply of, increase your need for, or interfere with the activity of:

- Potassium

Additional Ways This Drug May Upset Your Nutritional Balance

Caspofungin can cause abdominal pain, nausea, and vomiting, all of which can upset your eating habits and possibly interfere with good nutrition. It can also cause diarrhea, which can hamper nutrient absorption.

Restoring Your Nutritional Balance

To compensate for the nutrient loss caused by this drug, speak to your physician about taking 100–300 mg potassium per day.

You can also eat foods that contain the depleted nutrient:

- Potassium: dried figs, California avocado, papaya, banana, dates

Consult with your physician before making any changes to your diet or supplemental regimen.

CELECOXIB (sel-e-KOKS-ib)

Brand Name: Celebrex

About Celecoxib

Aspirin and other NSAIDs (nonsteroidal anti-inflammatory drugs) like ibuprofen and ketoprofen have long been mainstays of treatment for osteoarthritis, rheumatoid arthritis, menstrual cramps, and other painful conditions. These drugs often work well, but they can extract a price, literally, in blood.

The NSAIDs work by interfering with the actions of a substance called COX (cyclooxygenase). For a long time, we thought that COX had two primary duties: encouraging inflammation and protecting the lining of the stomach. It seemed there was no way to inhibit COX in order to get the good effect—ending unnecessary inflammation—without also getting the bad effect—an ulcer that left the lining of your stomach inflamed and bleeding. Then we learned that there are two COXs: COX-1, which is primarily responsible for protecting the stomach lining, and COX-2, which focuses on promoting inflammation. Now we had a way to reduce inflammation without having to put up with bleeding ulcers. All we had to do was find a drug that would inhibit COX-2 while leaving COX-1 alone.

Although we don't yet have a drug that does this perfectly, celecoxib is much more likely to target COX-2 and reduce inflammation, while bypassing the stomach-protecting COX-1. In fact, it's 375 times more likely to go after COX-2 than COX-1. There's still a danger of developing stomach ulcers with celecoxib, but it's much less likely than with other NSAIDs.

Celecoxib is used to treat osteoarthritis, rheumatoid arthritis, painful menstruation, and other forms of pain.

Possible Side Effects

The drug's side effects include insomnia, back pain, and upper respiratory tract infections.

Which Nutrients Are Robbed

Taking this medicine may deplete your supply of, increase your need for, or interfere with the activity of:

- Folic acid
- Sodium
- Potassium

Additional Ways This Drug May Upset Your Nutritional Balance

Celecoxib can cause hypoglycemia, dyspepsia, abdominal pain, and nausea, all of which can upset your eating habits and possibly interfere with good nutrition. It can also cause diarrhea, which can hamper nutrient absorption.

Restoring Your Nutritional Balance

To compensate for the nutrient loss caused by this drug, speak to your physician about taking 400–800 mcg folic acid and 100–300 mg potassium per day. And ask your physician to consider the potential effects of sodium depletion.

You can also eat foods that contain the depleted nutrients:

- Folic acid: beef liver, fortified breakfast cereals, spinach, great northern beans, asparagus
- Potassium: dried figs, California avocado, papaya, banana, dates

Consult with your physician before making any changes to your diet or supplemental regimen.

THE CEPHALOSPORINS (sef-a-loe-SPOR-in)

GENERIC NAME	PRONUNCIATION	BRAND NAME (EXAMPLE)
Cefaclor	SEF-a-klor	Ceclor
Cefadroxil	sef-uh-DROKS-il	Duricef
Cefamandole	sef-uh-MAN-dole	Mandol
Cefazolin	sef-A-zoe-lin	Ancef, Kefzol
Cefdinir	sef-DI-neer	Omnicef
Cefditoren	sef-da-TOR-en	Spectracef
Cefepime	SEF-e-peem	Maxipime
Cefonicid	se-FON-i-sid	Monocid
Cefoperazone	sef-oh-PER-a-zohn	Cefobid
Cefotaxime	sef-oh-TAKS-eem	Claforan
Cefotetan	SEF-oh-tee-tan	Cefotan
Cefoxitin	se-FOKS-i-tin	Mefoxin
Cefpodoxime	sef-pode-OKS-eem	Vantin
Cefprozil	sef-PROE-zil	Cefzil
Ceftazidime	SEF-tay-zi-deem	Ceptaz, Fortaz, Tazidime
Ceftibuten	sef-TYE-byoo-ten	Cedax
Ceftizoxime	sef-ti-ZOKS-eem	Cefizox
Ceftriaxone	sef-trye-AKS-ohn	Rocephin
Cefuroxime	se-fyoor-OKS-eem	Ceftin, Kefurox, Zinacef
Cephalexin	sef-uh-LEX-in	Biocef, Keftab
Cephalothin	sef-A-loe-thin	Ceporacin
Cephapirin	sef-uh-PYE-rin	Cefadyl
Cephradine	SEF-ruh-deen	Velosef
Loracarbef	lor-uh-KAR-bef	Lorabi

About the Cephalosporins

The cephalosporins are a large group of antibiotics that can be divided into four different generations, or subgroups, that were developed one after another. Each new generation has a somewhat different spectrum of action or group of bacteria it can combat, and each drug within each generation is more effective against some bacteria than others, works better in one part of the body than another, and so on. The various cephalosporins may be used to treat skin, urinary tract, joint, respiratory tract, and other infections.

Possible Side Effects

Side effects of the various cephalosporins may include headache, rash, stomach upset, dizziness, and fever. There's also a possibility, especially with the second- and third-generation cephalosporins, of developing a super-infection. This can happen if the cephalosporin kills off some bacteria but not others, upsetting the normal balance between organisms and allowing the survivors to grow unchecked.

Which Nutrients Are Robbed

Taking these medicines may deplete your supply of, increase your need for, or interfere with the activity of:

- Biotin
- Inositol
- Thiamin
- Riboflavin
- Niacin
- Vitamin B_6
- Vitamin B_{12}
- Vitamin K
- *Bifidobacterium bifidum*
- *Lactobacillus acidophilus*

Additional Ways This Drug May Upset Your Nutritional Balance

Various cephalosporins can cause nausea, vomiting, loss of appetite, and abdominal pain, all of which can upset your eating habits and possibly inter-fere with good nutrition. They can also cause diarrhea, which can hamper nu-trient absorption.

Restoring Your Nutritional Balance

To compensate for the nutrient losses caused by these drugs, speak to your physician about taking 500–1,000 mcg biotin, 250–1,000 mg inositol, 25–100 mg thiamin, 25–100 mg riboflavin, 50–100 mg niacin, 50–100 mg vi-tamin B_6, 500–1,000 mcg vitamin B_{12}, 60–80 mcg vitamin K, 15 billion live *Bifidobacterium bifidum* organisms, and 15 billion live *Lactobacillus acidophilus* or-ganisms per day.

You can also eat foods that contain the depleted nutrients:

- Biotin: beef liver, soybeans, rice bran, peanut butter, barley
- Inositol: cantaloupe, oranges, green beans, grapefruit juice, limes
- Thiamin: braised liver, turkey heart, roasted chicken, gefilte fish, sardines
- Riboflavin: dried sunflower seeds, orange juice, bulgur, spinach noodles, pine nuts
- Niacin: chicken breast, beef liver, mackerel, barley, bulgur
- Vitamin B_6: potato, banana, garbanzo beans, chicken breast, fortified oatmeal
- Vitamin B_{12}: beef liver, rainbow trout, sockeye salmon, beef, haddock
- Vitamin K: kale, broccoli, parsley, Swiss chard, spinach

- *Bifidobacterium bifidum*: Jerusalem artichokes, asparagus, garlic, and onions may stimulate the growth or activity of this probiotic
- *Lactobacillus acidophilus*: yogurt containing live lactobacillus cultures, kefir, acidophilus milk

Consult with your physician before making any changes to your diet or supplemental regimen.

CHLORAMPHENICOL (klor-am-FEN-i-kole)

Brand Names: Chloromycetin, Chloroptic, Diochloram, Ocu-Chlor, Pentamycetin

About Chloramphenicol

The *Rickettsiae* bacteria are unusual in that they can survive and reproduce only when they're inside the cells of another organism. They're usually passed from animals to humans via the bites of ticks, lice, fleas, and mites that have already fed on the animals.

One form of this kind of bacteria, the *Rickettsia rickettsii,* causes Rocky Mountain spotted fever. The bacteria migrate to the cells lining the blood vessels in your skin, heart, kidney, brain, lungs, and elsewhere. Symptoms take at least a few days to appear, but when they do, they can hit hard. The disease may begin with a high fever that can last a week or two. You may develop a dry cough, body-wide rashes, and little purplish areas caused by bleeding under the skin. Depending on where the bacteria have taken up residence in your body, you may suffer from headaches, insomnia, delirium, abdominal pain, vomiting, heart damage, anemia, and pneumonia.

Rocky Mountain spotted fever can be fatal, but fortunately, antibiotics such as chloramphenicol can cut the risk of death significantly. Although it has largely been superseded by newer antibiotics, chloramphenicol still is used sometimes. It works by interferring with the ability of microbes to manufacture protein. This drug is also used to treat typhus, certain types of eye infection, and diseases in which the invading bacteria are resistant to other antibacterial drugs. Chloramphenicol can be administered intravenously, through injection, via eye or ear drops, or as a cream that is applied to the skin.

Possible Side Effects

The drug's more common side effects can be listed according to the method of delivery. Injection or intravenous: Diarrhea, nausea, vomiting, bone marrow supression. Eyedrops: Burning or stinging, blurred vision, and allergic reactions. Topical cream: Allergic reactions.

Which Nutrients Are Robbed

Taking this medicine may deplete your supply of, increase your need for, or interfere with the activity of:

- Folic acid
- Vitamin B_{12}

Additional Ways This Drug May Upset Your Nutritional Balance

Chloramphenicol can cause nausea and vomiting, which can upset your eating habits and possibly interfere with good nutrition. It can also cause diarrhea, which can hamper nutrient absorption.

Restoring Your Nutritional Balance

To compensate for the nutrient loss caused by this drug, speak to your physician about taking 400–800 mcg folic acid and 500–1,000 mcg vitamin B_{12} per day.

You can also eat foods that contain the depleted nutrients:

- Folic acid: beef liver, fortified breakfast cereals, spinach, great northern beans, asparagus
- Vitamin B_{12}: beef liver, rainbow trout, sockeye salmon, beef, haddock

Consult with your physician before making any changes to your diet or supplemental regimen.

CHLOROTHIAZIDE AND RELATED DIURETICS

Chlorothiazide, Methyclothiazide, Polythiazide, Trichlormethiazide (klor-oh-THYE-uh-zide, meth-i-kloe-THYE-uh-zide, pol-ee-THYE-uh-zide, trye-klor-meth-EYE-uh-zide)

Brand Names: Chlorothiazide: Diuril
Methyclothiazide: Aquatensen, Duretic, Enduron

Polythiazide: Renese

Trichlormethiazide: Metahydrin, Naqua

About Chlorothiazide and Related Diuretics

Chlorothiazide, developed in the late 1950s, was a powerful new addition to the nation's medicine chest. This drug was the first strong, reliable diuretic, a medicine designed to flush expendable fluid out of the body. Chlorothiazide belongs to a group of medicines known as the thiazide diuretics, which work by interfering with the movement of salt and water across certain areas within the kidneys, making them excrete more fluid.

Since the introduction of chlorothiazide several decades ago, other thiazide and thiazide-like diuretics have been developed. They all have similar actions in the body but are metabolized somewhat differently. These drugs are used to treat elevated blood pressure, congestive heart failure, and other conditions that can be improved by drawing fluid out of the body. One of these ailments is acute tubular necrosis, which is doctor-speak for rapid kidney failure caused by damage to the tubules where urine is processed. This can occur if the fresh blood supplying the tubules is suddenly interrupted, something like what happens to the heart during a heart attack. Chlorothiazide is one of the diuretics used in such cases to help ensure that the urine keeps flowing.

Possible Side Effects

These drugs' side effects include weakness, fatigue, elevated cholesterol, and decreased blood levels of potassium.

Which Nutrients Are Robbed

Taking these drugs may deplete your supply of, increase your need for, or interfere with the activity of:

- Magnesium
- Phosphorus
- Potassium
- Sodium
- Zinc
- Coenzyme Q_{10}

Restoring Your Nutritional Balance

To compensate for the nutrient loss caused by these drugs, speak to your physician about taking 500–1,000 mg magnesium, 700 mg phosophorus, 50–200 mg zinc, and 30–100 mg coenzyme Q_{10} per day. And ask your physician to consider the potential effects of sodium depletion.

A Note on Potassium: "Regular" diuretics lower potassium levels, while potassium-sparing diuretics do not—they may increase levels instead. It is not uncommon for doctors to prescribe two different diuretics. That's why you should speak to your physician about your potassium levels, and whether it is appropriate for you to take supplements or eat potassium-rich foods.

You can also eat foods that contain the depleted nutrients:

- Magnesium: Florida avocado, toasted wheat germ, almonds, shredded wheat cereal, pumpkin seeds
- Phosphorus: plain nonfat yogurt, lentils, salmon, milk, halibut
- Zinc: oysters, beef shank, chicken, pork tenderloin, plain yogurt
- Coenzyme Q_{10}: beef, chicken, trout, salmon, oranges, broccoli

Consult with your physician before making any changes to your diet or supplemental regimen.

CHLORPROMAZINE (klor-PROE-mah-zeen)

Brand Name: Thorazine

About Chlorpromazine

Chlorpromazine is a fairly famous drug: many people know it by its trade name of Thorazine and know that it's used to treat schizophrenia. In fact, chlorpromazine was one of the first truly useful drugs to be developed for this disorder.

"Disorder" is perhaps the best single word to use in describing schizophrenia, which can cause major disorders in your thinking, mood, and behavior. These are some of the changes that may occur with schizophrenia:

- Your physical appearance may range from uncared for and bland, to mildly unusual, to outright bizarre.
- You may have perceptual distortions, like seeing or hearings things that aren't there.
- Your thought patterns may range from having few thoughts at all to a flood of delusional ideas.
- Your ability to interact with others may suffer as you withdraw, have problems with interpersonal relationships, and find it difficult or impossible to derive pleasure.
- It may be difficult to engage in conversation for you may be mute, ram-

ble on about unrelated topics, make up words, repeat words and phrases that don't make sense, or literally repeat what others are saying.

- Your motor activity (physical movements) may be completely absent (catatonic stupor) or frenzied.
- You may be depressed.
- You may have feelings of dread, intense fear, and depersonalization (of being apart from yourself).

The treatment for schizophrenia includes medications such as chlorpromazine—although this pioneer drug is being superseded by newer medicines. Chlorpromazine has multiple effects on neurotransmitters, hormones, and brain activity. It is also used to treat mania, persistent hiccups, nausea, and vomiting.

Possible Side Effects

The drug's more common side effects include low blood pressure upon arising; allergic reactions; repetitive, involuntary, purposeless movements; and symptoms resembling Parkinson's disease (motor retardation, a wooden facial expression, and an unsteady gait).

Which Nutrients Are Robbed

Taking this medicine may deplete your supply of, increase your need for, or interfere with the activity of:

- Riboflavin
- Coenzyme Q_{10}

Additional Ways This Drug May Upset Your Nutritional Balance

Chlorpromazine can cause low blood sugar (hypoglycemia) and nausea, which can upset your eating habits and possibly interfere with good nutrition.

Restoring Your Nutritional Balance

To compensate for the nutrient loss caused by this drug, speak to your physician about taking 25–100 mg riboflavin and 30–100 mg coenzyme Q_{10} per day.

You can also eat foods that contain the depleted nutrients:

- Riboflavin: dried sunflower seeds, orange juice, bulgur, spinach noodles, pine nuts
- Coenzyme Q_{10}: beef, chicken, trout, salmon, oranges, broccoli

Consult with your physician before making any changes to your diet or supplemental regimen.

CHLORPROPAMIDE (klor-PROE-pah-mide)

Brand Names: Apo-Chlorpropamide, Diabinese, Novo-Propamide

About Chlorpropamide

Diabetes, a potentially fatal disease afflicting some 15 million Americans, has to do with sugar (glucose) in the blood. Specifically, there's too much of it—and it doesn't simply float around, like extra bubbles in a bath. Over time, high levels of blood glucose can lead to a buildup of plaque in the arteries in the heart, brain, legs, and penis (among other areas), contributing to heart disease, stroke, gangrene, impotence, and infections. It can also damage blood vessels in the retina, leading to blindness, or in the kidney, leading to kidney failure. By interfering with normal glucose metabolism and the blood supply, diabetes can damage the nerves and lead to weakness in the legs, pain in the hands and feet, and other problems. It can even suppress the immune system, increasing the odds of developing various infections.

Chlorpropamide is used to treat type 2 diabetes, which is caused by the failure of normal amounts of insulin to move glucose out of the bloodstream and into the cells where it can be used for fuel or storage.

Chlorpropamide stimulates the pancreas to produce extra insulin, which, in effect, "puts more men on the job" to help round up excess blood sugar and get it into the cells where it belongs.

Possible Side Effects

The drug's side effects include tingling and/or weakness of the hands and feet, and yellowing of the skin or whites of the eyes.

Which Nutrients Are Robbed

Taking this medicine may deplete your supply of, increase your need for, or interfere with the activity of:

- Sodium
- Coenzyme Q_{10}

Additional Ways This Drug May Upset Your Nutritional Balance

Chlorpropamide can cause loss of appetite, stomach upset, nausea, and vomiting, all of which can upset your eating habits and possibly interfere with good nutrition.

Restoring Your Nutritional Balance

To compensate for the nutrient loss caused by this drug, speak to your physician about taking 30–100 mg coenzyme Q_{10} per day. And ask your physician to consider the potential effects of sodium depletion.

You can also eat foods that contain the depleted nutrient:

- Coenzyme Q_{10}: beef, chicken, trout, salmon, oranges, broccoli

Consult with your physician before making any changes to your diet or supplemental regimen.

CHLORTHALIDONE (klor-THAL-i-dohn)

Brand Names: Apo-Chlorthalidone, Hygroton, Thalitone

About Chlorthalidone

If your bathtub overfills, you simply pull the plug and let some of the water drain out. And when your body becomes "overfilled" with fluid, diuretics like chlorthalidone act as "plug pullers" to let that extra water drain away. This is very helpful, because sometimes just reducing body fluid can do much to ease vexing problems. For example, if you have elevated blood pressure, reducing body fluid will also reduce the volume of the blood. This means there is less blood for your heart to pump, which automatically lowers your blood pressure. With congestive heart failure, fluid can gather in your lungs, making breathing difficult. If your liver is malfunctioning, fluid can accumulate in your abdomen, making you extremely bloated and uncomfortable. These are times you may want to pull the plug and release more water than usual via the kidneys.

Chlorthalidone is a diuretic that forces fluid out of the body by increasing the kidneys' production of urine. This makes chlorthalidone helpful in treating mildly to moderately elevated blood pressure, as well as accumulations of fluid due to congestive heart failure and certain kidney ailments.

Possible Side Effects

The drug's side effects include low blood pressure, dizziness, weakness, and drowsiness.

Which Nutrients Are Robbed

Taking this medicine may deplete your supply of, increase your need for, or interfere with the activity of:

- Magnesium
- Potassium
- Phosphorus
- Zinc

Additional Ways This Drug May Upset Your Nutritional Balance

Chlorthalidone may cause nausea and vomiting, which can upset your eating habits and possibly interfere with good nutrition.

Restoring Your Nutritional Balance

To compensate for the nutrient loss caused by this drug, speak to your physician about taking 500–1,000 mg magnesium, 700 mg phosphorus, and 50–200 mg zinc per day.

A Note on Potassium: "Regular" diuretics lower potassium levels, while potassium-sparing diuretics do not—they may increase levels instead. It is not uncommon for doctors to prescribe two different diuretics. That's why you should speak to your physician about your potassium levels, and whether it is appropriate for you to take supplements or eat potassium-rich foods.

You can also eat foods that contain the depleted nutrients:

- Magnesium: Florida avocado, toasted wheat germ, almonds, shredded wheat cereal, pumpkin seeds
- Phosphorus: plain nonfat yogurt, lentils, salmon, milk, halibut
- Zinc: oysters, beef shank, chicken, pork tenderloin, plain yogurt

Consult with your physician before making any changes to your diet or supplemental regimen.

CHOLESTYRAMINE (koe-less-TEER-uh-meen)

Brand Names: LoCHOLEST, Novo-Cholamine, Prevalite, PMS-Cholestyramine, Questran, Questran Light Sugar Free

About Cholestyramine

Cholestyramine, which is used to reduce elevated LDL "bad" cholesterol, is a bile acid sequestrant. This means that it "latches" on to bile in the intestines, sequesters it (sets it apart), and carries it out of the body along with other wastes.

How does eliminating bile help reduce cholesterol? Bile, which is manufactured from cholesterol, is released by the gallbladder into the digestive system to help the body absorb vitamins, fats, and cholesterol from the foods we eat. Normally, over 90 percent of the bile that's used for this purpose is reabsorbed by the body. But when cholestyramine is used, much of the bile is bound up and swept out of the body—and therefore must be replaced. If larger than usual amounts of bile are swept out of the body, then larger than usual amounts of cholesterol must be used to make new bile. So levels of circulating cholesterol, including the LDL, will drop.

Unfortunately, this process interferes with the absorption of fats and fat-soluble nutrients and can result in decreased absorption of vitamin A, vitamin D, and vitamin E, among other nutrients.

Cholestyramine is used to reduce cholesterol and to treat diarrhea and itching associated with excess bile acids, as well as other problems.

Possible Side Effects

The drug's more common side effects include nausea, vomiting, constipation, stomach pain, and heartburn.

Which Nutrients Are Robbed

Taking this medicine may deplete your supply of, increase your need for, or interfere with the activity of:

- Beta-carotene
- Folic acid
- Vitamin A
- Vitamin B_{12}
- Vitamin D
- Vitamin E
- Vitamin K
- Calcium
- Iron
- Magnesium
- Phosphorus
- Zinc

Additional Ways This Drug May Upset Your Nutritional Balance

Cholestyramine can cause bloating, which can upset your eating habits and possibly interfere with good nutrition. It can also cause diarrhea, which can hamper nutrient absorption.

Restoring Your Nutritional Balance

To compensate for the nutrient loss caused by this drug, speak to your physician about taking 25,000 IU beta-carotene, 400–800 mcg folic acid, 5,000 IU vitamin A, 500–1,000 mcg vitamin B_{12}, 400 IU vitamin D, 400 IU vitamin E, 60–80 mcg vitamin K, 1,200 mg calcium, 500–1,000 mg magnesium, 700 mg phosphorus, and 50–200 mg zinc per day. Ask your physician to consider the potential effects of iron depletion.

You can also eat foods that contain the depleted nutrients:

- Beta-carotene: carrot, spinach, mango, cantaloupe, apricot nectar
- Folic acid: beef liver, fortified breakfast cereals, spinach, great northern beans, asparagus
- Vitamin A: beef liver, chicken liver, cheese pizza, whole milk, cheddar cheese
- Vitamin B_{12}: beef liver, rainbow trout, sockeye salmon, beef, haddock
- Vitamin D: salmon, mackerel, sardines, eel, fortified milk
- Vitamin E: wheat germ oil, almonds, safflower oil, corn oil, soybean oil
- Vitamin K: kale, broccoli, parsley, Swiss chard, spinach
- Calcium: milk, dried figs, Swiss cheese, yogurt, tofu
- Magnesium: Florida avocado, toasted wheat germ, almonds, shredded wheat cereal, pumpkin seeds
- Phosphorus: plain nonfat yogurt, lentils, salmon, milk, halibut
- Zinc: oysters, beef shank, chicken, pork tenderloin, plain yogurt

Consult with your physician before making any changes to your diet or supplemental regimen.

CHOLINE MAGNESIUM TRISALICYLATE (KOE-leen mag-NEE-zee-um trye-suh-LISS-uh-late)

Brand Names: Tricosal, Trilisate

About Choline Magnesium Trisalicylate

Choline magnesium trisalicylate is a chemical cousin to aspirin, one of our oldest and most durable medicines. You can tell from their names that they're related: Choline magnesium tri*salicylate* and acetyl*salicylic* acid (which is the technical name for aspirin) are both salicylates.

Salicylates dampen the symptoms of inflammation. Typically, the most noticeable of these symptoms are pain and, if the inflammation is in a joint, difficulty in moving that part of the body. Salicylates work primarily by slowing the production of prostaglandins, hormone-like substances that play a crucial role in the inflammation process. You can think of prostaglandins as being like a team of advance people for a politician, staging a huge, noisy rally in town hall. The advance people get hundreds of specialized workers to arrive first, setting the stage for the later arrival of thousands. All the hustle and bustle jams the hall with bodies for a while, although soon everyone will leave and things will get back to normal again.

But suppose the rally was over, and the politician and advance people had left—but new advance people kept arriving, bringing more people with them. There's no need for a rally anymore, but these new advance people want to keep the hoopla going forever. You'd need a way to prevent the new advance teams from getting to town hall. That's something like what choline magnesium trisalicylate does; it cuts back on the body's production of prostaglandins, the "advance people" for inflammation, allowing the site to clear up and return to normal. This makes it helpful in dealing with inflammatory diseases such as rheumatoid arthritis. Although choline magnesium salicylate is a chemical cousin to aspirin, it does not thin the blood as well as aspirin and therefore is not used to prevent heart attacks or strokes.

Possible Side Effects

The drug's more common side effects include ringing in the ears, nausea, vomiting, constipation, heartburn, and diarrhea.

Which Nutrients Are Robbed

Taking this medicine may deplete your supply of, increase your need for, or interfere with the activity of:

- Folic acid
- Vitamin C
- Iron
- Potassium
- Sodium

Additional Ways This Drug May Upset Your Nutritional Balance

Choline magnesium trisalicylate can cause nausea, vomiting, and heartburn, all of which can upset your eating habits and possibly interfere with good nutrition. It can also cause diarrhea, which can hamper nutrient absorption.

Restoring Your Nutritional Balance

To compensate for the nutrient loss caused by this drug, speak to your physician about taking 400–800 mcg folic acid, 250–1,500 mg vitamin C, and 100–300 mg potassium per day. And ask your physician to consider the potential effects of iron and sodium depletion.

You can also eat foods that contain the depleted nutrients:

- Folic acid: beef liver, fortified breakfast cereals, spinach, great northern beans, asparagus

- Vitamin C: papaya, guava, red pepper, cantaloupe, black currants
- Potassium: dried figs, California avocado, papaya, banana, dates

Consult with your physician before making any changes to your diet or supplemental regimen.

CHOLINE SALICYLATE (KOE-leen sa-LISS-uh-late)

Brand Names: Arthropan, Teejel

About Choline Salicylate

Sometimes you just can't handle taking pills to quell your pain or inflammation. That's when a liquid painkiller and anti-inflammatory like choline salicylate comes in handy. This fluid cousin to aspirin is used to treat osteoarthritis, rheumatoid arthritis, and other inflammatory conditions. It's also helpful for teething babies who have tender gums and thus trouble with eating and sleeping. (Needless to say, when your children have trouble sleeping, so do you!)

Choline salicylate works by interfering with a substance called COX (cyclooxygenase) that plays a key role in the inflammation process. Unfortunately, COX also protects the stomach, which is why choline salicylate can cause ulcers.

Possible Side Effects

The drug's more common side effects include stomach upset, nausea, heartburn, fatigue, weakness, and difficulty breathing. This drug crosses the placenta and gets into breast milk, so if you're pregnant or breastfeeding, consider its effects on your child and consult your physician before taking it.

Which Nutrients Are Robbed

Taking this medicine may deplete your supply of, increase your need for, or interfere with the activity of:

- Folic acid
- Vitamin C
- Iron
- Potassium
- Sodium

Additional Ways This Drug May Upset Your Nutritional Balance

Choline salicylate can cause heartburn, stomach pain, and nausea, all of which can upset your eating habits and possibly interfere with good nutrition.

Restoring Your Nutritional Balance

To compensate for the nutrient loss caused by this drug, speak to your physician about taking 400–800 mcg folic acid, 250–1,500 mg vitamin C, and 100–300 mg potassium per day. And ask your physician to consider the potential effects of iron and sodium depletion.

You can also eat foods that contain the depleted nutrients:

- Folic acid: beef liver, fortified breakfast cereals, spinach, great northern beans, asparagus
- Vitamin C: papaya, guava, red pepper, cantaloupe, black currants
- Potassium: dried figs, California avocado, papaya, banana, dates

Consult with your physician before making any changes to your diet or supplemental regimen.

CIDOFOVIR (si-DOFF-uh-veer)

Brand Name: Vistide

About Cidofovir

Cytomegalovirus, known as CMV for short, is a herpes virus that can be detected in the saliva, urine, blood, vaginal secretions, and breast milk. It produces a disease quite similar to infectious mononucleosis and can also attack the nervous system, eyes, lungs, liver, and other parts of the body.

Many healthy people don't suffer at all when attacked by CMV, for their immune systems are strong enough to keep the virus under control. But in those with compromised immune systems (especially in the case of acquired immunodeficiency syndrome [AIDS]), a CMV infection can be devastating. It tends to strike those with weakened immune systems over and over again, often causing retinitis, an inflammation of the retina of the eye, which can leave you blind.

Cidofovir is used to treat CMV retinitis in patients with AIDS. It works by interfering with the ability of the virus to manufacture DNA and replicate itself.

Possible Side Effects

The drug's more common side effects include fever, chills, headache, stomach upset, hair loss, discoloration of the skin, asthma, and bronchitis.

Which Nutrients Are Robbed

Taking this medicine may deplete your supply of, increase your need for, or interfere with the activity of:

- Calcium
- Potassium

Additional Ways This Drug May Upset Your Nutritional Balance

Cidofovir can cause changes in taste, loss of appetite, abdominal pain, heartburn, nausea, and vomiting, all of which can upset your eating habits and possibly interfere with good nutrition. It can also cause diarrhea, which can hamper nutrient absorption.

Restoring Your Nutritional Balance

To compensate for the nutrient loss caused by this drug, speak to your physician about taking 1,200 mg calcium and 100–300 mg potassium per day.

You can also eat foods that contain the depleted nutrients:

- Calcium: milk, dried figs, Swiss cheese, yogurt, tofu
- Potassium: dried figs, California avocado, papaya, banana, dates

Consult with your physician before making any changes to your diet or supplemental regimen.

CIMETIDINE (sye-MET-i-deen)

Brand Names: Apo-Cimetidine, Gen-Cimetidine, Novo-Cimetidine, Nu-Cimet, Peptol, PMS-Cimetidine, Tagamet, Tagamet HB

About Cimetidine

A gnawing or burning pain just below the breastbone (sternum), aching or soreness, hunger, and a feeling of emptiness in your stomach: these are all symptoms of a duodenal ulcer, an erosion of the lining of the duodenum, the first part of the small intestines lying just beyond the stomach. These symptoms are more likely to hit when your stomach is empty, and they tend to recede when you take antacids, drink milk, or eat food—but they come back in a few hours. The pain may strike daily for a week or several weeks, then disappear on its own, but it will most likely return within months.

Very different symptoms are seen with a gastric ulcer, an erosion of the tissues lining the stomach. There's pain, yes, but it may be caused, not relieved, by eating. Swelling of the stomach lining makes it difficult for food to move from the stomach to the duodenum, leading to bloating, nausea, and vomiting.

A delicate balance exists between the acid needed to digest food and the body's protective mechanisms that defend the GI (gastrointestinal) tract against that same acid. When the balance is upset and tissues in the stomach or duodenum lose their protection, they can be eaten away by the acid. This can happen for various reasons: not enough mucous is being produced to protect the lining, the intestines are infected by the *Helicobacter pylori* bacteria, or certain drugs are irritating the stomach lining. If left unchecked, ulcers can cause very serious problems including internal bleeding, narrowing of the passageway between the stomach and the duodenum, narrowing of the duodenum itself, or even perforation of the linings of these vital organs.

Cimetidine, one of the drugs used to treat duodenal and gastric ulcers, works by reducing the amount of acid produced by the stomach. With less acid to irritate the linings, ulcers have a chance to heal.

Cimetidine is used to treat active duodenal ulcers and certain gastric ulcers. It's also used for gastroesophageal reflux disease and to prevent bleeding in the upper GI tract in critically ill people.

Possible Side Effects

The drug's side effects include headache, drowsiness, and dizziness.

Which Nutrients Are Robbed

Taking this medicine may deplete your supply of, increase your need for, or interfere with the activity of:

- Thiamin
- Folic acid
- Vitamin B_{12}
- Vitamin D
- Calcium
- Iron
- Zinc

Additional Ways This Drug May Upset Your Nutritional Balance

Cimetidine can cause nausea and vomiting, which can upset your eating habits and possibly interfere with good nutrition. It can also cause diarrhea, which can hamper nutrient absorption.

Restoring Your Nutritional Balance

To compensate for the nutrient loss caused by this drug, speak to your physician about taking 25–100 mg thiamin, 400–800 mcg folic acid, 500–1,000 mcg vitamin B_{12}, 400 IU vitamin D, 1,200 mg calcium, and 50–200 mg zinc per day. And ask your physician to consider the potential effects of iron depletion.

You can also eat foods that contain the depleted nutrients:

- Thiamin: braised liver, turkey heart, roasted chicken, gefilte fish, sardines
- Folic acid: beef liver, fortified breakfast cereals, spinach, great northern beans, asparagus
- Vitamin B_{12}: beef liver, rainbow trout, sockeye salmon, beef, haddock
- Vitamin D: salmon, mackerel, sardines, eel, fortified milk
- Calcium: milk, dried figs, Swiss cheese, yogurt, tofu
- Zinc: oysters, beef shank, chicken, pork tenderloin, plain yogurt

Consult with your physician before making any changes to your diet or supplemental regimen.

CINOXACIN (sin-OKS-uh-sin)

Brand Name: Cinobac

About Cinoxacin

Cinoxacin is an older antibiotic with limited action. It is still used occasionally to treat infections of the lower urinary tract (bladder and ureter).

Possible Side Effects

The drug's side effects include headache, dizziness, stomach upset, rash, facial swelling, and difficulty breathing.

Which Nutrients Are Robbed

Taking this medicine may deplete your supply of, increase your need for, or interfere with the activity of:

- Biotin
- Inositol
- Thiamin
- Vitamin B_6
- Vitamin B_{12}
- Vitamin K

- Riboflavin
- Niacin

- *Bifidobacterium bifidum*
- *Lactobacillus acidophilus*

Additional Ways This Drug May Upset Your Nutritional Balance

Cinoxacin can cause stomach upset, which can upset your eating habits and possibly interfere with good nutrition.

Restoring Your Nutritional Balance

To compensate for the nutrient loss caused by this drug, speak to your physician about taking 500–1,000 mcg biotin, 250–1,000 mg inositol, 25–100 mg thiamin, 25–100 mg riboflavin, 50–100 mg niacin, 50–100 mg vitamin B_6, 500–1,000 mcg vitamin B_{12}, 60–80 mcg vitamin K, 15 billion live *Bifidobacterium bifidum* organisms, and 15 billion live *Lactobacillus acidophilus* organisms per day.

You can also eat foods that contain the depleted nutrients:

- Biotin: beef liver, soybeans, rice bran, peanut butter, barley
- Inositol: cantaloupe, oranges, green beans, grapefruit juice, limes
- Thiamin: braised liver, turkey heart, roasted chicken, gefilte fish, sardines
- Riboflavin: dried sunflower seeds, orange juice, bulgur, spinach noodles, pine nuts
- Niacin: chicken breast, beef liver, mackerel, barley, bulgur
- Vitamin B_6: potato, banana, garbanzo beans, chicken breast, fortified oatmeal
- Vitamin B_{12}: beef liver, rainbow trout, sockeye salmon, beef, haddock
- Vitamin K: kale, broccoli, parsley, Swiss chard, spinach
- *Bifidobacterium bifidum*: Jerusalem artichokes, asparagus, garlic, and onions may stimulate the growth or activity of this probiotic
- *Lactobacillus acidophilus*: yogurt containing live lactobacillus cultures, kefir, acidophilus milk

Consult with your physician before making any changes to your diet or supplemental regimen.

CIPROFLOXACIN (sip-roe-FLOKS-uh-sin)

Brand Names: Ciloxan, Cipro, Cipro XR

About Ciprofloxacin

In 2001, with the horrors of September 11 still fresh in our minds, we were suddenly struck by a new source of terror. Some people were receiving envelopes through the mail that contained anthrax powder.

Anthrax is a bacteria-borne infectious disease caused by exposure to the *Bacillus anthracis* spores. It usually strikes cattle, goats, camels, sheep, and other herbivores, but it can also infect humans who are exposed to these diseased animals or to the spores themselves.

The symptoms of anthrax may include a fever of 100 degrees or more, muscle aches, fatigue, cough, headache, loss of appetite, nausea, vomiting, and sores on the skin that turn into ulcerations. Some people with anthrax think they just have the flu, so they don't seek treatment.

These bacteria harm us by secreting three toxic substances that work together. The first, protective antigen, latches on to selected cells and opens up a channel that allows the other two, edema factor and lethal factor, to rush in. Once inside the cells, edema factor triggers an excessive buildup of fluid. This can cause a dangerous accumulation of fluid in the cavity around the lungs, as well as interfere with the immune system. Meanwhile, lethal factor disrupts the cells' self-regulation processes, either killing them or making it impossible for them to function.

Ciprofloxacin, the FDA-approved treatment for anthrax, fights bacteria by interfering with their ability to synthesize their DNA. This prevents the bacterial army from growing.

In addition to anthrax, ciprofloxacin is used to treat infections of the urinary tract, lower respiratory tract, sinuses, and other parts of the body.

Possible Side Effects

The drug's side effects include restlessness, headache, and kidney failure.

Which Nutrients Are Robbed

Taking this medicine may deplete your supply of, increase your need for, or interfere with the activity of:

- Biotin
- Inositol
- Vitamin B_{12}
- Vitamin K

- Thiamin
- Riboflavin
- Niacin
- Vitamin B$_6$

- Zinc
- *Bifidobacterium bifidum*
- *Lactobacillus acidophilus*

Additional Ways This Drug May Upset Your Nutritional Balance

Ciprofloxacin can cause nausea, vomiting, and abdominal pain, all of which can upset your eating habits and possibly interfere with good nutrition. It can also cause diarrhea, which can hamper nutrient absorption.

Restoring Your Nutritional Balance

To compensate for the nutrient loss caused by this drug, speak to your physician about taking 500–1,000 mcg biotin, 250–1,000 mg inositol, 25–100 mg thiamin, 25–100 mg riboflavin, 50–100 mg niacin, 50–100 mg vitamin B$_6$, 500–1,000 mcg vitamin B$_{12}$, 60–80 mcg vitamin K, 50–200 mg zinc, 15 billion live *Bifidobacterium bifidum* organisms, and 15 billion live *Lactobacillus acidophilus* organisms per day.

You can also eat foods that contain the depleted nutrients:

- Biotin: beef liver, soybeans, rice bran, peanut butter, barley
- Inositol: cantaloupe, oranges, green beans, grapefruit juice, limes
- Thiamin: braised liver, turkey heart, roasted chicken, gefilte fish, sardines
- Riboflavin: dried sunflower seeds, orange juice, bulgur, spinach noodles, pine nuts
- Niacin: chicken breast, beef liver, mackerel, barley, bulgur
- Vitamin B$_6$: potato, banana, garbanzo beans, chicken breast, fortified oatmeal
- Vitamin B$_{12}$: beef liver, rainbow trout, sockeye salmon, beef, haddock
- Vitamin K: kale, broccoli, parsley, Swiss chard, spinach
- Zinc: oysters, beef shank, chicken, pork tenderloin, plain yogurt
- *Bifidobacterium bifidum*: Jerusalem artichokes, asparagus, garlic, and onions may stimulate the growth or activity of this probiotic
- *Lactobacillus acidophilus*: yogurt containing live lactobacillus cultures, kefir, acidophilus milk

Consult with your physician before making any changes to your diet or supplemental regimen.

CISPLATIN (SIS-plat-in)

Brand Names: Platinol, Platinol-AQ

About Cisplatin

The discovery of the anticancer drug cisplatin could be described as a fortunate accident. Researchers happened to notice that certain formulations of platinum made it difficult for bacterial cells called *Escherichia coli* (*E. coli*) to divide, and caused unusual growth in these cells. From this discovery came the drug cisplatin, which interferes with the manufacture of DNA and is particularly good at killing cells that replicate rapidly, such as cancer cells.

Cisplatin is used to treat a variety of cancers, including those of the breast, testicles, head, neck, and bladder.

The first symptom of bladder cancer is usually blood in the urine, although a small percentage of people will first notice burning upon urination or a frequent and urgent need to urinate. The odds of surviving this cancer— that is, the five-year survival rate—vary according to the cancer's characteristics and how far advanced it is. With a slow-growing tumor that has not pushed into the bladder's muscle layer, the odds are above 90 percent. But if the tumor has pushed deep into the muscle layer, the five-year survival rate drops to 60 percent or less.

Bladder cancer affects more men than women and tends to strike after the age of 60. Smoking, industrial chemicals, and chronic irritation due to bladder stones or certain parasitic infections are linked to the development of the disease.

Cisplatin attacks cells by interfering with their ability to manufacture new DNA.

Possible Side Effects

The drug's more common side effects include nausea and vomiting, nerve damage, loss of hair, inhibited blood cell production, kidney failure, and high-frequency hearing loss.

Which Nutrients Are Robbed

Taking this medicine may deplete your supply of, increase your need for, or interfere with the activity of:

- Calcium
- Magnesium
- Potassium
- Sodium

Additional Ways This Drug May Upset Your Nutritional Balance

Cisplatin causes more nausea and vomiting than just about any other chemotherapy drug, affecting 76 percent to 100 percent of patients. Nausea and vomiting can last up to one week after therapy is concluded. Obviously, this greatly upsets your eating habits and interferes with good nutrition.

Restoring Your Nutritional Balance

To compensate for the nutrient loss caused by this drug, speak to your physician about taking 1,200 mg calcium, 500–1,000 mg magnesium, and 100–300 mg potassium per day. And ask your physician to consider the potential effects of sodium depletion.

You can also eat foods that contain the depleted nutrients:

- Calcium: milk, dried figs, Swiss cheese, yogurt, tofu
- Magnesium: Florida avocado, toasted wheat germ, almonds, shredded wheat cereal, pumpkin seeds
- Potassium: dried figs, California avocado, papaya, banana, dates

Consult with your physician before making any changes to your diet or supplemental regimen.

CLARITHROMYCIN (kluh-RITH-roe-mye-sin)

Brand Names: Biaxin, Biaxin XL

About Clarithromycin

Doctors call the throat the pharynx, so an infection of the throat is known as pharyngitis. Viruses—the same ones that cause colds—can trigger pharyngitis. So can bacteria, although they are less likely to do so.

Antibiotics can't fight viral pharyngitis, but they can treat the kind that stems from bacteria, which bring about a sore throat; pain when swallowing; inflammation of the throat tissues; enlarged, pus-filled tonsils; and sometimes abscesses in the nearby tissues. There can even be ear pain, because the throat and ears share certain nerve pathways.

Some cases of bacterial pharyngitis clear up on their own, thanks to a healthy immune system. But there's always the risk of an infection worsening or spreading, so doctors often prescribe an antibiotic such as clarithromycin. Clarithromycin has just about the same bacteria-fighting abilities as its better-known chemical cousin erythromycin, but it's less likely to cause gastrointestinal problems. It also lasts longer than erythromycin, so you don't have to take it as often.

In addition to pharyngitis, clarithromycin is used to treat a wide variety of bacterial problems, including certain skin infections, pneumonia, and certain kinds of duodenal ulcers.

Possible Side Effects

The drug's most common side effects include abnormal taste sensation, diarrhea, abdominal pain, vomiting, headache, and rash.

Which Nutrients Are Robbed

Taking this medicine may deplete your supply of, increase your need for, or interfere with the activity of:

- Biotin
- Inositol
- Thiamin
- Riboflavin
- Niacin
- Vitamin B_6
- Vitamin B_{12}
- Vitamin K
- *Bifidobacterium bifidum*
- *Lactobacillus acidophilus*

Additional Ways This Drug May Upset Your Nutritional Balance

Clarithromycin can cause low blood sugar (hypoglycemia), nausea, vomiting, changes in taste, heartburn, and abdominal pain, all of which can upset your eating habits and possibly interfere with good nutrition. It can also cause diarrhea, which can hamper nutrient absorption.

Restoring Your Nutritional Balance

To compensate for the nutrient loss caused by this drug, speak to your physician about taking 500–1,000 mcg biotin, 250–1,000 mg inositol, 25–100 mg thiamin, 25–100 mg riboflavin, 50–100 mg niacin, 50–100 mg vitamin B_6, 500–1,000 mcg vitamin B_{12}, 60–80 mcg vitamin K, 15 billion live *Bifidobacterium bifidum* organisms, and 15 billion live *Lactobacillus acidophilus* organisms per day.

You can also eat foods that contain the depleted nutrients:

- Biotin: beef liver, soybeans, rice bran, peanut butter, barley
- Inositol: cantaloupe, oranges, green beans, grapefruit juice, limes
- Thiamin: braised liver, turkey heart, roasted chicken, gefilte fish, sardines
- Riboflavin: dried sunflower seeds, orange juice, bulgur, spinach noodles, pine nuts

- Niacin: chicken breast, beef liver, mackerel, barley, bulgur
- Vitamin B$_6$: potato, banana, garbanzo beans, chicken breast, fortified oatmeal
- Vitamin B$_{12}$: beef liver, rainbow trout, sockeye salmon, beef, haddock
- Vitamin K: kale, broccoli, parsley, Swiss chard, spinach
- *Bifidobacterium bifidum*: Jerusalem artichokes, asparagus, garlic, and onions may stimulate the growth or activity of this probiotic
- *Lactobacillus acidophilus*: yogurt containing live lactobacillus cultures, kefir, acidophilus milk

Consult with your physician before making any changes to your diet or supplemental regimen.

CLINDAMYCIN (klin-duh-MYE-sin)

Brand Names: Alti-Clindamycin, Cleocin, Cleocin HCL, Cleocin Pediatric, Cleocin Phosphate, Clindagel, Clindets, Dalacin C

About Clindamycin

The human heart is wrapped in a protective lining called the endocardium, and when bacteria infect that lining, you'll suffer from bacterial endocarditis. The word "endocarditis" is a little misleading, for the infection doesn't usually remain confined to the heart's outer lining. Instead, it generally moves right into the heart muscle and heart valves.

Endocarditis can be a major illness, triggering fever, rapid heart rate, weight loss, anemia, joint pain, and serious damage to the heart valves. Little clumps of bacteria and blood clots can accumulate at the infected valves, break off, and travel through the bloodstream until they become stuck in an artery. If the artery happens to be in your heart, you may suffer a heart attack; if it's in your brain, you may be hit with a stroke.

One of the medicines used for bacterial endocarditis is clindamycin. This drug works by preventing bacteria from forming the proteins they need to replicate themselves.

Clindamycin is also used to prevent endocarditis in people who are particularly at risk. For example, those who have congenital heart defects or preexisting problems with heart valves may be given clindamycin before undergoing surgery, dental work, or any other procedure that might allow bacteria to enter the body. The drug is also used to treat bacterial vaginosis.

Clindamycin comes in several different forms: oral, IV, injection, topical cream, and intravaginal cream or suppositories.

Possible Side Effects

The drug's most common side effects in each of its different forms include:

Oral: diarrhea, abdominal pain
Injected: vein inflammation or abscess at injection site
Systemic: low blood pressure, nausea, vomiting, fungal overgrowth, rash
Topical: dryness, burning, itching of the skin
Vaginal: yeast infections, painful intercourse

Which Nutrients Are Robbed

Taking this medicine may deplete your supply of, increase your need for, or interfere with the activity of:

- Vitamin K
- *Bifidobacterium bifidum*
- *Lactobacillus acidophilus*

Additional Ways This Drug May Upset Your Nutritional Balance

Clindamycin can cause abdominal pain, nausea, and vomiting, which can upset your eating habits and possibly interfere with good nutrition. It can also cause diarrhea, which can hamper nutrient absorption.

Restoring Your Nutritional Balance

To compensate for the nutrient loss caused by this drug, speak to your physician about taking 60–80 mcg vitamin K, 15 billion live *Bifidobacterium bifidum* organisms, and 15 billion live *Lactobacillus acidophilus* organisms per day.

You can also eat foods that contain the depleted nutrients:

- Vitamin K: kale, broccoli, parsley, Swiss chard, spinach
- *Bifidobacterium bifidum:* Jerusalem artichokes, asparagus, garlic, and onions may stimulate the growth or activity of this probiotic
- *Lactobacillus acidophilus:* yogurt containing live lactobacillus cultures, kefir, acidophilus milk

Consult with your physician before making any changes to your diet or supplemental regimen.

CLOFIBRATE (kloe-FYE-brate)

Brand Names: Abitrate, Atromid-S, Claripex

About Clofibrate

Most of us are aware of the dangers of total cholesterol, and have probably heard about the LDL "bad" cholesterol and the HDL "good" cholesterol. Another form of cholesterol, called VLDL, is not as well known but does concern doctors when it rises too high.

VLDL, which stands for very low density lipoprotein, is made in the liver out of fat and cholesterol. (It contains a lot of fats—triglycerides—so it's not very dense.) VLDL's job is to carry those fats to various cells in the body. After it deposits enough fats, it is transformed into an LDL particle and busies itself delivering cholesterol to the cells.

Medical researchers have not yet mapped out the link between elevated VLDL and the arterial damage seen with coronary heart disease. They do know, however, that if you have more VLDL, you're likely to have less of the protective HDL, and your risk of developing heart disease rises.

Clofibrate is used along with diet therapy to treat people with elevated VLDL and blood fat levels. The drug is thought to interfere with the production of cholesterol in the liver.

Possible Side Effects

The drug's side effects include nausea, diarrhea, fever, irregular heartbeat, muscle weakness, and decreased libido.

Which Nutrients Are Robbed

Taking this medicine may deplete your supply of, increase your need for, or interfere with the activity of:

- Beta-carotene
- Vitamin E
- Vitamin B_{12}
- Iron

Additional Ways This Drug May Upset Your Nutritional Balance

Clofibrate can cause abdominal distress, heartburn, nausea, and vomiting, all of which can upset your eating habits and possibly interfere with good nutrition. It can also cause diarrhea, which can hamper nutrient absorption.

This drug can also trigger hyperkalemia, or too much potassium in the blood.

Restoring Your Nutritional Balance

To compensate for the nutrient loss caused by this drug, speak to your physician about taking 25,000 IU beta-carotene, 500–1,000 mcg vitamin B_{12}, and 400 IU vitamin E per day. And ask your physician to consider the potential effects of iron depletion.

You can also eat foods that contain the depleted nutrients:

- Beta-carotene: carrot, spinach, mango, cantaloupe, apricot nectar
- Vitamin B_{12}: beef liver, rainbow trout, sockeye salmon, beef, haddock
- Vitamin E: wheat germ oil, almonds, safflower oil, corn oil, soybean oil

Consult with your physician before making any changes to your diet or supplemental regimen.

CLOMIPRAMINE (kloe-MIP-rah-meen)

Brand Names: Anafranil, Apo-Clomipramine, Gen-Clomipramine, Novo-Clopramine

About Clomipramine

Do you know someone who washes her hands over and over again for no obvious reason? Have you seen someone in a restaurant spending an awful lot of time arranging the food on his plate, making it look just right before he begins eating?

How about someone who checks the doors over and over again at night, even when she knows she locked them five minutes earlier? Or counts certain things over and over again, perhaps the number of sidewalk squares from point X to point Y, or the number of steps to each landing of the staircase?

These may be the symptoms of obsessive-compulsive disorder (OCD). The obsessive part of the disorder is the recurrence of intrusive and unwanted ideas. You may, for example, keep worrying about getting germs from touching things, continually fret that the toaster is still on, or fear that you will get hurt or hurt someone else. The compulsive part is the incessant desire to perform some act over and over again to ward off what's worrying you—such as washing your hands to get rid of germs that you fear will make you sick or constantly checking the locks to keep burglars from breaking in. Most of the people with OCD know there's no real danger and that their rituals don't really solve any problems, but they can't stop their obsessive thoughts and compulsive behaviors.

If you have such symptoms, a psychotherapist may help you gain control of OCD by slowly exposing you to the things you fear. Physicians approach the problem by prescribing drugs such as clomipramine. An antidepressant, clomipramine apparently helps control OCD by keeping the "feel-good" neurotransmitter serotonin in play in the nervous system for longer than usual.

Clomipramine is also used to treat panic attacks, depression, and chronic pain.

Possible Side Effects

The drug's more common side effects include drowsiness, dizziness, headache, nervousness, stomach upset, fatigue, and tremor.

Which Nutrients Are Robbed

Taking this medicine may deplete your supply of, increase your need for, or interfere with the activity of:

- Riboflavin
- Sodium
- Coenzyme Q_{10}

Additional Ways This Drug May Upset Your Nutritional Balance

Clomipramine can cause nausea, vomiting, loss of appetite, and abdominal pain, all of which can upset your eating habits and possibly interfere with good nutrition. It can also cause diarrhea, which can hamper nutrient absorption.

Restoring Your Nutritional Balance

To compensate for the nutrient loss caused by this drug, speak to your physician about taking 25–100 mg riboflavin and 30–100 mg coenzyme Q_{10} per day. And ask your physician to consider the potential effects of sodium depletion.

You can also eat foods that contain the depleted nutrients:

- Riboflavin: dried sunflower seeds, orange juice, bulgur, spinach noodles, pine nuts
- Coenzyme Q_{10}: beef, chicken, trout, salmon, oranges, broccoli

Consult with your physician before making any changes to your diet or supplemental regimen.

CLONIDINE (KLON-i-deen)

Brand Names: Apo-Clonidine, Catapres, Catapres TTS-1, Catapres TTS-2, Catapres TTS-3, Dixarit, Duraclon, Novo-Clonidine, Nu-Clonidine

About Clonidine

Getting hooked on narcotics is relatively easy, but getting off can be a major battle. The symptoms of withdrawal are often harsh: crying, rapid breathing, profuse perspiration, tremors, hot and cold flashes, generalized aching, diarrhea, elevated temperature, a rapid heart rate, and more. These symptoms may begin several hours after you've stopped taking the drug and can take a few days to reach their peak.

Clonidine is used to relieve some of the symptoms of narcotic withdrawal and reduce the intensity of others. The drug has several actions, including lowering the blood pressure and slowing the heart rate. Clonidine is also used to treat elevated blood pressure and relieve cancer pain that does not respond to opioids.

Possible Side Effects

The drug's more common side effects include drowsiness, dizziness, itchy, inflamed patches on the skin, and dry mouth.

Which Nutrients Are Robbed

Taking this medicine may deplete your supply of, increase your need for, or interfere with the activity of:

- Coenzyme Q_{10}

Additional Ways This Drug May Upset Your Nutritional Balance

Clonidine can cause nausea, vomiting, dry mouth, loss of appetite, and changes in taste, all of which can upset your eating habits and possibly interfere with good nutrition.

Restoring Your Nutritional Balance

To compensate for the nutrient loss caused by this drug, speak to your physician about taking 30–100 mg coenzyme Q_{10} per day.

You can also eat foods that contain the depleted nutrient:

- Coenzyme Q_{10}: beef, chicken, trout, salmon, oranges, broccoli

Consult with your physician before making any changes to your diet or supplemental regimen.

CLOXACILLIN (kloks-uh-SIL-in)

Brand Names: Apo-Cloxi, Cloxapen, Novo-Cloxin, Nu-Cloxi, Tegopen

About Cloxacillin

A staphylococcal (staph) infection can be mild, middling, or potentially fatal, depending on your general health and where the infection settles. Should the sphere-shaped staph bacteria get into the bloodstream, they can infect the heart, bones, or other parts of the body, with the symptoms they trigger depending on where they take up residence.

Most of the time, however, the germs just sit on your skin and in your nasal membranes or live in your intestinal, urinary, or upper respiratory tracts, causing no harm. The problems arise when a cut, burn, or other break in the skin allows them to enter your body, or your immune system weakens and allows them to spread.

Staph infections can be hard to get rid of because the bacteria have evolved to the point where they can produce "anti-antibiotic enzymes." These enzymes are weapons evolved by the bacteria over time that have rendered several antibiotics useless against staph infections.

Cloxacillin is one of the antibiotics prescribed to treat certain staph infections because it is able to resist such enzymes.

Possible Side Effects

The drug's side effects include rashes, allergic reactions, and seizures.

Which Nutrients Are Robbed

Taking this medicine may deplete your supply of, increase your need for, or interfere with the activity of:

- Biotin
- Inositol
- Thiamin
- Riboflavin
- Niacin
- Vitamin B_6
- Vitamin B_{12}
- Vitamin K
- Potassium
- *Bifidobacterium bifidum*
- *Lactobacillus acidophilus*

Restoring Your Nutritional Balance

To compensate for the nutrient loss caused by this drug, speak to your physician about taking 500–1,000 mcg biotin, 250–1,000 mg inositol, 25–100

mg thiamin, 25–100 mg riboflavin, 50–100 mg niacin, 50–100 mg vitamin B_6, 500–1,000 mcg vitamin B_{12}, 60–80 mcg vitamin K, 100–300 mg potassium, 15 billion live *Bifidobacterium bifidum* organisms, and 15 billion live *Lactobacillus acidophilus* organisms per day.

You can also eat foods that contain the depleted nutrients:

- Biotin: beef liver, soybeans, rice bran, peanut butter, barley
- Inositol: cantaloupe, oranges, green beans, grapefruit juice, limes
- Thiamin: braised liver, turkey heart, roasted chicken, gefilte fish, sardines
- Riboflavin: dried sunflower seeds, orange juice, bulgur, spinach noodles, pine nuts
- Niacin: chicken breast, beef liver, mackerel, barley, bulgur
- Vitamin B_6: potato, banana, garbanzo beans, chicken breast, fortified oatmeal
- Vitamin B_{12}: beef liver, rainbow trout, sockeye salmon, beef, haddock
- Vitamin K: kale, broccoli, parsley, Swiss chard, spinach
- Potassium: dried figs, California avocado, papaya, banana, dates
- *Bifidobacterium bifidum:* Jerusalem artichokes, asparagus, garlic, and onions may stimulate the growth or activity of this probiotic
- *Lactobacillus acidophilus:* yogurt containing live lactobacillus cultures, kefir, acidophilus milk

Consult with your physician before making any changes to your diet or supplemental regimen.

COLCHICINE (KOL-chi-seen)

Brand Names: This drug is sold under its generic name.

About Colchicine

Gout often strikes without warning. You go to sleep one night feeling fine, only to be awakened by excruciating pain in the bunion joint of your big toe. The joint is "hot" due to inflammation, the skin is tight, red, and shiny, and the slightest touch is too painful to bear. You may also have a fever, chills, and an overall feeling of sickness. The problem could subside on its own, or it may go away and return (in some cases, over and over again), eventually destroying so much tissue that the joint is permanently damaged.

Gout tortures some 2 million Americans—most of them male. It's caused by excess uric acid in the blood, which crystallizes in the joint, triggering an attack. Immune system "soldiers" rush to the scene, attempting to get rid of the uric acid buildup, but the cleanup process triggers inflammation, which causes even more pain.

Colchicine helps quell inflammation in the area, reducing the pain without slowing the cleanup process. Within 12 to 24 hours of taking this drug, gout-related pain levels can fall significantly.

Colchicine used to be the standard treatment for gout, but because it can cause diarrhea and other side effects, other drugs (particularly nonsteroidal anti-inflammatory drugs [NSAIDs]) may be tried first. However, colchicine is still used to prevent future attacks of gout in people who are at risk. It may also be prescribed to treat Mediterranean fever and some cases of cirrhosis of the liver.

Possible Side Effects

The drug's more common side effects include bone marrow depression, diarrhea, nausea, vomiting, and abdominal pain.

Which Nutrients Are Robbed

Taking this medicine may deplete your supply of, increase your need for, or interfere with the activity of:

- Beta-carotene
- Folic acid
- Vitamin B$_{12}$
- Calcium
- Magnesium
- Potassium
- Sodium

Additional Ways This Drug May Upset Your Nutritional Balance

Colchicine can cause nausea, vomiting, abdominal pain, and loss of appetite, all of which can upset your eating habits and possibly interfere with good nutrition. It can also cause diarrhea, which can hamper nutrient absorption.

Restoring Your Nutritional Balance

To compensate for the nutrient loss caused by this drug, speak to your physician about taking 25,000 IU beta-carotene, 400–800 mcg folic acid, 500–1,000 mcg vitamin B$_{12}$, 1,200 mg calcium, 500–1,000 mg magnesium, and 100–300 mg potassium per day. And ask your physician to consider the potential effects of sodium depletion.

You can also eat foods that contain the depleted nutrients:

- Beta-carotene: carrot, spinach, mango, cantaloupe, apricot nectar
- Folic acid: beef liver, fortified breakfast cereals, spinach, great northern beans, asparagus
- Vitamin B_{12}: beef liver, rainbow trout, sockeye salmon, beef, haddock
- Calcium: milk, dried figs, Swiss cheese, yogurt, tofu
- Magnesium: Florida avocado, toasted wheat germ, almonds, shredded wheat cereal, pumpkin seeds
- Potassium: dried figs, California avocado, papaya, banana, dates

Consult with your physician before making any changes to your diet or supplemental regimen.

COLCHICINE PLUS PROBENECID (KOL-chi-seen, proe-BEN-e-sid)

Brand Names: ColBenemid, Proben-C

About Colchicine plus Probenecid

Gout is a twofold problem, causing pain and inflammation. The pain (which can be intense) starts when uric acid crystals form within a joint, often the bunion joint of the big toe. When the immune system sets off a major inflammation response as it attempts to clear away the uric acid, the pain can become excruciating.

Nonsteroidal anti-inflammatory drugs (NSAIDs) are often given to ease pain and inflammation, and colchicine or corticosteroids may be used to reduce inflammation even further. Some doctors also prescribe a uricosuric drug called probenecid to lower uric acid levels. Uricosuric drugs slow the reabsorption of uric acid by the kidneys, so more is allowed to flow out of the body with the urine.

Probenecid is used for those who have already had several gout attacks, whose blood levels of uric acid are very high, or who have little stones made of uric acid in their body tissues. Probenecid is not used for gout attacks in progress.

Possible Side Effects

Colchicine's more common side effects include nausea and vomiting, abdominal pain, and diarrhea. Probenecid's side effects include painful urination, rash, itching, kidney stones, and liver damage.

Which Nutrients Are Robbed

Taking this medicine may deplete your supply of, increase your need for, or interfere with the activity of:

- Beta-carotene
- Potassium
- Vitamin B$_{12}$
- Sodium

Additional Ways This Drug May Upset Your Nutritional Balance

Colchicine can cause nausea, vomiting, abdominal pain, and loss of appetite, while probenecid can trigger loss of appetite, nausea, vomiting, and sore gums. All of this can upset your eating habits and possibly interfere with good nutrition. Colchicine can also cause diarrhea, which can hamper nutrient absorption.

Restoring Your Nutritional Balance

To compensate for the nutrient loss caused by this drug, speak to your physician about taking 25,000 IU beta-carotene, 500–1,000 mcg vitamin B$_{12}$, and 100–300 mg potassium per day. And ask your physician to consider the potential effects of sodium depletion.

You can also eat foods that contain the depleted nutrients:

- Beta-carotene: carrot, spinach, mango, cantaloupe, apricot nectar
- Vitamin B$_{12}$: beef liver, rainbow trout, sockeye salmon, beef, haddock
- Potassium: dried figs, California avocado, papaya, banana, dates

Consult with your physician before making any changes to your diet or supplemental regimen.

COLESEVELAM (koe-le-SEV-e-lam)

Brand Name: WelChol

About Colesevelam

Colesevelam is a bile acid sequestrant, a medicinal way of forcing the body to use up some of its cholesterol instead of letting large amounts float through the arteries and possibly cause damage.

Using colesevelam to reduce cholesterol is a once-removed approach. To understand how it works, imagine that you have to babysit a very energetic child. You can't reach into her body to turn down the energy switch, so instead you take her to a hilly park and let her run up and down the hills for a couple of hours. You get her to use up most of her energy, so she gets tired and calms down.

Colesevelam does something similar in the body, binding to bile acids as a way of getting the body to use up cholesterol. Bile acids help the body break down and absorb fat, fat-soluble vitamins, and other nutrients that are found in the fatty parts of food. Normally, once the bile acids have done their job, they're reabsorbed by the body and recycled. But colesevelam prevents the bile acids from being reused by binding to them so they are carried out of the body along with other wastes.

When the supply of bile acids begins to run low, the body has no choice but to make more. And because it takes cholesterol to make bile acids, the body must use some of its cholesterol to do so. This drives down the levels of blood cholesterol, particularly LDL "bad" cholesterol.

Colesevelam is used to treat elevated cholesterol, either by itself or in conjunction with a statin drug.

Possible Side Effects

The drug's more common side effects include constipation, stomach upset, weakness and inflammation of the pharynx.

Which Nutrients Are Robbed

Taking this medicine may deplete your supply of, increase your need for, or interfere with the activity of:

- Beta-carotene
- Folic acid
- Vitamin A
- Vitamin B$_{12}$
- Vitamin D
- Vitamin E
- Vitamin K
- Iron

Additional Ways This Drug May Upset Your Nutritional Balance

Colesevelam can cause heartburn, bloating, and nausea, which can upset your eating habits and possibly interfere with good nutrition.

Restoring Your Nutritional Balance

To compensate for the nutrient loss caused by this drug, speak to your physician about taking 25,000 IU beta-carotene, 400–800 mcg folic acid,

5,000 IU vitamin A, 500–1,000 mcg vitamin B$_{12}$, 400 IU vitamin D, 400 IU vitamin E, and 60–80 mcg vitamin K per day. And ask your physician to consider the potential effects of iron depletion.

You can also eat foods that contain the depleted nutrients:

- Beta-carotene: carrot, spinach, mango, cantaloupe, apricot nectar
- Folic acid: beef liver, fortified breakfast cereals, spinach, great northern beans, asparagus
- Vitamin A: beef liver, chicken liver, cheese pizza, whole milk, cheddar cheese
- Vitamin B$_{12}$: beef liver, rainbow trout, sockeye salmon, beef, haddock
- Vitamin D: salmon, mackerel, sardines, eel, fortified milk
- Vitamin E: wheat germ oil, almonds, safflower oil, corn oil, soybean oil
- Vitamin K: kale, broccoli, parsley, Swiss chard, spinach

Consult with your physician before making any changes to your diet or supplemental regimen.

COLESTIPOL (koe-LESS-ti-pole)

Brand Name: Colestid

About Colestipol

Doctors would love to be able to turn the cholesterol meter up or down at will. When you need more cholesterol to make cell walls, nerve cells, or bile, they would turn the meter up. And when you have too much cholesterol circulating in your bloodstream, they would turn the meter down.

If only it were so.

But it's not. We don't have such easy ways of fine-tuning the amount of cholesterol produced in the body, so the millions of Americans with high cholesterol need to find another way to handle the problem. That's where colestipol can help.

Colestipol does not make the body produce less cholesterol. Instead, it binds to bile acids in the digestive tract. Bile acids are secreted by the gallbladder when we eat to help us break down and absorb fats, fat-soluble vitamins, and other fatty substances from our food.

After they've completed their job, most bile acids are reabsorbed so that they can be used over again. But colestipol grabs hold of bile acids so that they can be swept out of the body with other waste products. Then the body must use some of its cholesterol supply to replace those bile acids, which lowers the amount of cholesterol circulating in the blood.

That's the good part. The bad part is that the bile acids bound up by colestipol aren't able to help absorb the fat-soluble vitamins and other beneficial nutrients in the fatty parts of food, so you may run short of vitamins A, D, and E, among other nutrients.

Colestipol is used to treat elevated cholesterol and related problems.

Possible Side Effects

The drug's more common side effects include constipation, vertigo, fatigue, abdominal pain and distention, and flatulence.

Which Nutrients Are Robbed

Taking this medicine may deplete your supply of, increase your need for, or interfere with the activity of:

- Beta-carotene
- Folic acid
- Vitamin A
- Vitamin B_{12}
- Vitamin D
- Vitamin E
- Vitamin K
- Calcium
- Iron

Additional Ways This Drug May Upset Your Nutritional Balance

Colestipol can cause abdominal pain and distension, nausea, and vomiting, all of which can upset your eating habits and possibly interfere with good nutrition. It can also cause diarrhea, which can hamper nutrient absorption.

Restoring Your Nutritional Balance

To compensate for the nutrient loss caused by this drug, speak to your physician about taking 25,000 IU beta-carotene, 400–800 mcg folic acid, 5,000 IU vitamin A, 500–1,000 mcg vitamin B_{12}, 400 IU vitamin D, 400 IU vitamin E, 60–80 mcg vitamin K, and 1,200 mg calcium per day. And ask your physician to consider the potential effects of iron depletion.

You can also eat foods that contain the depleted nutrients:

- Beta-carotene: carrot, spinach, mango, cantaloupe, apricot nectar
- Folic acid: beef liver, fortified breakfast cereals, spinach, great northern beans, asparagus

- Vitamin A: beef liver, chicken liver, cheese pizza, whole milk, cheddar cheese
- Vitamin B$_{12}$: beef liver, rainbow trout, sockeye salmon, beef, haddock
- Vitamin D: salmon, mackerel, sardines, eel, fortified milk
- Vitamin E: wheat germ oil, almonds, safflower oil, corn oil, soybean oil
- Vitamin K: kale, broccoli, parsley, Swiss chard, spinach
- Calcium: milk, dried figs, Swiss cheese, yogurt, tofu

Consult with your physician before making any changes to your diet or supplemental regimen.

CORTISONE (KOR-ti-sohn)

Brand Name: Cortone

About Cortisone

There are two adrenal glands in your body, one sitting atop each of your kidneys. The outer layer of the adrenal gland, called the adrenal cortex, synthesizes and releases a number of important substances, including the glucocorticoids that affect fat, protein, and carbohydrate metabolism, and helps the body produce glucose to keep the blood sugar stable between meals.

But sometimes the adrenal cortex stops producing sufficient amounts of these vital substances. Doctors call this adrenocortical insufficiency. The problem may take the form of Addison's disease, in which the adrenal glands have been almost completely destroyed by cancer, a tuberculosis infection, or another ailment. Or the problem may be due to an infection by HIV or another virus, an autoimmune disease, or something else that has harmed the adrenal cortex. Adrenocortical insufficiency can cause weakness, fever, low blood pressure, and abdominal pain.

Cortisone is used to treat adrenocortical insufficiency. In a sense, the drug replaces what the body can no longer manufacture on its own. Cortisone (a glucocorticoid) is not a perfect substitute for healthy adrenal glands, and it does have potentially serious side effects, but it can keep you going.

Possible Side Effects

The drug's more common side effects include insomnia, nervousness, indigestion, and increased appetite.

Which Nutrients Are Robbed

Taking this medicine may deplete your supply of, increase your need for, or interfere with the activity of:

- Vitamin A
- Folic acid
- Vitamin B$_6$
- Vitamin C
- Vitamin D
- Vitamin K
- Calcium
- Magnesium
- Phosphorus
- Potassium
- Selenium
- Zinc

Additional Ways This Drug May Upset Your Nutritional Balance

Cortisone can cause indigestion, which can upset your eating habits and possibly interfere with good nutrition.

Restoring Your Nutritional Balance

To compensate for the nutrient loss caused by this drug, speak to your physician about taking 5,000 IU vitamin A, 400–800 mcg folic acid, 50–100 mg vitamin B$_6$, 250–1,500 mg vitamin C, 400 IU vitamin D, 60–80 mcg vitamin K, 1,200 mg calcium, 500–1,000 mg magnesium, 700 mg phosphorus, 100–300 mg potassium, 20–100 mcg selenium, and 50–200 mg zinc per day.

You can also eat foods that contain the depleted nutrients:

- Vitamin A: beef liver, chicken liver, cheese pizza, whole milk, cheddar cheese
- Folic acid: beef liver, fortified breakfast cereals, spinach, great northern beans, asparagus
- Vitamin B$_6$: potato, banana, garbanzo beans, chicken breast, fortified oatmeal
- Vitamin C: papaya, guava, red pepper, cantaloupe, black currants
- Vitamin D: salmon, mackerel, sardines, eel, fortified milk
- Vitamin K: kale, broccoli, parsley, Swiss chard, spinach
- Calcium: milk, dried figs, Swiss cheese, yogurt, tofu
- Magnesium: Florida avocado, toasted wheat germ, almonds, shredded wheat cereal, pumpkin seeds
- Phosphorus: plain nonfat yogurt, lentils, salmon, milk, halibut
- Potassium: dried figs, California avocado, papaya, banana, dates
- Selenium: Brazil nuts, tuna, beef liver, turkey breast, spaghetti with meat sauce

- Zinc: oysters, beef shank, chicken, pork tenderloin, plain yogurt

Consult with your physician before making any changes to your diet or supplemental regimen.

CYCLOPHOSPHAMIDE (sye-kloe-FOSS-fuh-mide)

Brand Names: Cytoxan, Neosar, Procytox

About Cyclophosphamide

Your good health depends on a constant and plentiful supply of red blood cells, white blood cells, and other blood components. Various blood cells are born in the bone marrow, then released into the bloodstream when they're mature and ready to take on their duties. But sometimes this process falters and the marrow doesn't produce enough cells, leading to a disease called aplastic anemia. Radiation, certain drugs, toxins, and chemotherapy can trigger this disease, but the most common cause is an errant immune system that suppresses the birthing process of the new cells.

With aplastic anemia, you have too few red blood cells to ferry oxygen through the body and too few white blood cells to fight off infection. You feel tired and weak, and tend to succumb to infections that your body would ordinarily fight off. You may bruise and bleed easily. If the problem is severe and not treated quickly, death is inevitable.

Blood transfusions can supply you with fresh red blood cells and other blood components, but that doesn't solve the underlying problem. The larger solution is to suppress the overactive immune system, prevent it from attacking the bone marrow, then transplant new bone marrow or stem cells from a compatible donor. In older folks and those for whom a suitable donor cannot be found, treatment is based solely on suppressing the immune system.

Cyclophosphamide is given to weaken the immune system and suppress its attacks on the bone marrow. Given in high doses, it may bring about remission in difficult cases. Cyclophosphamide may also be used to treat lymphoma and leukemia and to prevent the body from rejecting transplanted tissues.

Possible Side Effects

The drug's more common side effects include loss of hair, sterility, nausea and vomiting, anemia, and a potentially fatal inflammation of the bladder called acute hemorrhagic cystitis.

Which Nutrients Are Robbed

Taking this medicine may deplete your supply of, increase your need for, or interfere with the activity of:

- Potassium
- Sodium

Additional Ways This Drug May Upset Your Nutritional Balance

Cyclophosphamide can cause nausea, vomiting, and loss of appetite, all of which can upset your eating habits and possibly interfere with good nutrition. It can also cause diarrhea, which can hamper nutrient absorption.

Restoring Your Nutritional Balance

To compensate for the nutrient loss caused by this drug, speak to your physician about taking 100–300 mg potassium per day. And ask your physician to consider the potential effects of sodium depletion.

You can also eat foods that contain the depleted nutrient:

- Potassium: dried figs, California avocado, papaya, banana, dates

Consult with your physician before making any changes to your diet or supplemental regimen.

CYCLOSERINE (sye-kloe-SER-een)

Brand Name: Seromycin Pulvules

About Cycloserine

Tuberculosis, or TB, used to be a major killer in the United States. Entire wards in hospitals were devoted to its treatment, and there were special TB sanatoriums where patients went to rest and keep away from others, so they wouldn't spread the infection.

TB is caused by the *Mycobacterium tuberculosis* bacteria, which spreads from person to person through the air. Your immune system will kill most of the TB germs that get into your body, and literally capture and hold others inside white blood cells. Most of the time, these captive TB germs remain safely in "prison," but sometimes they can begin to multiply and spread. Perhaps it's because your immune system has been weakened through age, disease, or the use of certain medicines. Whatever the cause, the "prison guards" can no longer do their job, and the bacteria that escape run rampant.

Typically, the TB bacteria infect the lungs, causing coughing, a lack of energy, loss of appetite, night sweats, a general "blah" feeling, and, in later stages, shortness of breath.

If the bacteria move to other parts of the body, any number of symptoms can develop. If they go to your bladder, there may be blood in your urine and pain when you urinate. If they go to your reproductive organs, there may be swelling in this area, or sterility. If they go to your joints, there may be pain and arthritis-like problems. If they go to your abdominal cavity, there may be swelling, tenderness, and pain.

TB is treated with antibiotics such as cycloserine. It works by preventing the *Mycobacterium tuberculosis* from building their cell walls. These half-built bacteria cannot survive.

Possible Side Effects

The drug's side effects include irregular heartbeat, headache, drowsiness, convulsions, and tremors.

Which Nutrients Are Robbed

Taking this medicine may deplete your supply of, increase your need for, or interfere with the activity of:

- Folic acid
- Vitamin B_{12}
- Vitamin B_6

Restoring Your Nutritional Balance

To compensate for the nutrient loss caused by this drug, speak to your physician about taking 400–800 mcg folic acid, 50–100 mg vitamin B_6, and 500–1,000 mcg vitamin B_{12} per day.

You can also eat foods that contain the depleted nutrients:

- Folic acid: beef liver, fortified breakfast cereals, spinach, great northern beans, asparagus
- Vitamin B_6: potato, banana, garbanzo beans, chicken breast, fortified oatmeal
- Vitamin B_{12}: beef liver, rainbow trout, sockeye salmon, beef, haddock

Consult with your physician before making any changes to your diet or supplemental regimen.

CYCLOSPORINE (sye-kloe-SPOR-een)

Brand Names: Neoral, Sandimmune, Restasis, SangCya

About Cyclosporine

The body has a very clear sense of what is "me" and what is "not-me." It also knows that "me" organs, tissues, and cells belong to the body, but "not-me" parts do not. In fact, "not-me" is, by definition, dangerous. Therefore, the body mounts an aggressive attack designed to destroy any version of "not-me" that it finds.

This works to your advantage, unless you deliberately put "not-me" tissue inside your body, as is the case with an organ transplant. Doctors will match the organ carefully, trying to ensure its compatibility. But even if the organ was donated by your brother or sister, your body will most likely recognize it as foreign and mount an attack (a process called rejection). You may suffer from fatigue, changes in blood pressure, fever, chills, and other problems as your body tries to destroy the transplanted organ.

Doctors have no way of informing your body that the new organ is acceptable. All they can do is use cyclosporine or other immunosuppressant drugs to squelch the immune system and make it difficult for your body to recognize it as "not-me." The downside of this is that you will become more vulnerable to a host of ailments, ranging from colds to cancer.

Its immune-suppressing properties also make cyclosporine useful in treating severe cases of rheumatoid arthritis, as well as psoriasis that has not been helped by other drugs.

Possible Side Effects

The drug's side effects include high blood pressure, headache, nausea, and excessive body hair.

Which Nutrients Are Robbed

Taking this medicine may deplete your supply of, increase your need for, or interfere with the activity of:

- Magnesium
- Potassium

Additional Ways This Drug May Upset Your Nutritional Balance

Cyclosporine can cause low blood sugar (hypoglycemia), changes in taste, nausea, and vomiting, which can upset your eating habits and possibly interfere with good nutrition. It can also cause diarrhea, which can hamper nutrient absorption.

In those taking it following a transplant, this drug can also trigger hyperkalemia, or too much potassium in the blood.

Restoring Your Nutritional Balance

To compensate for the nutrient loss caused by this drug, speak to your physician about taking 500–1,000 mg magnesium per day. And ask your physician to monitor your potassium status.

You can also eat foods that contain the depleted nutrient:

- Magnesium: Florida avocado, toasted wheat germ, almonds, shredded wheat cereal, pumpkin seeds

Consult with your physician before making any changes to your diet or supplemental regimen.

DACTINOMYCIN (dak-ti-noe-MYE-sin)

Brand Name: Cosmegen

About Dactinomycin

Children under the age of five are the typical targets of a kind of kidney cancer called Wilm's tumor. The first indication of the tumor might be a mass in the child's abdomen or symptoms such as pain in the abdomen, nausea, vomiting, poor appetite, or blood in the urine.

Fortunately, the disease can be cured in three-quarters or more of those who get it. (The survival rate depends on how far the cancer has spread before it's treated.) The afflicted kidney is surgically removed, then chemotherapy drugs are used to kill any remaining cancer cells.

Dactinomycin is an antibiotic used to combat Wilm's tumor and other forms of cancer. To imagine how it works, think of a developer building a tract of new houses. Before doing so, he must unroll the blueprints to figure out how many boards to cut, how many windows to make, and so on. If you prevent those blueprints from unrolling, no new houses can be built. Dactinomycin does something similar to cancer cells, binding to their coiled-up DNA strands and preventing them from unrolling. If the DNA coil can't unroll, it can't produce RNA and the proteins the cells need to stay alive and reproduce.

Possible Side Effects

The drug's more common side effects include unusual fatigue, severe nausea and vomiting, anemia, liver toxicity, fever, and hair loss.

Which Nutrients Are Robbed

Taking this medicine may deplete your supply of, increase your need for, or interfere with the activity of:

• Calcium

Additional Ways This Drug May Upset Your Nutritional Balance

Dactinomycin can cause nausea, vomiting, loss of appetite, abdominal pain, and altered taste, all of which can upset your eating habits and possibly interfere with good nutrition. It can also cause diarrhea, which can hamper nutrient absorption.

Restoring Your Nutritional Balance

To compensate for the nutrient loss caused by this drug, speak to your physician about taking 1,200 mg calcium per day.

You can also eat foods that contain the depleted nutrient:

• Calcium: milk, dried figs, Swiss cheese, yogurt, tofu

Consult with your physician before making any changes to your diet or supplemental regimen.

DEFEROXAMINE (de-fer-OKS-uh-meen)

Brand Name: Desferal

About Deferoxamine

Inside each red blood cell are a couple of hundred molecules of hemoglobin, an iron-protein compound that carries oxygen from the lungs to the cells and carbon dioxide back to the lungs for disposal. Most of the body's iron supply is found in hemoglobin. When a red blood cell dies, the iron is sent to the bone marrow for recycling, where it becomes part of newly formed red blood cells.

This is a good system for preserving iron, but unfortunately, we don't have an equally good system for getting rid of an iron buildup. Iron excess, which can stem from taking in too much iron (via supplements or other therapy), from a hereditary disorder called hemochromatosis, or from other problems, can cause nausea, vomiting, and damage to the intestines and coronary arteries.

While bloodletting is an old-fashioned way of getting rid of excess iron, deferoxamine offers a more modern approach. Injected into the body, it latches on to iron in the blood. The iron/deferoxamine complex is then plucked out of the blood by the kidneys and disposed of via the urine. (In the process, the drug may give the urine an orange-red tinge.)

Possible Side Effects

The drug's side effects include shock, low blood pressure, stomach upset, acute respiratory distress, fever, and dizziness.

Which Nutrients Are Robbed

Taking this medicine may deplete your supply of, increase your need for, or interfere with the activity of:

- Calcium

Additional Ways This Drug May Upset Your Nutritional Balance

Deferoxamine can cause diarrhea, which can hamper nutrient absorption.

Restoring Your Nutritional Balance

To compensate for the nutrient loss caused by this drug, speak to your physician about taking 1,200 mg calcium per day.

You can also eat foods that contain the depleted nutrient:

- Calcium: milk, dried figs, Swiss cheese, yogurt, tofu

Consult with your physician before making any changes to your diet or supplemental regimen.

DELAVIRDINE (de-luh-VIR-deen)

Brand Name: Rescriptor

About Delavirdine

Viruses don't attack body cells or tissues directly. Instead, they go through a complicated process designed to get you to do the dirty work and harm yourself.

But first, the virus must enter your body. Perhaps you inhale it, or it's passed to you when you touch an infected person and then touch your mouth or nose. Inside the body, the virus attaches itself to a likely cell, works its way through the cell's wall, and burrows inside. There it drops its outer coating to reveal its nucleic acids, and takes over and enslaves this captive cell. New virus parts are made within this hijacked cell and assembled into copies of the virus. These new viruses burst out of the original cell and go on the prowl themselves, looking for other cells to invade.

Delavirdine is used in combination with two or more other antiviral drugs to treat HIV-1 infection. It slows the progression of the virus by interfering with the manufacture of viral DNA inside the infected cells.

Possible Side Effects

The drug's more common side effects include rash, itching, headache, fatigue, nausea, vomiting, and diarrhea.

Which Nutrients Are Robbed

Taking this medicine may deplete your supply of, increase your need for, or interfere with the activity of:

- Vitamin B$_{12}$
- Zinc
- Copper
- Carnitine

Additional Ways This Drug May Upset Your Nutritional Balance

Delavirdine can cause nausea and vomiting, which can upset your eating habits and possibly interfere with good nutrition. It can also cause diarrhea, which can hamper nutrient absorption.

Restoring Your Nutritional Balance

To compensate for the nutrient loss caused by this drug, speak to your physician about taking 500–1,000 mcg vitamin B$_{12}$, 2 mcg copper, 50–200 mg zinc, and 250–1,000 mg carnitine per day.

You can also eat foods that contain the depleted nutrients:

- Vitamin B_{12}: beef liver, rainbow trout, sockeye salmon, beef, haddock
- Copper: beef liver, almonds, raw mushrooms, hazelnuts, lentils
- Zinc: oysters, beef shank, chicken, pork tenderloin, plain yogurt
- Carnitine: ground beef, pork, Canadian bacon, whole milk, cod

Consult with your physician before making any changes to your diet or supplemental regimen.

DEMECLOCYCLINE (dem-e-kloe-SYE-kleen)

Brand Name: Declomycin

About Demeclocycline

Your skin is a vital part of your body's defensive system. You can think of your skin as a fort, a tremendous physical barrier to infection. At the natural openings in the skin, such as the mouth, nose, and eyes, your body stations specialized immune system cells, which stand like guards. And when germs enter through an unnatural opening in the skin—a cut, scrape, or burn—your body rushes immune system cells to the area to do battle with the invaders.

Most of the time the body wins, and the battle is so quick and uneventful that you don't even know it has occurred. But occasionally the body has trouble fighting off an invader and may need help in the form of an antibiotic. Demeclocycline, a broad-spectrum antibiotic, is designed to combat a large number of bacteria by preventing them from manufacturing proteins.

Demeclocycline is used to treat acne, a respiratory disease called pertussis, urinary tract infections, gonorrhea, and other infections.

Possible Side Effects

The drug's more common side effects include sore mouth, sensitivity to light, nausea, and diarrhea.

Which Nutrients Are Robbed

Taking this medicine may deplete your supply of, increase your need for, or interfere with the activity of:

- Biotin
- Folic acid
- Inositol
- Thiamin
- Riboflavin
- Niacin
- Vitamin B$_6$
- Vitamin B$_{12}$

- Vitamin C
- Vitamin K
- Calcium
- Iron
- Magnesium
- Zinc
- *Bifidobacterium bifidum*
- *Lactobacillus acidophilus*

Additional Ways This Drug May Upset Your Nutritional Balance

Demeclocycline can cause nausea, which can upset your eating habits and possibly interfere with good nutrition. It can also cause diarrhea, which can hamper nutrient absorption.

Restoring Your Nutritional Balance

To compensate for the nutrient loss caused by this drug, speak to your physician about taking 500–1,000 mcg biotin, 400–800 mcg folic acid, 250–1,000 mg inositol, 25–100 mg thiamin, 25–100 mg riboflavin, 50–100 mg niacin, 50–100 mg vitamin B$_6$, 500–1,000 mcg vitamin B$_{12}$, 250–1,500 mg vitamin C, 60–80 mcg vitamin K, 1,200 mg calcium, 500–1,000 mg magnesium, 15 billion live *Bifidobacterium bifidum* organisms, and 15 billion live *Lactobacillus acidophilus* organisms per day. And ask your physician to consider the potential effects of iron and zinc depletion.

You can also eat foods that contain the depleted nutrients:

- Biotin: beef liver, soybeans, rice bran, peanut butter, barley
- Folic acid: beef liver, fortified breakfast cereals, spinach, great northern beans, asparagus
- Inositol: cantaloupe, oranges, green beans, grapefruit juice, limes
- Thiamin: braised liver, turkey heart, roasted chicken, gefilte fish, sardines
- Riboflavin: dried sunflower seeds, orange juice, bulgur, spinach noodles, pine nuts
- Niacin: chicken breast, beef liver, mackerel, barley, bulgur
- Vitamin B$_6$: potato, banana, garbanzo beans, chicken breast, fortified oatmeal
- Vitamin B$_{12}$: beef liver, rainbow trout, sockeye salmon, beef, haddock
- Vitamin C: papaya, guava, red pepper, cantaloupe, black currants
- Vitamin K: kale, broccoli, parsley, Swiss chard, spinach
- Calcium: milk, dried figs, Swiss cheese, yogurt, tofu
- Magnesium: Florida avocado, toasted wheat germ, almonds, shredded wheat cereal, pumpkin seeds

- *Bifidobacterium bifidum*: Jerusalem artichokes, asparagus, garlic, and onions may stimulate the growth or activity of this probiotic
- *Lactobacillus acidophilus*: yogurt containing live lactobacillus cultures, kefir, acidophilus milk

Consult with your physician before making any changes to your diet or supplemental regimen.

DENILEUKIN DIFTITOX (DEN-i-loo-kin DIFF-ti-toks)

Brand Name: ONTAK

About Denileukin Diftitox

Tunneling throughout your body is a system of tubes and gathering points, kind of like the subway tracks and subway stations that run throughout New York City. This is your lymph system, a collection of vessels, valves, ducts, and nodes that transports fluid and performs other functions. Certain white blood cells called lymphocytes inhabit the lymph system. These lymphocytes are like the subway police, always on the lookout for trouble—which, in the lymph system, can take the form of infections.

If the lymphocytes themselves become cancerous, the resulting disease is called lymphoma. These cancerous cells may remain in a lymph node or may spread to the bone marrow or almost any organ.

Depending on the type of lymphoma you have, you may notice a swelling in the lymph nodes under your arms, in your groin, or in your neck. If lymph nodes in the chest become enlarged, they may interfere with breathing and bring about a cough. If lymph nodes in the abdomen enlarge, they may press on nearby organs, causing pain, constipation, and other symptoms. If the bone marrow is attacked, the resulting destruction of immune-system cells may leave you open to recurring infections.

Denileukin diftitox is a high-tech drug that's used to treat a form of this disease called cutaneous T-cell lymphoma. It's actually a fusion protein that works like a smart bomb targeting cancer cells. It plugs into specific receptor sites on the cancer cells and delivers toxins that burrow inside the cells and prevent them from making their proteins, which results in their death.

Possible Side Effects

The drug's more common side effects include water retention, low blood pressure, nausea, vomiting, weakness, fever, chills, and allergic reactions.

Which Nutrients Are Robbed

Taking this medicine may deplete your supply of, increase your need for, or interfere with the activity of:

- Calcium
- Potassium

Additional Ways This Drug May Upset Your Nutritional Balance

Denileukin diftitox can cause loss of appetite, heartburn, bloating, nausea, and vomiting, all of which can upset your eating habits and possibly interfere with good nutrition. It can also cause diarrhea, which can hamper nutrient absorption.

Restoring Your Nutritional Balance

To compensate for the nutrient loss caused by this drug, speak to your physician about taking 1,200 mg calcium, and 100–300 mg potassium per day.

You can also eat foods that contain the depleted nutrients:

- Calcium: milk, dried figs, Swiss cheese, yogurt, tofu
- Potassium: dried figs, California avocado, papaya, banana, dates

Consult with your physician before making any changes to your diet or supplemental regimen.

DESIPRAMINE (des-IP-rah-meen)

Brand Names: Norpramin, Alti-Desipramine, Apo-Desipramine, Novo-Desipramine, Pertofrane, PMS-Desipramine

About Desipramine

Acute pain, the kind you get when you stub your toe or slice your finger, is fairly easy to handle. A variety of medicines, from aspirin to narcotics, can ease such pain for hours on end. And, assuming you can tolerate the side effects, you can keep using these painkillers until the source of your pain goes away.

Chronic pain, however, is a different story. As far as your doctor can tell, there's no underlying cause. Yet you're not crazy and you're not faking it; the pain is real. But why does it exist? And why do so many of us suffer? According to the American Pain Foundation, over 50 million Americans suffer from chronic pain.

While our standard painkillers aren't much help for chronic pain, desipramine may be. An antidepressant that's also used for ADHD (attention deficit hyperactivity disorder), desipramine has an unlabeled use as a treatment for chronic pain. (Although it hasn't been officially approved to treat chronic pain, doctors use it anyway because it seems to work.) The drug has several effects on the central nervous system and alters the concentrations of the brain chemicals serotonin and norepinephrine, but we don't know exactly how it quells chronic pain.

Possible Side Effects

The drug's side effects include dizziness, delirium, agitation, stomach upset, blurred vision, and excessive sweating.

Which Nutrients Are Robbed

Taking this medicine may deplete your supply of, increase your need for, or interfere with the activity of:

- Riboflavin
- Sodium
- Coenzyme Q_{10}

Additional Ways This Drug May Upset Your Nutritional Balance

Desipramine can cause nausea, an unpleasant taste, loss of appetite, and heartburn, all of which can upset your eating habits and possibly interfere with good nutrition. It can also cause diarrhea, which can hamper nutrient absorption.

Restoring Your Nutritional Balance

To compensate for the nutrient loss caused by this drug, speak to your physician about taking 25–100 mg riboflavin and 30–100 mg coenzyme Q_{10} per day. And ask your physician to consider the potential effects of sodium depletion.

You can also eat foods that contain the depleted nutrients:

- Riboflavin: dried sunflower seeds, orange juice, bulgur, spinach noodles, pine nuts
- Coenzyme Q_{10}: beef, chicken, trout, salmon, oranges, broccoli

Consult with your physician before making any changes to your diet or supplemental regimen.

DEXAMETHASONE (deks-uh-METH-uh-sohn)

Brand Names: Cortastat, Decadron, Decadron Phosphate, Dexamethasone Intensol, Dexasone, Diodex, Hexadrol Phosphate, Maxidex, Solurex

About Dexamethasone

Dexamethasone helps quell inflammation, which is why it's prescribed to treat several diseases involving inflammation. It's also used in cases of a little-known condition known as infantile spasms, or salaam seizures.

It's a very scary experience for parents to see their little one go from lying quietly on her back to throwing her upper body and neck forward and bending her arms at the elbows while thrusting her legs out straight. This involuntary movement is all over in a few seconds, although it may happen several times a day.

Infantile spasms usually strike during the first three years of life. Unfortunately, the problem doesn't end there, because most of these youngsters suffer from mental retardation and slow neurological development. And it's common for them to suffer from one seizure disorder or another later in life.

Dexamethasone is one of the drugs used to treat infantile spasms. Although it doesn't cure them and doesn't prevent problems later in life, it does help to control the spasms. Dexamethasone is also prescribed for septic shock, certain autoimmune diseases, allergies, and other ailments in which inflammation is a concern, and to help control nausea and vomiting.

Possible Side Effects

The drug's more common side effects include nervousness, insomnia, increased appetite, and indigestion.

Which Nutrients Are Robbed

Taking this medicine may deplete your supply of, increase your need for, or interfere with the activity of:

- Vitamin A
- Vitamin B_6
- Folic acid
- Vitamin C
- Vitamin D
- Vitamin K
- Calcium
- Magnesium
- Phosphorus
- Potassium
- Selenium
- Zinc

Additional Ways This Drug May Upset Your Nutritional Balance

Dexamethasone can cause indigestion, which can upset your eating habits and possibly interfere with good nutrition.

Restoring Your Nutritional Balance

To compensate for the nutrient loss caused by this drug, speak to your physician about taking 5,000 IU vitamin A, 50–100 mg vitamin B_6, 250–1,500 mg vitamin C, 400 IU vitamin D, 60–80 mcg vitamin K, 1,200 mg calcium, 500–1,000 mg magnesium, 700 mg phosphorus, 100–300 mg potassium, 20–100 mcg selenium, and 50–200 mg zinc per day.

Taking folic acid can increase the risk of seizures in some people, so discuss the use of this nutrient with your physician.

You can also eat foods that contain the depleted nutrients:

- Vitamin A: beef liver, chicken liver, cheese pizza, whole milk, cheddar cheese
- Vitamin B_6: potato, banana, garbanzo beans, chicken breast, fortified oatmeal
- Vitamin C: papaya, guava, red pepper, cantaloupe, black currants
- Vitamin D: salmon, mackerel, sardines, eel, fortified milk
- Vitamin K: kale, broccoli, parsley, Swiss chard, spinach
- Calcium: milk, dried figs, Swiss cheese, yogurt, tofu
- Magnesium: Florida avocado, toasted wheat germ, almonds, shredded wheat cereal, pumpkin seeds
- Phosphorus: plain nonfat yogurt, lentils, salmon, milk, halibut
- Potassium: dried figs, California avocado, papaya, banana, dates
- Selenium: Brazil nuts, tuna, beef liver, turkey breast, spaghetti with meat sauce
- Zinc: oysters, beef shank, chicken, pork tenderloin, plain yogurt

Consult with your physician before making any changes to your diet or supplemental regimen.

DICLOFENAC, DICLOFENAC PLUS MISOPROSTOL
(dye-KLOE-fen-ak, mye-soe-PROST-ole)

Brand Names: Diclofenac: Apo-Diclo, Cataflam, Novo-Difenac, Nu-Diclo, Solaraze, Voltaren, Voltaren Ophthalmic, Voltaren-XR
Diclofenac plus misoprostol: Arthrotec

About Diclofenac, Diclofenac plus Misoprostol

Diclofenac is an NSAID (nonsteroidal anti-inflammatory drug) and a cousin to ibuprofen and aspirin. Normally when we think of the NSAIDs, we think of popping a pill to relieve the pain or inflammation of arthritis or maybe menstrual cramps. Diclofenac is certainly helpful in those cases, and it also comes in a liquid form that can be used in the eyes following cataract removal.

Cataracts, which can cause blindness, are common in the United States, often appearing in people in their mid-60s to mid-70s. Caused by the clouding of the lens of the eye, they can lead to blurred vision, halos, difficulty reading, and even blindness. An injury to the eye can cause a cataract, as can corticosteroids and other drugs, X-rays, eye diseases, and diabetes. The cause of most cataracts, however, is unknown.

Fortunately, cataract surgery is fairly safe and successful. The usual approach is to cut into the eye, break up the cataract with ultrasound, remove the pieces, and replace the lens with an artificial one. If all goes well, your vision improves within a few weeks. During the immediate postsurgical period, you may be given a liquid form of diclofenac to put into your eyes to quell any inflammation.

The pill form of diclofenac, used to quell pain and inflammation, can cause ulcers and gastrointestinal bleeding. That's why diclofenac may be combined with misoprostol, a drug that protects the mucosal lining of the stomach from such damage.

Possible Side Effects

The drug's more common side effects include:

Eye drops: burning and tearing of the eyes
Topical gel: itching, rash, and dry skin
Oral: stomach upset, headache, dizziness

Which Nutrients Are Robbed

Taking this medicine may deplete your supply of, increase your need for, or interfere with the activity of:

- Folic acid

Additional Ways This Drug May Upset Your Nutritional Balance

Diclofenac can cause abdominal pain and cramps, indigestion, nausea, peptic ulcer, and gastrointestinal bleeding, all of which can upset your eating habits and possibly interfere with good nutrition. It can also cause diarrhea, which can hamper nutrient absorption.

Diclofenac plus misoprostol can cause diarrhea, which can hamper nutrient absorption.

Restoring Your Nutritional Balance

To compensate for the nutrient loss caused by this drug, speak to your physician about taking 400–800 mcg folic acid per day.

You can also eat foods that contain the depleted nutrient:

- Folic acid: beef liver, fortified breakfast cereals, spinach, great northern beans, asparagus

Consult with your physician before making any changes to your diet or supplemental regimen.

DICLOXACILLIN (dye-kloks-uh-SIL-in)

Brand Names: Dycill, Dynapen, Pathocil

About Dicloxacillin

Dicloxacillin is a jack-of-all-trades antibiotic that is used to treat ailments such as:

- Itching, discolored, crusty skin on the face and elsewhere (impetigo)
- Heat rash, or burning and itching skin (miliaria)
- Areas of redness and heat on the skin, with fever, chills, and general malaise (erysipelas)
- Painful inflammation of the hair follicles and adjacent areas (furunculosis)

- Nasal infection (nasal vestibulitis)
- Breast abscesses that develop during nursing
- Infections resulting from animal or human bites

Why this collection of apparently unrelated ailments? They all may be caused by staphylococci bacteria, which make enzymes that destroy many forms of penicillin. However, dicloxacillin is not affected by many of these enzymes and is thus an effective treatment for such infections.

Possible Side Effects

The drug's most common side effects include abdominal pain, nausea, and diarrhea.

Which Nutrients Are Robbed

Taking this medicine may deplete your supply of, increase your need for, or interfere with the activity of:

- Biotin
- Inositol
- Thiamin
- Riboflavin
- Niacin
- Vitamin B$_6$
- Vitamin B$_{12}$
- Vitamin K
- Potassium
- *Bifidobacterium bifidum*
- *Lactobacillus acidophilus*

Additional Ways This Drug May Upset Your Nutritional Balance

Dicloxacillin can cause vomiting, nausea, and abdominal pain, which can upset your eating habits and possibly interfere with good nutrition. It can also cause diarrhea, which can hamper nutrient absorption.

Restoring Your Nutritional Balance

To compensate for the nutrient loss caused by this drug, speak to your physician about taking 500–1,000 mcg biotin, 250–1,000 mg inositol, 25–100 mg thiamin, 25–100 mg riboflavin, 50–100 mg niacin, 50–100 mg vitamin B$_6$, 500–1,000 mcg vitamin B$_{12}$, 60–80 mcg vitamin K, 100–300 mg potassium, 15 billion live *Bifidobacterium bifidum* organisms, and 15 billion live *Lactobacillus acidophilus* organisms per day.

You can also eat foods that contain the depleted nutrients:

- Biotin: beef liver, soybeans, rice bran, peanut butter, barley
- Inositol: cantaloupe, oranges, green beans, grapefruit juice, limes

- Thiamin: braised liver, turkey heart, roasted chicken, gefilte fish, sardines
- Riboflavin: dried sunflower seeds, orange juice, bulgur, spinach noodles, pine nuts
- Niacin: chicken breast, beef liver, mackerel, barley, bulgur
- Vitamin B_6: potato, banana, garbanzo beans, chicken breast, fortified oatmeal
- Vitamin B_{12}: beef liver, rainbow trout, sockeye salmon, beef, haddock
- Vitamin K: kale, broccoli, parsley, Swiss chard, spinach
- Potassium: dried figs, California avocado, papaya, banana, dates
- *Bifidobacterium bifidum*: Jerusalem artichokes, asparagus, garlic, and onions may stimulate the growth or activity of this probiotic
- *Lactobacillus acidophilus*: yogurt containing live lactobacillus cultures, kefir, acidophilus milk

Consult with your physician before making any changes to your diet or supplemental regimen.

DIDANOSINE (dye-DAN-oh-seen)

Brand Names: Videx, Videx EC

About Didanosine

Kaposi's sarcoma is a cancer that takes hold in the blood vessels and spreads throughout the body. Its most prominent feature is colored, sometimes raised areas of skin. In the past, Kaposi's sarcoma was known for striking older Italian or Jewish men. It was relatively rare in the United States until the early 1980s, when it began cropping up with surprising frequency in younger men. Medical researchers soon realized that Kaposi's is a hallmark of acquired immunodeficiency disease (AIDS), the stealthy disease that steadily destroys the immune system, leaving its victims susceptible to diseases that were formerly confined to small numbers or small groups of people.

The "older" form of Kaposi's, the one that attacks seniors, can sometimes simply be monitored, or the afflicted tissue can be destroyed with X-rays, freezing, or electricity. But when Kaposi's strikes those with AIDS, it can be much more dangerous. First appearing as colored spots on the skin, it can spread to the lymph nodes and internal organs, causing bleeding and other problems.

There is no cure for AIDS-related Kaposi's. The best treatment is to attack the human immunodeficiency virus (HIV) that cripples the immune system and triggers AIDS. To do that, doctors turn to a variety of drugs, including didanosine, an antiretroviral agent designed to combat HIV, a retrovirus. (HIV is called a retrovirus because it stores its genetic information in the form of RNA, rather than as DNA.) The drug attacks the HIV after the virus has burrowed into the body's cells and is about to get the hijacked cells to churn out new copies of the virus.

Didanosine is always used in combination with other medicines to treat HIV infection.

Possible Side Effects

The drug's most common side effects include abdominal pain, diarrhea, and inflammation of the nerves in the hands and feet (peripheral neuropathy).

Which Nutrients Are Robbed

Taking this medicine may deplete your supply of, increase your need for, or interfere with the activity of:

- Vitamin B_{12}
- Zinc
- Copper
- Carnitine

Additional Ways This Drug May Upset Your Nutritional Balance

Didanosine can cause diarrhea, which can hamper nutrient absorption.

Restoring Your Nutritional Balance

To compensate for the nutrient loss caused by this drug, speak to your physician about taking 500–1,000 mcg vitamin B_{12}, 2 mcg copper, 50–200 mg zinc, and 250–1,000 mg carnitine per day.

You can also eat foods that contain the depleted nutrients:

- Vitamin B_{12}: beef liver, rainbow trout, sockeye salmon, beef, haddock
- Copper: beef liver, almonds, raw mushrooms, hazelnuts, lentils
- Zinc: oysters, beef shank, chicken, pork tenderloin, plain yogurt
- Carnitine: ground beef, pork, Canadian bacon, whole milk, cod

Consult with your physician before making any changes to your diet or supplemental regimen.

DIFLORASONE (dye-FLOR-uh-sohn)

Brand Names: Florone, Maxiflor, Psorcon

About Diflorasone

Lichen simplex chronicus and circumscribed neurodermatitis are two fancy names that essentially mean you've scratched an itch so much that you've made it a lot worse.

Perhaps you had a mosquito bite, or some chemical irritated your skin, and you began to scratch it. Whatever the cause of the initial itch, you've scratched it so much that the skin has thickened, causing more itching and scratching. This has begun a nasty cycle that leaves your skin in worse and worse shape, perhaps to the point of becoming leathery and brownish. The overly scratched itches commonly arise on the neck, forearms, inner elbows, wrists, thighs, back of the knees, lower legs, ankles, head, and the anal/rectal area.

The best way to solve the problem is to stop scratching, but that's not always as easy as it sounds. For some people, the solution may be diflorasone, a corticosteroid that helps ease itching.

Possible Side Effects

The drug's side effects include joint pain, a burning sensation, and dryness of the skin.

Which Nutrients Are Robbed

Taking this medicine may deplete your supply of, increase your need for, or interfere with the activity of:

- Folic acid
- Vitamin C
- Vitamin D
- Calcium
- Magnesium
- Potassium
- Selenium
- Zinc
- Melatonin

Restoring Your Nutritional Balance

To compensate for the nutrient loss caused by this drug, speak to your physician about taking 400–800 mcg folic acid, 250–1,500 mg vitamin C, 400 IU vitamin D, 1,200 mg calcium, 500–1,500 magnesium, 100–300 mg potassium, 20–100 mcg selenium, 50–200 mg zinc, and 1–3 mg melatonin per day.

You can also eat foods that contain the depleted nutrients:

- Folic acid: beef liver, fortified breakfast cereals, spinach, great northern beans, asparagus
- Vitamin C: papaya, guava, red pepper, cantaloupe, black currants
- Vitamin D: salmon, mackerel, sardines, eel, fortified milk
- Calcium: milk, dried figs, Swiss cheese, yogurt, tofu
- Magnesium: Florida avocado, toasted wheat germ, almonds, shredded wheat cereal, pumpkin seeds
- Potassium: dried figs, California avocado, papaya, banana, dates
- Selenium: Brazil nuts, tuna, beef liver, turkey breast, spaghetti with meat sauce
- Zinc: oysters, beef shank, chicken, pork tenderloin, plain yogurt

Consult with your physician before making any changes to your diet or supplemental regimen.

DIFLUNISAL (dye-FLOO-ni-sal)

Brand Names: Dolobid, Apo-Diflunisal, Novo-Diflunisal, Nu-Diflunisal

About Diflunisal

To those who suffer from it, acute pain is very simple. You stub your toe, cut yourself, or fall down, and it hurts. You pull a muscle at the gym or hold downward-facing dog position too long in yoga class, and it hurts. The source of the pain is completely obvious, and the pain eventually fades away.

But pain itself is a very complex phenomenon that is still not well understood. It begins with a stimulus, like stubbing your toe. Cell membranes in the area release substances that begin a rapid-fire biochemical cascade. Phospholipids give way to arachidonic acid and then to cyclooxygenase (COX). From COX we get the prostaglandins, thromboxane, and other substances that call white blood cells to the damaged area. These are early steps in the inflammation process, which can be painful in itself. And that's just one of the pathways to pain. There are others in play at the same time.

In some ways, it's good that pain is such a complex phenomenon. Because it is a multistep procedure, pain can be attacked by various medicines at many points along the way between burning your hand and still feeling the sting two days later.

Diflunisal, a chemical cousin of aspirin, attacks pain by interfering with the action of COX. The medicine is easily absorbed, begins easing pain within an hour, and lasts for a third to half a day.

Possible Side Effects

The drug's more common side effects include chest pain, irregular heartbeat, fluid retention, stomach upset, and vaginal bleeding.

Which Nutrients Are Robbed

Taking this medicine may deplete your supply of, increase your need for, or interfere with the activity of:

- Folic acid

Additional Ways This Drug May Upset Your Nutritional Balance

Diflunisal can cause abdominal cramps, bloating, indigestion, nausea, and vomiting, all of which can upset your eating habits and possibly interfere with good nutrition. It can also cause diarrhea, which can hamper nutrient absorption.

Restoring Your Nutritional Balance

To compensate for the nutrient loss caused by this drug, speak to your physician about taking 400–800 mcg folic acid per day.

You can also eat foods that contain the depleted nutrient:

- Folic acid: beef liver, fortified breakfast cereals, spinach, great northern beans, asparagus

Consult with your physician before making any changes to your diet or supplemental regimen.

DIGOXIN (di-JOKS-in)

Brand Names: Digitek, Lanoxicaps, Lanoxin

About Digoxin

If you've ever watched *ER* or another medical show on television, you've undoubtedly noticed a heart monitor hanging on the wall, tracing a squiggly line and beeping. You can follow the line as it moves across the monitor, bouncing up and down, creating hills and valleys, as it records the action of a patient's heart.

Normally, the line rises and falls in a very regular pattern as it moves across the screen. Often you can tell what's wrong with the heart by looking at changes in the pattern. With atrial fibrillation, for example, the two atria (the smaller of the heart's four chambers), begin to contract rapidly and randomly. This upsets the heart's electrical activity, and you can see on the monitor that the peaks in each pattern are now much taller, and they are not equidistant apart. Some are closer to each other, some farther. Atrial fibrillation may be caused by heart failure, problems with the heart valves, or other ailments.

With another kind of irregular heartbeat, called atrial flutter, very deep and thin valleys appear on the monitor, instead of the shallow, barely discernible valleys seen with a healthy heart. Atrial flutter may be triggered by heart failure, a blood clot in the lungs, and problems with the heart valves.

Digoxin is used to treat atrial fibrillation, atrial flutter, and other types of irregular heartbeat. It works by increasing the force with which the heart contracts, then increasing the amount of time the heart rests at critical junctures. It also makes it more difficult for the electrical impulse that commands the heart to beat to pass through certain areas of the heart. The net effect is a slower heart rate and a more normal heart rhythm.

Possible Side Effects

The drug's side effects include dizziness, mental disturbances, nausea, diarrhea, slow heartbeat, headache, and weakness.

Which Nutrients Are Robbed

Taking this medicine may deplete your supply of, increase your need for, or interfere with the activity of:

- Thiamin
- Calcium
- Magnesium
- Phosphorus
- Potassium

Additional Ways This Drug May Upset Your Nutritional Balance

Digoxin can cause nausea, vomiting, and abdominal pain, all of which can upset your eating habits and possibly interfere with good nutrition. It can also cause diarrhea, which can hamper nutrient absorption.

Restoring Your Nutritional Balance

To compensate for the nutrient loss caused by this drug, speak to your physician about taking 25–100 mg thiamin, 1,200 mg calcium, 500–1,000 mg magnesium, and 700 mg phosphorus per day. And ask your physician to consider the potential effects of potassium depletion.

You can also eat foods that contain the depleted nutrients:

- Thiamin: braised liver, turkey heart, roasted chicken, gefilte fish, sardines
- Calcium: milk, dried figs, Swiss cheese, yogurt, tofu
- Magnesium: Florida avocado, toasted wheat germ, almonds, shredded wheat cereal, pumpkin seeds
- Phosphorus: plain nonfat yogurt, lentils, salmon, milk, halibut

Consult with your physician before making any changes to your diet or supplemental regimen.

DIGOXIN IMMUNE FAB (di-JOKS-in i-MYOON fab)

Brand Names: Digibind, Digi-Fab

About Digoxin Immune Fab

Digoxin immune fab is an antidote used for serious overdoses of digoxin. It works by binding to digoxin in your body, preventing the medicine from triggering dangerous changes in your heart's action.

Possible Side Effects

The drug's side effects include the reappearance of irregular heartbeat and chronic heart failure (symptoms that were controlled by digoxin), low blood levels of potassium, and allergic reactions.

Which Nutrients Are Robbed

Taking this medicine may deplete your supply of, increase your need for, or interfere with the activity of:

- Potassium

Restoring Your Nutritional Balance

To compensate for the nutrient loss caused by this drug, speak to your physician about taking 100–300 mg potassium per day.

You can also eat foods that contain the depleted nutrient:

• Potassium: dried figs, California avocado, papaya, banana, dates

Consult with your physician before making any changes to your diet or supplemental regimen.

DIRITHROMYCIN (dye-RITH-roe-mye-sin)

Brand Name: Dynabac

About Dirithromycin

If your pharynx, otherwise known as your throat, is attacked by streptococci bacteria, you'll have what's commonly called strep throat. (Doctors refer to it as streptococcal pharyngitis.) The disease tends to hit fast, causing soreness and tenderness, pain when swallowing, and a generally "blah" feeling. The throat, tonsils, and soft palate are red and swollen. Various complications can arise, including infections of the sinuses and ears, and rheumatic fever.

Dirithromycin is one of the drugs that's been approved to treat streptococcal pharyngitis. (Actually, its main purpose is to prevent the complications of strep throat.) The drug works by preventing bacteria from manufacturing certain proteins.

Possible Side Effects

The drug's side effects include headache, skin rash, difficulty swallowing, and wheezing.

Which Nutrients Are Robbed

Taking this medicine may deplete your supply of, increase your need for, or interfere with the activity of:

• Biotin
• Inositol
• Thiamin

• Vitamin B_6
• Vitamin B_{12}
• Vitamin K

- Riboflavin
- Niacin

- *Bifidobacterium bifidum*
- *Lactobacillus acidophilus*

Additional Ways This Drug May Upset Your Nutritional Balance

Dirithromycin can cause stomach cramps, upset stomach, and vomiting, all of which can upset your eating habits and possibly interfere with good nutrition. It can also cause diarrhea, which can hamper nutrient absorption.

Restoring Your Nutritional Balance

To compensate for the nutrient loss caused by this drug, speak to your physician about taking 500–1000 mcg biotin, 250–1,000 mg inositol, 25–100 mg thiamin, 25–100 mg riboflavin, 50–100 mg niacin, 50–100 mg vitamin B_6, 500–1,000 mcg vitamin B_{12}, 60–80 mcg vitamin K, 15 billion live *Bifidobacterium bifidum* organisms, and 15 billion live *Lactobacillus acidophilus* organisms per day. You can also eat foods that contain the depleted nutrients:

- Biotin: beef liver, soybeans, rice bran, peanut butter, barley
- Inositol: cantaloupe, oranges, green beans, grapefruit juice, limes
- Thiamin: braised liver, turkey heart, roasted chicken, gefilte fish, sardines
- Riboflavin: dried sunflower seeds, orange juice, bulgur, spinach noodles, pine nuts
- Niacin: chicken breast, beef liver, mackerel, barley, bulgur
- Vitamin B_6: potato, banana, garbanzo beans, chicken breast, fortified oatmeal
- Vitamin B_{12}: beef liver, rainbow trout, sockeye salmon, beef, haddock
- Vitamin K: kale, broccoli, parsley, Swiss chard, spinach
- *Bifidobacterium bifidum*: Jerusalem artichokes, asparagus, garlic, and onions may stimulate the growth or activity of this probiotic
- *Lactobacillus acidophilus*: yogurt containing live acidophilus cultures, kefir, acidophilus milk

Consult with your physician before making any changes to your diet or supplemental regimen.

DISOPYRAMIDE (dye-soe-PEER-uh-mide)

Brand Names: Norpace, Norpace CR, Rythmodan, Rythmodan-LA

About Disopyramide

Cardiac arrhythmias can take the form of the heart beating too fast, too slow, or irregularly—like singing a song in fits and starts, running some notes together and holding others for too long.

Some people think of the heartbeat as a single thing; that is, that the entire heart contracts at once to push the blood through the arteries. But actually the heart is made up of four separate chambers that must contract in a certain rhythm to produce a single heartbeat. If any part of the process goes wrong, the heart can get into trouble.

In a condition called *atrial fibrillation*, the two chambers called the atria in the top part of the heart beat randomly and too rapidly. This throws the ventricles, the two chambers at the bottom of the heart, out of sync. It's as if the tuba players in an orchestra are keeping one beat, while the violinists keep another. Obviously, you can't make music that way.

Disopyramide is used to treat several types of irregular heartbeat, including atrial fibrillation.

Possible Side Effects

The drug's more common side effects include dry mouth, blurred vision, constipation, and urinary hesitancy.

Which Nutrients Are Robbed

Taking this medicine may deplete your supply of, increase your need for, or interfere with the activity of:

- Potassium

Additional Ways This Drug May Upset Your Nutritional Balance

Disopyramide can cause abdominal bloating, loss of appetite, nausea, and vomiting, all of which can upset your eating habits and possibly interfere with good nutrition. It can also cause diarrhea, which can hamper nutrient absorption.

Restoring Your Nutritional Balance

To compensate for the nutrient loss caused by this drug, speak to your physician about taking 100–300 mg potassium per day.

You can also eat foods that contain the depleted nutrient:

- Potassium: dried figs, California avocado, papaya, banana, dates

Consult with your physician before making any changes to your diet or supplemental regimen.

DOXEPIN (DOKS-e-pin)

Brand Names: Adapin, Alti-Doxepin, Apo-Doxepin, Novo-Doxepin, Prudoxin, Sinequan, Triadapin, Zonalon

About Doxepin

Many drugs have more than one use, but doxepin's dual actions are particularly impressive because they are so different.

Taken in pill form, it's an antidepressant that works by preventing the reabsorption of serotonin in the nervous system. Serotonin is a neurotransmitter—a chemical messenger—that carries a "things-are-good" message throughout the nervous system. The body continually manufactures and breaks down this neurotransmitter, but sometimes the body breaks down more than it makes, resulting in low levels of serotonin, which is believed to be a major cause of depression. Most antidepressants are designed to pump up the serotonin supply by either increasing the amount that's manufactured or delaying its breakdown.

Doxepin works in the second way, by inhibiting the normal breakdown of serotonin to ensure that there will be enough of this neurotransmitter available to keep sending the "things-are-good" message.

Doxepin is also used in cream form to relieve the itching in some forms of dermatitis.

Possible Side Effects

The drug's side effects include drowsiness, low blood pressure, stomach upset, blurred vision, and ringing in the ears.

Which Nutrients Are Robbed

Taking this medicine may deplete your supply of, increase your need for, or interfere with the activity of:

- Riboflavin   • Coenzyme Q_{10}
- Sodium

Additional Ways This Drug May Upset Your Nutritional Balance

Doxepin can cause vomiting, indigestion, loss of appetite, nausea, an unpleasant taste, and heartburn, all of which can upset your eating habits and possibly interfere with good nutrition. It can also cause diarrhea, which can hamper nutrient absorption.

Restoring Your Nutritional Balance

To compensate for the nutrient loss caused by this drug, speak to your physician about taking 25–100 mg riboflavin and 30–100 mg coenzyme Q_{10} per day. And ask your physician to consider the potential effects of sodium depletion.

You can also eat foods that contain the depleted nutrients:

- Riboflavin: dried sunflower seeds, orange juice, bulgur, spinach noodles, pine nuts
- Coenzyme Q_{10}: beef, chicken, trout, salmon, oranges, broccoli

Consult with your physician before making any changes to your diet or supplemental regimen.

DOXORUBICIN, DOXORUBICIN LIPOSOMAL (doks-oh-ROO-bi-sin, lip-uh-SOE-mal)

Brand Names: Doxorubicin: Adriamycin, Adriamycin PFS, Adriamycin RDF, Caelyx, Rubex
Doxorubicin Liposomal: Doxil

About Doxorubicin

A special kind of cloning routinely carried out in your body helps to keep you healthy. In your bone marrow, lymph nodes, and elsewhere, plasma cells produce antibodies designed to fight off specific invading organisms. Each plasma cell reproduces itself many times to form what's known as a clone, with all the cells in the clone manufacturing copies of that one antibody. There are thousands of different clones in your body, each churning out one particular antibody.

Sometimes, for reasons we don't necessarily understand, the cells in a particular clone go on a birthing spree, reproducing themselves wildly. With a form of cancer called multiple myeloma, the irresponsible clone multiplies to such an extent that it starts to crowd out other blood cells growing in the bone marrow. It manufactures proteins to suppress the growth of the red blood cells, white blood cells, and platelets needed to maintain good health. Not only that, the errant clone produces vast amounts of its own antibody, leaving less raw material available for other clones to make other antibodies. That's kind of like a crazy weapons supplier to the U.S. Army making billions of rifles, but no bazookas and no bayonets.

Many times, cells from the errant clone will move to other parts of the body, settle in, and continue multiplying rapidly, developing into tumors that can damage the surrounding tissue. The upshot of all of this can be anemia, fatigue, weakness, heart problems, fever, chills, one infection after another, kidney damage, loss of bone density, and other problems.

Medical scientists have not yet developed a cure for multiple myeloma, although we do have drugs that slow the disease progression and reduce its symptoms. One of the drugs used is doxorubicin. In advanced cases of multiple myeloma, doxorubicin in combination with other drugs helps some 75 percent of patients, relieving their symptoms significantly and prolonging their lives.

Doxorubicin is also used to treat cancer of the lungs, breast, stomach, pancreas, liver, prostate, and other parts of the body. It works by preventing the synthesis of DNA and RNA inside cancerous and other rapidly growing cells. It's also used to treat the Kaposi's sarcoma seen in acquired immunodeficiency disease (AIDS).

Possible Side Effects

The drug's more common side effects include heart abnormalities, hair loss, severe nausea and vomiting, decreased white blood cells, and anemia.

Which Nutrients Are Robbed

Taking this medicine may deplete your supply of, increase your need for, or interfere with the activity of:

- Riboflavin
- Carnitine

Additional Ways This Drug May Upset Your Nutritional Balance

Doxorubicin can cause loss of appetite, nausea, and vomiting, while doxorubicin liposomal can cause nausea and vomiting. These side effects can upset your eating habits and possibly interfere with good nutrition.

Doxorubicin can also cause diarrhea, which can hamper nutrient absorption.

Doxorubicin liposomal can cause nausea and vomiting, which can upset your eating habits and possibly interfere with good nutrition.

Restoring Your Nutritional Balance

To compensate for the nutrient loss caused by this drug, speak to your physician about taking 25–100 mg riboflavin and 250–1,000 mg carnitine per day.

You can also eat foods that contain the depleted nutrients:

- Riboflavin: dried sunflower seeds, orange juice, bulgur, spinach noodles, pine nuts
- Carnitine: ground beef, pork, Canadian bacon, whole milk, cod

Consult with your physician before making any changes to your diet or supplemental regimen.

DOXYCYCLINE (doks-i-SYE-kleen)

Brand Names: Adoxa, Apo-Doxy, Doryx, Doxycin, Doxy-100, Monodox, Vibramycin, Vibra-Tabs

About Doxycycline

Doxycycline is a member of the tetracycline group of drugs, which are broad-spectrum antibiotics effective against a wide variety of bacteria. They work by preventing the bacteria from manufacturing proteins and reproducing themselves. In a sense, doxycycline and the other tetracyclines prevent the bacterial troops from being reinforced, making it easier for the immune system to destroy those that already exist. (In technical terms, doxycycline is *bacteriostatic,* which means it prevents bacteria from replicating, rather than *bactericidal,* which would mean that it kills them.)

Doxycycline is used to treat mycoplasmal pneumonia, which triggers a form of pneumonia that can begin by mimicking the flu, with a mild cough, sore throat, and fatigue. The symptoms can progress to anemia, joint pain, rash, and a severe cough. After a week or two, symptoms usually begin to subside, and those who are otherwise healthy can often recover without treatment.

When treatment is appropriate, doxycycline may be used. The antibiotic doesn't immediately cure the pneumonia, but it does shorten the duration of the symptoms and promote healing. Doxycycline is used to treat a number of other ailments, including syphilis.

Possible Side Effects

The drug's side effects include sensitivity to light, loss of appetite, diarrhea, anemia, and worsening of existing lupus.

Which Nutrients Are Robbed

Taking this medicine may deplete your supply of, increase your need for, or interfere with the activity of:

- Biotin
- Folic acid
- Inositol
- Thiamin
- Riboflavin
- Niacin
- Vitamin B_6
- Vitamin B_{12}
- Vitamin C
- Vitamin K
- Calcium
- Iron
- Magnesium
- Zinc
- *Bifidobacterium bifidum*
- *Lactobacillus acidophilus*

Additional Ways This Drug May Upset Your Nutritional Balance

Doxycycline can cause loss of appetite, heartburn, bloating, and nausea, which can upset your eating habits and possibly interfere with good nutrition. It can also cause diarrhea, which can hamper nutrient absorption.

Restoring Your Nutritional Balance

To compensate for the nutrient loss caused by this drug, speak to your physician about taking 500–1,000 mcg biotin, 400–800 mcg folic acid, 250–1,000 mg inositol, 25–100 mg thiamin, 25–100 mg riboflavin, 50–100 mg niacin, 50–100 mg vitamin B_6, 500–1,000 mcg vitamin B_{12}, 250–1,500 mg vitamin C, 60–80 mcg vitamin K, 1,200 mg calcium, 500–1,000 mg magnesium, 15 billion live *Bifidobacterium bifidum* organisms, and 15 billion live *Lactobacillus acidophilus* organisms per day. And ask your physician to consider the potential effects of iron depletion, as well as the effects of zinc and doxycycline on each other.

You can also eat foods that contain the depleted nutrients:

- Biotin: beef liver, soybeans, rice bran, peanut butter, barley
- Folic acid: beef liver, fortified breakfast cereals, spinach, great northern beans, asparagus

- Inositol: cantaloupe, oranges, green beans, grapefruit juice, limes
- Thiamin: braised liver, turkey heart, roasted chicken, gefilte fish, sardines
- Riboflavin: dried sunflower seeds, orange juice, bulgur, spinach noodles, pine nuts
- Niacin: chicken breast, beef liver, mackerel, barley, bulgur
- Vitamin B_6: potato, banana, garbanzo beans, chicken breast, fortified oatmeal
- Vitamin B_{12}: beef liver, rainbow trout, sockeye salmon, beef, haddock
- Vitamin C: papaya, guava, red pepper, cantaloupe, black currants
- Vitamin K: kale, broccoli, parsley, Swiss chard, spinach
- Calcium: milk, dried figs, Swiss cheese, yogurt, tofu
- Magnesium: Florida avocado, toasted wheat germ, almonds, shredded wheat cereal, pumpkin seeds
- *Bifidobacterium bifidum*: Jerusalem artichokes, asparagus, garlic, and onions may stimulate the growth or activity of this probiotic
- *Lactobacillus acidophilus*: yogurt containing live lactobacillus cultures, kefir, acidophilus milk

Consult with your physician before making any changes to your diet or supplemental regimen.

ENALAPRIL, ENALAPRIL PLUS FELODIPINE, ENALAPRIL PLUS HYDROCHLOROTHIAZIDE (e-NAL-uh-pril, fe-LOE-di-peen, hye-droe-klor-oh-THYE-uh-zide)

Brand Names: Enalapril: Vasotec, Vasotec I.V.
Enalapril plus felodipine: Lexxel
Enalapril plus hydrochlorothiazide: Vaseretic

About Enalapril, Enalapril plus Felodipine, Enalapril plus Hydrochlorothiazide

Heart failure is a very serious condition. Simply put, it means that your heart can't do its job well anymore; it cannot pump enough blood to satisfy your body's demand for oxygen and nutrients. As your heart begins to fail, you can suffer from swelling of the ankles, a backup of fluid into your lungs, and shortness of breath.

This potentially fatal condition can be caused by elevated blood pressure, coronary artery disease, infection of the heart muscle, diabetes, kidney failure, problems with the heart valves, an overactive thyroid gland, or other problems. According to a study that appeared in the American Heart Association's journal, *Circulation*, people over the age of 40 have a 1 in 5 chance of developing heart failure.[1]

Many types of drugs are used to treat heart failure, including enalapril, which works by allowing the blood vessels to open wider, thereby reducing the heart's workload. (When the blood vessels are fully open, the heart doesn't have to work as hard to pump the blood through these passageways.) Enalapril also helps to rid the body of excess sodium and water, which means that there's less blood volume, or less fluid, for the tired heart to push through the body.

Thanks to these and other actions, enalapril is used to treat heart failure, elevated blood pressure, and problems with the heart's left ventricle after a heart attack.

You can take enalapril on its own or in combination with a calcium channel blocker called felodipine. Calcium channel blockers help lower blood pressure by depriving the muscles surrounding the blood vessels of calcium, which they need in order to contract. With less calcium present, they are more likely to remain relaxed and open, allowing blood to flow through them more easily. This opening-wide action reduces resistance to the flow of blood, which lowers blood pressure.

Enalapril may also be combined with the diuretic called hydrochlorothiazide. (See page 304 for more on hydrochlorothiazide.)

Possible Side Effects

Enalapril's more common side effects include headache, fainting, low blood pressure, stomach upset, weakness, and allergic reactions. Felodipine's more common side effects include headache, rapid heartbeat, and flushing. Hydrochlorothiazide's more common side effects include low blood pressure and skin sensitivity to light.

Which Nutrients Are Robbed

Taking enalapril or enalapril plus felodipine may deplete your supply of, increase your need for, or interfere with the activity of:

- Zinc

Taking enalapril plus hydrochlorothiazide may deplete your supply of, increase your need for, or interfere with the activity of:

- Vitamin B_6
- Sodium
- Magnesium
- Zinc

- Phosphorus   • Coenzyme Q_{10}
- Potassium

Additional Ways These Drugs May Upset Your Nutritional Balance

Enalapril can cause changes in taste, abdominal pain, nausea, vomiting, and loss of appetite; and hydrochlorothiazide can trigger loss of appetite. These side effects can upset your eating habits and possibly interfere with good nutrition. Enalapril can also cause diarrhea, which can hamper nutrient absorption, and trigger hyperkalemia, or too much potassium in the blood. This is more liked to happen in people who are taking nonsteroidal anti-inflammatory drugs (NSAIDs) or who have renal insufficiency, a kidney problem.

Restoring Your Nutritional Balance

To compensate for the nutrient loss caused by enalapril or enalapril plus felodipine, speak to your physician about taking 50–200 mg zinc per day.

You can also eat foods that contain the depleted nutrient:

- Zinc: oysters, beef shank, chicken, pork tenderloin, plain yogurt

To compensate for the nutrient loss caused by enalapril plus hydrochlorothiazide, speak to your physician about taking 50–100 mg vitamin B_6, 500–1,000 mg magnesium, 700 mg phosphorus, 50–200 mg zinc, and 30–100 mg coenzyme Q_{10} per day. And ask your physician to consider the potential effects of sodium depletion.

A Note on Potassium: "Regular" diuretics lower potassium levels, while potassium-sparing diuretics do not—they may increase levels instead. It is not uncommon for doctors to prescribe two different diuretics. That's why you should speak to your physician about your potassium levels, and whether it is appropriate for you to take supplements or eat potassium-rich foods.

You can also eat foods that contain the depleted nutrients:

- Vitamin B_6: potato, banana, garbanzo beans, chicken breast, fortified oatmeal
- Magnesium: Florida avocado, toasted wheat germ, almonds, shredded wheat cereal, pumpkin seeds
- Phosphorus: plain nonfat yogurt, lentils, salmon, milk, halibut
- Zinc: oysters, beef shank, chicken, pork tenderloin, plain yogurt
- Coenzyme Q_{10}: beef, chicken, trout, salmon, oranges, broccoli

Consult with your physician before making any changes to your diet or supplemental regimen.

ENOXACIN (en-OKS-uh-sin)

Brand Name: Penetrex

About Enoxacin

DNA is the blueprint for life, a set of detailed instructions for the construction of every single organ, tissue, cell, protein, and enzyme in your body. The DNA "blueprint" must be read continually if the cells are to reproduce themselves correctly. Bacteria also have DNA blueprints that they must read to make proteins, enzymes, and the countless other substances that they need to stay alive.

Interfering with the reading of the DNA blueprints is one of the pharmacological strategies for slaying bacteria. DNA is wrapped up in a tight coil, and before a portion of it can be read, it must relax and uncoil. Enoxacin, a member of the fluoroquinolone group of antibiotics, prevents this from happening. Unable to read its DNA instructions, the bacteria cannot make new proteins and other substances, so they die. Enoxacin is useful in treating a variety of bacterial infections.

Possible Side Effects

The drug's side effects include nausea, vomiting, dizziness, insomnia, and headache.

Which Nutrients Are Robbed

Taking this medicine may deplete your supply of, increase your need for, or interfere with the activity of:

- Vitamin B_6
- Zinc
- Magnesium
- Coenzyme Q_{10}
- Potassium

Additional Ways This Drug May Upset Your Nutritional Balance

Enoxacin can cause abdominal pain, changes in taste, nausea, and vomiting, which can upset your eating habits and possibly interfere with good nutrition. It can also cause diarrhea, which can hamper nutrient absorption.

Restoring Your Nutritional Balance

To compensate for the nutrient loss caused by this drug, speak to your physician about taking 50–100 mg vitamin B_6, 500–1,000 mg magnesium, 100–300 mg potassium, 50–200 mg zinc, and 30–100 mg coenzyme Q_{10} per day.

You can also eat foods that contain the depleted nutrients:

- Vitamin B$_6$: potato, banana, garbanzo beans, chicken breast, fortified oatmeal
- Magnesium: Florida avocado, toasted wheat germ, almonds, shredded wheat cereal, pumpkin seeds
- Potassium: dried figs, California avocado, papaya, banana, dates
- Zinc: oysters, beef shank, chicken, pork tenderloin, plain yogurt
- Coenzyme Q$_{10}$: beef, chicken, trout, salmon, oranges, broccoli

Consult with your physician before making any changes to your diet or supplemental regimen.

EPOPROSTENOL (e-poe-PROST-en-ole)

Brand Name: Flolan

About Epoprostenol

After the blood has delivered oxygen to the cells and collected waste products (carbon dioxide), it's returned to the right side of the heart. From there it's pumped into the lungs, where it exchanges the carbon dioxide for another load of fresh oxygen. Then it's returned to the left side of the heart and pumped throughout the body.

Normally, blood pressure is about 120/80. The pressure is lower in the arteries in the lungs (pulmonary arteries), averaging about 25/15. That's because it doesn't take much pressure to move the blood the short distance from the heart to the lungs and back again.

When blood pressure rises to an abnormal level in the lungs (a condition called pulmonary hypertension), the walls of the pulmonary arteries become damaged and thickened, which hinders the exchange of carbon dioxide and oxygen. Your bone marrow may try to compensate for the lack of oxygen in the blood by producing more red blood cells, but this only makes the blood thicker and harder for the heart to pump. Then the right side of your heart must work harder to keep the blood flowing to the lungs and back. Eventually this extra workload causes the heart to enlarge and thicken, and possibly fail.

If you have pulmonary hypertension, you're most likely short of breath. You may feel generally weak because you're not able to get enough oxygen into your red blood cells. Your chest may hurt and you might feel light-headed when you exert yourself.

Epoprostenol is one of the treatments for pulmonary hypertension. This drug is a powerful vasodilator, which means it relaxes the muscles in the blood vessel walls. This allows the blood vessels to open wider, lowering their resistance to the flow of blood. The heart is then able to do its job without exerting as much force, and blood pressure falls. Epoprostenol also helps thin the blood by keeping the platelets from clumping together.

Possible Side Effects

The drug's more common side effects include flushing, rapid heartbeat, fever, chills, tremor, stomach upset, and heart failure.

Which Nutrients Are Robbed

Taking this medicine may deplete your supply of, increase your need for, or interfere with the activity of:

- Potassium

Additional Ways This Drug May Upset Your Nutritional Balance

Epoprostenol can cause loss of appetite, abdominal pain, nausea, and vomiting, all of which can upset your eating habits and possibly interfere with good nutrition. It can also cause diarrhea, which can hamper nutrient absorption.

Restoring Your Nutritional Balance

To compensate for the nutrient loss caused by this drug, speak to your physician about taking 100–300 mg potassium per day.

You can also eat foods that contain the depleted nutrient:

- Potassium: dried figs, California avocado, papaya, banana, dates

Consult with your physician before making any changes to your diet or supplemental regimen.

ERYTHROMYCIN (e-rith-roe-MYE-sin)

Brand Names: Apo-Erythro E-C, Diomycin, E-mycin, EryPed, Ery-Tab, Erythrocin, Romycin, Staticin, Theramycin Z

About Erythromycin

In 1976, the country was thrown into a panic when a new disease seemed to spread like wildfire among people attending an American Legion convention in Philadelphia. It was dubbed Legionnaires' disease, and the bacterium responsible was named *Legionella pneumophilia.*

Legionnaires' disease can begin with a cough and fever, and perhaps muscle aches, fatigue, or a headache. A chest X-ray may show pneumonia (infection or inflammation of the lungs, in which the air sacs fill with pus and other liquid), and other tests may show that the kidneys are not working well.

Today we know that the disease strikes in two forms: the more severe Legionnaires' disease, which is accompanied by pneumonia, and the milder Pontiac fever. Between 8,000 and 18,000 people contract Legionnaires' disease every year—and of those, 5 to 30 percent die, making it crucial to diagnose and treat this disease as soon as possible. Anyone can get Legionnaires' disease, although it typically strikes middle age or older people.

According to the Centers for Disease Control, erythromycin is the antibiotic currently recommended for treating Legionnaires' disease. It's also used to treat a variety of bacterial infections, including those that cause pneumonia, diphtheria, inflammation of the urethra, and syphilis.

Possible Side Effects

The drug's more common side effects include abdominal pain, nausea, diarrhea, headache, rash, and cough.

Which Nutrients Are Robbed

Taking this medicine may deplete your supply of, increase your need for, or interfere with the activity of:

- Biotin
- Folic acid
- Inositol
- Thiamin
- Riboflavin
- Niacin
- Vitamin B_6
- Vitamin B_{12}
- Vitamin K
- *Bifidobacterium bifidum*
- *Lactobacillus acidophilus*

Additional Ways This Drug May Upset Your Nutritional Balance

Erythromycin can cause abdominal pain, nausea, vomiting, heartburn, bloating, and loss of appetite, all of which can upset your eating habits and possibly interfere with good nutrition. It can also cause diarrhea, which can hamper nutrient absorption.

Restoring Your Nutritional Balance

To compensate for the nutrient loss caused by this drug, speak to your physician about taking 500–1,000 mcg biotin, 400–800 mg folic acid, 250–1,000 mg inositol, 25–100 mg thiamin, 25–100 mg riboflavin, 50–100 mg niacin, 50–100 mg vitamin B_6, 500–1,000 mcg vitamin B_{12}, 60–80 mcg vitamin K, 15 billion live *Bifidobacterium bifidum* organisms, and 15 billion live *Lactobacillus acidophilus* organisms per day.

You can also eat foods that contain the depleted nutrients:

- Biotin: beef liver, soybeans, rice bran, peanut butter, barley
- Folic acid: beef liver, fortified breakfast cereals, spinach, great northern beans, asparagus
- Inositol: cantaloupe, oranges, green beans, grapefruit juice, limes
- Thiamin: braised liver, turkey heart, roasted chicken, gefilte fish, sardines
- Riboflavin: dried sunflower seeds, orange juice, bulgur, spinach noodles, pine nuts
- Niacin: chicken breast, beef liver, mackerel, barley, bulgur
- Vitamin B_6: potato, banana, garbanzo beans, chicken breast, fortified oatmeal
- Vitamin B_{12}: beef liver, rainbow trout, sockeye salmon, beef, haddock
- Vitamin K: kale, broccoli, parsley, Swiss chard, spinach
- *Bifidobacterium bifidum*: Jerusalem artichokes, asparagus, garlic, and onions may stimulate the growth or activity of this probiotic
- *Lactobacillus acidophilus*: yogurt containing live lactobacillus cultures, kefir, acidophilus milk

Consult with your physician before making any changes to your diet or supplemental regimen.

ESMOLOL (ES-moe-lol)

Brand Name: Brevibloc

About Esmolol

Esmolol is a very short-acting drug with a half-life of only about 10 minutes. This means that 10 minutes after it's been administered, half of it has been "deactivated" by the body and no longer has medicinal effects.

Esmolol helps to prevent irregular heartbeat and keeps blood pressure under control. But, you may be wondering, what's the point of a drug that's half used up in just 10 minutes? Wouldn't you want something that lasts for several hours or a whole day?

Short-acting drugs like esmolol come in handy when it's too dangerous to use the long-acting versions. For example, during surgery doctors may want to ensure that a critically ill patient's heart doesn't start racing. They could give the patient a long-acting, powerful medication, but it would keep working long after the surgery was completed and could send the patient into crisis mode. Instead, they give a continuous intravenous infusion of the short-lived esmolol, which protects the heart but is quickly cleared from the body once the infusion is stopped.

In short, esmolol is a carefully targeted dose of medicine that leaves the body as soon as it's no longer needed—but even brief exposure to this drug can rob you of nutrients.

Possible Side Effects

The drug's more common side effects include low blood pressure, profuse sweating, stomach upset, dizziness, excessive sleepiness, confusion, and headache.

Which Nutrients Are Robbed

Taking this medicine may deplete your supply of, increase your need for, or interfere with the activity of:

- Coenzyme Q_{10}
- Melatonin

Additional Ways This Drug May Upset Your Nutritional Balance

Esmolol can cause nausea and vomiting, which can upset your eating habits and possibly interfere with good nutrition.

Restoring Your Nutritional Balance

To compensate for the nutrient loss caused by this drug, speak to your physician about taking 30–100 mg coenzyme Q_{10} and 1–3 mg melatonin per day.

You can also eat foods that contain the depleted nutrient:

- Coenzyme Q_{10}: beef, chicken, trout, salmon, oranges, broccoli

Consult with your physician before making any changes to your diet or supplemental regimen.

ESOMEPRAZOLE (ess-oh-MEP-rah-zole)

Brand Name: Nexium

About Esomeprazole

The esophagus (the food tube that runs from the mouth to the stomach) has muscular walls that contract and relax rhythmically, pushing the food down the tube, through the lower esophageal sphincter, and into the stomach.

Ideally, the esophagus is a one-way tube: Food goes down into the stomach, but the contents of the stomach do not flow back up into the esophagus, thanks to the lower esophageal sphincter, the tube's exit door. The sphincter is normally kept shut by differences in pressure between the stomach and esophagus. But sometimes the pressure inside the stomach becomes so great that it blows the door open and allows the food—plus some very powerful stomach acid—to back up into the esophagus, a condition called gastroesophageal reflux disease (GERD), more commonly known as heartburn.

A protective mucous membrane lines the esophagus, but it can't ward off the tissue damage caused by repeated exposure to powerful stomach acid. The acid inflames the lining of the esophagus (a condition called esophagitis) and, in severe cases, actually burns holes in the lining (a very serious problem called erosive esophagitis).

Esomeprazole is used to treat erosive esophagitis, gastroesophageal reflux disease and, in combination with other drugs, duodenal ulcers caused by *Helicobacter pylori* bacteria. Although it doesn't keep the exit door shut, it does reduce the production of stomach acid.

Possible Side Effects

The drug's side effects include headache, flatulence, allergic reactions, and asthma.

Which Nutrients Are Robbed

Taking this medicine may deplete your supply of, increase your need for, or interfere with the activity of:

- Vitamin B_{12}
- Sodium
- Iron

Additional Ways This Drug May Upset Your Nutritional Balance

Esomeprazole can cause abdominal pain and nausea, which can upset your eating habits and possibly interfere with good nutrition. It can also cause diarrhea, which can hamper nutrient absorption.

Restoring Your Nutritional Balance

To compensate for the nutrient loss caused by this drug, speak to your physician about taking 500–1,000 mcg vitamin B_{12} per day. And ask your physician to consider the potential effects of iron and sodium depletion.

You can also eat foods that contain the depleted nutrient:

- Vitamin B_{12}: beef liver, rainbow trout, sockeye salmon, beef, haddock

Consult with your physician before making any changes to your diet or supplemental regimen.

ESTROGEN AND ESTROGEN DERIVATIVES (ESS-troe-jen)

Brand Names: Activella, Alesse, Alora, Api, Brevicon, Cenestin, Climacteron, Climara, CombiPatch, Congest, Cyclessa, Cyclen, Delestrogen, Depo-Estradiol, Depo-Testadiol, Enpresse, Estinyl, Estratab, Estratest, Estrogel, Estrace, FemHRT, Gynodiol, Kariva, Levlen, Levora, Marvelon, Menest, Min-ovral, Necon, Nortrel, Ogen, Ortho-Cept, Ortho-Cyclen, Ortho-Est, Premarin, Portia, Tri-Cyclen, Triphasil, Triquilar, Vagifem, Vivelle, Yasmin

About the Various Estrogens and Estrogen Derivatives

This category includes numerous medications containing estrogen or estrogen derivatives, which are often used in conjunction with other drugs, especially progestin. In their various formulations, estrogens are used for birth control and to treat menopausal symptoms, certain forms of cancer, and ovarian failure, and for other purposes.

Prempro is an example of an estrogen-progestin combination that may be prescribed for menopausal symptoms. Estraderm, Ortho Tri-Cyclen, and Loestrin are examples of estrogen-progestin combinations prescribed for birth control.

Possible Side Effects

The side effects of estrogen and estrogen derivatives are many and varied and include acne, breast tenderness, blood clots, depression, dizziness, altered blood pressure, irritability, pain in the muscles or joints, vaginal bleeding, water retention, premenstrual-like syndrome, and yeast infections (candidiasis).

Which Nutrients Are Robbed

Taking these medicines may deplete your supply of, increase your need for, or interfere with the activity of:

- *Estradiol; estradiol and testosterone; estradiol cypionate and medroxyprogesterone; estrogen and medroxyprogesterone:* folic acid, magnesium, riboflavin, vitamin B, vitamin C, and zinc
- *Estradiol and ethynodiol diacetate; ethinyl estradiol and desogestrel; ethinyl estradiol and levonorgesterel; ethinyl estradiol and norethindrone; ethinyl estradiol and norgestimate; ethinyl estradiol and norgestrel:* folic acid, magnesium, tyrosine, riboflavin, niacin, vitamin B_6, vitamin B_{12}, vitamin C, and zinc
- *Estradiol and norethindrone; ethinyl estradiol; ethinyl estradiol and fluoxymesterone:* folic acid, magnesium, riboflavin, vitamin B_6, vitamin B_{12}, vitamin C, zinc
- *Estrogens (conjugates A/synthetic); estrogens (conjugated); estrogens, esterified; estropipate; quinestrol:* magnesium, vitamin B_6
- *Estrogens and methyltestosterone:* magnesium, vitamin B_6, zinc

Additional Ways These Drugs May Upset Your Nutritional Balance

Various forms of estrogen and/or its derivatives can cause abdominal cramps, bloating, nausea, and vomiting, all of which can upset your eating habits and possibly interfere with good nutrition.

Various forms of estrogen, including ethinyl estradiol, can also trigger hypercalcemia, or too much calcium in the blood.

Restoring Your Nutritional Balance

To compensate for the nutrient loss caused by these drugs, speak to your physician about taking 400–800 mcg folic acid, 500–1,000 mg magnesium, 250–500 mg tyrosine, 25–100 mg riboflavin, 50–100 mg niacin, 50–100 mg vitamin B_6, 500–1,000 mcg vitamin B_{12}, 250–1,500 mg vitamin C, and 50–200 mg zinc per day.

You can also eat foods that contain the depleted nutrients:

- Folic acid: beef liver, fortified breakfast cereals, spinach, great northern beans, asparagus
- Magnesium: Florida avocado, toasted wheat germ, almonds, shredded wheat cereal, pumpkin seeds
- Tyrosine: soy, turkey, chicken, peanuts, banana
- Riboflavin: dried sunflower seeds, orange juice, bulgur, spinach noodles, pine nuts
- Niacin: chicken breast, beef liver, mackerel, barley, bulgur
- Vitamin B_6: potato, banana, garbanzo beans, chicken breast, fortified oatmeal
- Vitamin B_{12}: beef liver, rainbow trout, sockeye salmon, beef, haddock
- Vitamin C: papaya, guava, red pepper, cantaloupe, black currants
- Zinc: oysters, beef shank, chicken, pork tenderloin, plain yogurt

Consult with your physician before making any changes to your diet or supplemental regimen.

ETHACRYNIC ACID (eth-uh-KRIN-ik ASS-id)

Brand Name: Edecrin

About Ethacrynic Acid

Cirrhosis of the liver, heart failure, kidney failure, certain cancers, and other ailments can cause protein-laden fluid to gather in the abdominal cavity, a condition called ascites. If just a little fluid gathers, you may not have any symptoms. But if it continues creeping in, your abdomen can expand, feel uncomfortable, put pressure on the stomach, and interfere with your appetite. It can also press on your lungs, making breathing difficult. When your doctor taps on your abdomen, there will be a dull sound, something like what you'd hear if you tapped on a wooden keg of beer.

Part of the treatment for ascites is to put the kidneys into high gear, stimulating them to filter extra fluid out of the blood and send it to the bladder for excretion. Diuretics (water pills) like ethacrynic acid may be prescribed for this purpose.

Ethacrynic acid is used for ascites and other conditions that are treated by releasing excessive amounts of fluid from the body.

Possible Side Effects

The drug's side effects include loss of appetite, dry mouth, increased thirst, headache, dizziness, constipation, increased sensitivity to sunlight, rash, nausea, easy bleeding or bruising, and numbness in the hands or feet.

Which Nutrients Are Robbed

Taking this medicine may deplete your supply of, increase your need for, or interfere with the activity of:

- Thiamin
- Vitamin B_6
- Vitamin C
- Calcium
- Chloride
- Magnesium
- Potassium
- Sodium
- Zinc

Restoring Your Nutritional Balance

To compensate for the nutrient loss caused by this drug, speak to your physician about taking 25–100 mg thiamin, 50–100 mg vitamin B_6, 250–1,500 mg vitamin C, 1,200 mg calcium, 500–1,000 mg magnesium, and 50–200 mg zinc per day. And ask your physician to consider the potential effects of sodium and chloride depletion.

A Note on Potassium: "Regular" diuretics lower potassium levels, while potassium-sparing diuretics do not—they may increase levels instead. It is not uncommon for doctors to prescribe two different diuretics. That's why you should speak to your physician about your potassium levels, and whether it is appropriate for you to take supplements or eat potassium-rich foods.

You can also eat foods that contain the depleted nutrients:

- Thiamin: braised liver, turkey heart, roasted chicken, gefilte fish, sardines
- Vitamin B_6: potato, banana, garbanzo beans, chicken breast, fortified oatmeal

- Vitamin C: papaya, guava, red pepper, cantaloupe, black currants
- Calcium: milk, dried figs, Swiss cheese, yogurt, tofu
- Magnesium: Florida avocado, toasted wheat germ, almonds, shredded wheat cereal, pumpkin seeds
- Zinc: oysters, beef shank, chicken, pork tenderloin, plain yogurt

Consult with your physician before making any changes to your diet or supplemental regimen.

ETHAMBUTOL (e-THAM-byoo-tole)

Brand Names: Etibi, Myambutol

About Ethambutol

Imagine that a passel of rats has taken up residence in your house—big rats, little rats, strong rats, weak rats. So you set out traps baited with cheese to kill them. All the rats are lured by the cheese, all of them set off a trap and get smacked on the head as the bar crashes down on them, and soon only a few rats are left. But those left are the biggest, strongest rats, because they're the only ones who could get smacked on the head and still live. When these rats have babies, their offspring turn out to be just as big and strong as their parents, and pretty soon those traps just don't work anymore. All of the small, weak rats have been weeded out of the population, and only the big, strong ones remain.

Something similar can happen when medicines are used to destroy bacteria. A medicine may work at first, killing large numbers of the bacteria. But those that survive are the hardy ones, and they produce offspring that are equally strong. Soon all of the members of a particular bacterial colony will be resistant to the medicine. This often happens, and can happen very quickly. That's why doctors will often treat a bacterial infection with two or three drugs at once. This way, even if the bacteria rapidly develop a resistance to one of the drugs, one of the others may kill them.

Ethambutol is used in conjunction with other drugs to destroy the *Mycobacterum tuberculosis* that causes TB. It works by softening up the bacteria's cellular walls, making it easier for other drugs to get into the cells and destroy them.

Possible Side Effects

The drug's side effects include visual disturbances, confusion, headache, rash, stomach upset, and acute gout.

Which Nutrients Are Robbed

Taking this medicine may deplete your supply of, increase your need for, or interfere with the activity of:

- Copper
- Zinc

Additional Ways This Drug May Upset Your Nutritional Balance

Ethambutol can cause abdominal pain, loss of appetite, nausea, and vomiting, all of which can upset your eating habits and possibly interfere with good nutrition.

Restoring Your Nutritional Balance

To compensate for the nutrient loss caused by this drug, speak to your physician about taking 2 mcg copper and 50–200 mg zinc per day.

You can also eat foods that contain the depleted nutrients:

- Copper: beef liver, almonds, raw mushrooms, hazelnuts, lentils
- Zinc: oysters, beef shank, chicken, pork tenderloin, plain yogurt

Consult with your physician before making any changes to your diet or supplemental regimen.

ETHOSUXIMIDE (eth-oh-SUKS-i-mide)

Brand Name: Zarontin

About Ethosuximide

It's an odd kind of seizure that's not at all dramatic. You don't collapse, your limbs don't jerk, your head doesn't turn forcefully to one side, and your jaws don't lock shut.

It's a subtle seizure. Your eyelids flutter and your facial muscles may twitch. You stare without comprehending, and you're not aware of where you are or who's around you. It hits you all at once, lasts anywhere from a few seconds to half a minute, then disappears all at once. You don't even realize that something has happened. This is a petit mal seizure, also called an absence seizure.

Ethosuximide has been used since the early 1960s to treat petit mal seizures. Effective and relatively safe, it may work by altering the way that calcium is handled in the brain.

Possible Side Effects

The drug's more common side effects include lethargy, headache, dizziness, blurred vision, stomach upset, and hiccups.

Which Nutrients Are Robbed

Taking this medicine may deplete your supply of, increase your need for, or interfere with the activity of:

- Biotin
- Folic acid
- Vitamin D
- Vitamin K
- Calcium

Restoring Your Nutritional Balance

To compensate for the nutrient loss caused by this drug, speak to your physician about taking 500–1,000 mcg biotin, 400 IU vitamin D, 60–80 mcg vitamin K, and 1,200 mg calcium per day. Taking folic acid can increase the risk of seizures in some people, so discuss the use of this nutrient with your physician.

You can also eat foods that contain the depleted nutrients:

- Biotin: beef liver, soybeans, rice bran, peanut butter, barley
- Vitamin D: salmon, mackerel, sardines, eel, fortified milk
- Vitamin K: kale, broccoli, parsley, Swiss chard, spinach
- Calcium: milk, dried figs, Swiss cheese, yogurt, tofu

Consult with your physician before making any changes to your diet or supplemental regimen.

ETHOTOIN, MEPHENYTOIN (ETH-oh-toyn, me-FEN-i-toyn)

Brand Names: Ethotoin: Peganone
Mephenytoin: Mesantoin

About Ethotoin, Mephenytoin

These two antiseizure drugs are related to the drug phenytoin, and all three seem to be most effective at preventing partial and tonic-clonic seizures.

Seizures are brief periods in which the electrical activity of the brain goes haywire. Nerve cells fire off for no obvious reason. Depending on which parts of the brain are affected, this can cause something as simple as the trembling of a leg or as drastic as falling to the floor unconscious, shaking uncontrollably.

To imagine what's going on during a seizure, think of what would happen if all the electrical circuits in your car suddenly started firing randomly and uncontrollably. The headlights would flash on and off; the horn would honk; the windshield wipers would sweep back and forth a few times, stop, then start and stop again; the radio would turn on and off, becoming too loud, then too soft, then too loud. Something like that happens with a seizure.

With a simple partial seizure, only one side of your brain is affected, and you do not lose consciousness. With a tonic-clonic seizure—also called a grand mal seizure—you do lose consciousness and suffer from powerful muscle spasms.

Both ethotoin and mephenytoin are used to treat seizures. They have not been studied as much as some of the other seizure drugs, and are not used extensively. The two drugs appear to be less effective then their chemical cousin phenytoin.

Possible Side Effects

The more common side effects associated with ethotoin and mephenytoin include mild dizziness, drowsiness, stomach upset, constipation, bleeding, and swollen or tender gums.

Which Nutrients Are Robbed

Taking this medicine may deplete your supply of, increase your need for, or interfere with the activity of:

- Folic acid
- Vitamin D

Restoring Your Nutritional Balance

To compensate for the nutrient loss caused by this drug, speak to your physician about taking 400 IU vitamin D per day. Taking folic acid can increase the risk of seizures in some people, so discuss the use of this nutrient with your physician.

You can also eat foods that contain the depleted nutrient:

- Vitamin D: salmon, mackerel, sardines, eel, fortified milk

Consult with your physician before making any changes to your diet or supplemental regimen.

ETIDRONATE (e-ti-DROE-nate)

Brand Name: Didronel

About Etidronate

Throughout your childhood, your bones were in a constant state of change, growing longer, wider, and more dense. And they don't stop changing once you become an adult. They are continually broken down and rebuilt in a process called remodeling. Every day, some of your bone tissue is torn apart by cells called osteoclasts and some is rebuilt by other cells known as osteoblasts.

When you're young, there's more bone-building than breakdown. But when you're older (beginning around age 35), the balance tips and there begins to be more breakdown than building. If the breakdown processes greatly exceed the building, or if the bones are thin to begin with, the result is fragile, easily fractured bones, a condition known as osteoporosis.

But too much bone building isn't good either. In Paget's disease, the cellular teardown and rebuild crews both work at a furious pace. The result is the building of excessive amounts of bone, but this new bone tissue is of inferior quality. If this overbuilt, weakened bone tissue happens to reside near or inside a joint, it may push the joint out of alignment and cause osteoarthritis. If it's in the skull, it may trigger headaches—and, believe it or not, a bigger hat size. If it's in a leg or a hip, you may have difficulty walking. And no matter where it is, this poor-quality bone is more likely to fracture.

Etidronate is one of the medications used to treat Paget's disease. The drug works by slowing the rate at which bone is turned over, or torn down and rebuilt.

Possible Side Effects

The drug's more common side effects include diarrhea, nausea, and muscle or joint aches and soreness.

Which Nutrients Are Robbed

Taking this medicine may deplete your supply of, increase your need for, or interfere with the activity of:

- Calcium
- Magnesium
- Phosphorus
- Potassium

Additional Ways This Drug May Upset Your Nutritional Balance

Etidronate can cause changes in taste and nausea, which can upset your eating habits and possibly interfere with good nutrition. It can also cause diarrhea, which can hamper nutrient absorption.

Restoring Your Nutritional Balance

To compensate for the nutrient loss caused by this drug, speak to your physician about taking 1,200 mg calcium, 500–1,000 mg magnesium, 700 mg phosphorus, and 100–300 mg potassium per day.

You can also eat foods that contain the depleted nutrients:

- Calcium: milk, dried figs, Swiss cheese, yogurt, tofu
- Magnesium: Florida avocado, toasted wheat germ, almonds, shredded wheat cereal, pumpkin seeds
- Phosphorus: plain nonfat yogurt, lentils, salmon, milk, halibut
- Potassium: dried figs, California avocado, papaya, banana, dates

Consult with your physician before making any changes to your diet or supplemental regimen.

ETODOLAC (ee-TOE-doe-lak)

Brand Names: Apo-Etodolac, Gen-Etodolac, Lodine, Lodine XL, Utradol

About Etodolac

Etodolac is a nonsteroidal anti-inflammatory drug (NSAID) used to treat osteoarthritis and rheumatoid arthritis. New research suggests that it may also help combat colon cancer.

Like the other NSAIDs, etodolac reduces the production of substances called prostaglandins in the body. This reduction of prostaglandins helps to quell inflammation and its associated pain, which explains why the drug is helpful in treating osteoarthritis and rheumatoid arthritis. But etodolac doesn't interfere with the prostaglandins directly. Instead, it hampers the activity of COX (cyclooxygenase), which helps create the prostaglandins.

We've recently learned that there are two kinds of COX, called COX-1 and COX-2. We've also learned that COX-2 does more than produce prostaglandins. It also helps to convert healthy cells into colon cancer cells, then aids in their growth and spread.

One strategy for combating colon cancer—and possibly other forms of cancer—is to inhibit COX-2, which is exactly how etodolac works. But it's not a terribly selective drug; although it prefers to tackle COX-2, it also goes after the COX-1. Still, animal experiments have shown that it hampers COX-2 enough to interfere with the development and spread of colon cancer. This finding may explain why other studies have found that NSAIDs such as etodolac seem to reduce the rate of colorectal cancer.

Possible Side Effects

The drug's more common side effects include depression, abdominal cramps, stomach upset, rash, itching, and muscle weakness.

Which Nutrients Are Robbed

Taking this medicine may deplete your supply of, increase your need for, or interfere with the activity of:

- Folic acid

Additional Ways This Drug May Upset Your Nutritional Balance

Etodolac can cause abdominal cramps, nausea, vomiting, heartburn, and bloating, all of which can upset eating habits and possibly interfere with good nutrition. It can also cause diarrhea, which can hamper nutrient absorption.

Restoring Your Nutritional Balance

To compensate for the nutrient loss caused by this drug, speak to your physician about taking 400–800 mcg folic acid per day.

You can also eat foods that contain the depleted nutrient:

- Folic acid: beef liver, fortified breakfast cereals, spinach, great northern beans, asparagus

Consult with your physician before making any changes to your diet or supplemental regimen.

FAMOTIDINE (fa-MOE-ti-deen)

Brand Names: Alti-Famotidine, Apo-Famotidine, Gen-Famotidine, Novo-Famotidine, Nu-Famotidine, Pepcid, Pepcid AC

About Famotidine

Simply put, gastritis is an inflammation of the lining of the stomach. The problem may be caused by bacteria (such as *Helicobacter pylori*), illness, injury, severe burns, or bleeding elsewhere in the body. It can be triggered by aspirin or other drugs, radiation therapy, roundworms, an errant immune system reaction, or other problems.

The symptoms of gastritis include indigestion, heartburn, nausea, and upper abdominal pain. There can be bleeding of the stomach lining causing vomiting of blood, and the blood may turn the stool black. This bleeding can be slow and subtle or severe and fatal. It may go completely unnoticed or be completely obvious, as in the case of vomiting blood. Over time, gastritis and the problem that caused it may trigger ulcers, as well as the narrowing of passageways in the intestinal tract.

Famotidine is used to treat certain types of gastritis, as well as gastric and duodenal ulcers, heartburn, and related conditions. It works by reducing the secretion of gastric acid.

Possible Side Effects

The drug's side effects include dizziness, headache, a slow heartbeat, and elevated blood pressure.

Which Nutrients Are Robbed

Taking this medicine may deplete your supply of, increase your need for, or interfere with the activity of:

- Folic acid
- Thiamin
- Vitamin B_{12}
- Vitamin D
- Calcium
- Iron
- Zinc

Additional Ways This Drug May Upset Your Nutritional Balance

Famotidine can cause diarrhea, which can hamper nutrient absorption.

Restoring Your Nutritional Balance

To compensate for the nutrient loss caused by this drug, speak to your physician about taking 400–800 mcg folic acid, 25–100 mg thiamin, 500–1,000 mcg vitamin B_{12}, 400 IU vitamin D, 1,200 mg calcium, and 50–200 mg zinc per day. And ask your physician to consider the potential effects of iron depletion.

You can also eat foods that contain the depleted nutrients:

- Folic acid: beef liver, fortified breakfast cereals, spinach, great northern beans, asparagus
- Thiamin: braised liver, turkey heart, roasted chicken, gefilte fish, sardines
- Vitamin B$_{12}$: beef liver, rainbow trout, sockeye salmon, beef, haddock
- Vitamin D: salmon, mackerel, sardines, eel, fortified milk
- Calcium: milk, dried figs, Swiss cheese, yogurt, tofu
- Zinc: oysters, beef shank, chicken, pork tenderloin, plain yogurt

Consult with your physician before making any changes to your diet or supplemental regimen.

FENOFIBRATE (fen-oh-FYE-brate)

Brand Names: Apo-Fenofibrate, Apo-Feno-Micro, Gen-Fenofibrate Micro, Lipidil Micro, Lipidil Supra, TriCor

About Fenofibrate

Cholesterol is a key ingredient in cell membranes, brain cells, and nerve cells. It also forms the basis of bile, which we need to absorb fat and fat-soluble vitamins. Without cholesterol, we could not live.

However, too much cholesterol floating around in the bloodstream can be deadly and is a major problem in the United States, where millions of people rely on drugs to control their levels of total cholesterol, LDL (low density lipoprotein) cholesterol, and VLDL (very low density lipoprotein) cholesterol.

Although you don't hear much about it, it's just as important to control your VLDL as it is to control your total cholesterol and LDL "bad" cholesterol. VLDL is manufactured in the liver from cholesterol, blood fats, and protein. Its job is to transport blood fats from the liver to the fat cells for storage. A high VLDL is felt to contribute to the risk of heart disease. Unfortunately, due to heredity, diet, lifestyle, and other factors, some of us are too good at making VLDL. If your doctor gets particularly worried about elevations in your cholesterol or blood fat, he or she may prescribe fenofibrate.

Fenofibrate is believed to work by forcing the liver to produce less VLDL. It also lowers LDL and modestly raises HDL (high density lipoprotein), the "good" cholesterol.

Possible Side Effects

The drug's more common side effects include abdominal pain, constipation, respiratory disorders, and back pain.

Which Nutrients Are Robbed

Taking this medicine may deplete your supply of, increase your need for, or interfere with the activity of:

- Vitamin E
- Coenzyme Q_{10}
- Potassium

Additional Ways This Drug May Upset Your Nutritional Balance

Fenofibrate can cause low blood sugar (hypoglycemia) and abdominal pain, which can upset your eating habits and possibly interfere with good nutrition.

Restoring Your Nutritional Balance

To compensate for the nutrient loss caused by this drug, speak to your physician about taking 400 IU vitamin E, 100–300 mg potassium, and 30–100 mg coenzyme Q_{10} per day.

You can also eat foods that contain the depleted nutrients:

- Vitamin E: wheat germ oil, almonds, safflower oil, corn oil, soybean oil
- Potassium: dried figs, California avocado, papaya, banana, dates
- Coenzyme Q_{10}: beef, chicken, trout, salmon, oranges, broccoli

Consult with your physician before making any changes to your diet or supplemental regimen.

FENOLDOPAM (fe-NOL-doe-pam)

Brand Name: Corlopam

About Fenoldopam

Sometimes blood pressure has to be lowered right *now*, or else. Such is the case when the blood pressure jumps to 210/120 or higher (a condition known as malignant hypertension). If untreated, a hypertensive emergency like this can trigger a heart attack or stroke.

Fenoldopam is one of the newer drugs used for hypertensive emergencies, as well as for elevated blood pressure following surgery. The drug works by relaxing the muscles surrounding blood vessels and allowing these passageways to open wide. The newly widened vessels offer less resistance to the flow of blood, so blood pressure drops.

Fenoldopam works quickly and is rapidly metabolized in the body, so it must be taken continually via IV infusion.

Possible Side Effects

The drug's side effects include headache, rapid heartbeat, chest pain, dizziness, and stomach upset.

Which Nutrients Are Robbed

Taking this medicine may deplete your supply of, increase your need for, or interfere with the activity of:

• Potassium

Additional Ways This Drug May Upset Your Nutritional Balance

Fenoldopam can cause nausea and vomiting, which can upset your eating habits and possibly interfere with good nutrition. It can also cause diarrhea, which can hamper nutrient absorption.

Restoring Your Nutritional Balance

To compensate for the nutrient loss caused by this drug, speak to your physician about taking 100–300 mg potassium per day.

You can also eat foods that contain the depleted nutrient:

• Potassium: dried figs, California avocado, papaya, banana, dates

Consult with your physician before making any changes to your diet or supplemental regimen.

FENOPROFEN (fen-oh-PROE-fen)

Brand Name: Nalfon

About Fenoprofen

For most people, rheumatoid arthritis (RA) comes on gradually, attacking the smaller joints first (elbows and wrists, fingers and hands, ankles, feet, and toes), making them inflamed, stiff, and painful. Over time, these joints can become swollen, enlarged, twisted out of shape, and difficult to move. Swelling in the wrists can put pressure on the nerves and cause carpal tunnel syndrome. Cysts behind the knees can rupture, causing pain in the lower legs. Nodules, or bumps, can develop under the skin. And that's just what happens in the joints. In a small number of cases, RA can damage the blood vessels and interfere with the blood flow, or inflame the linings of the lungs and heart and scar the lungs themselves.

That's the bad news. The good news is that proper treatment can relieve symptoms in over 70 percent of those affected by RA.

Part of that treatment includes anti-inflammatory medicines such as fenoprofen. Although it doesn't cure the disease, fenoprofen helps relieve the inflammation that causes pain and swelling and contributes to difficulty in moving afflicted joints. Fenoprofen's ability to reduce pain and inflammation also makes it useful in treating other diseases, including osteoarthritis and mild to moderate pain triggered by other problems.

Possible Side Effects

The drug's more common side effects include dizziness, excessive sleepiness, stomach upset, loss of appetite, flatulence, headache, and constipation.

Which Nutrients Are Robbed

Taking this medicine may deplete your supply of, increase your need for, or interfere with the activity of:

- Folic acid

Additional Ways This Drug May Upset Your Nutritional Balance

Fenoprofen can cause heartburn, indigestion, nausea, abdominal cramps, loss of appetite, and vomiting, all of which can upset your eating habits and possibly interfere with good nutrition. It can also cause diarrhea, which can hamper nutrient absorption.

Restoring Your Nutritional Balance

To compensate for the nutrient loss caused by this drug, speak to your physician about taking 400–800 mcg folic acid per day.

You can also eat foods that contain the depleted nutrient:

- Folic acid: beef liver, fortified breakfast cereals, spinach, great northern beans, asparagus

Consult with your physician before making any changes to your diet or supplemental regimen.

FERRIC GLUCONATE (FER-ik GLOO-koe-nate)

Brand Name: Ferrlecit

About Ferric Gluconate

We need iron to make our red blood cells. Without sufficient iron, we suffer from iron deficiency anemia, a condition that causes fatigue, dizziness, irritability, drowsiness, difficulty concentrating, and shortness of breath.

Some groups are more likely than others to develop iron deficiency anemia because they have increased needs for the mineral. They include premature infants, rapidly growing children, pregnant and lactating women, women with heavy periods, and people with bowel disease, which interferes with the absorption of nutrients.

Loss of blood is the most common reason for iron deficiency in adults. In menstruating women, the cause of blood loss is usually obvious. In women who are not menstruating and in men, the cause may be subtle blood loss from a bleeding ulcer or another problem in the gastrointestinal tract.

Once the source of blood loss (if any) has been discovered and corrected, the next step is to replace the missing iron. Ferric gluconate is one of several supplements that can bring your iron stores back to normal.

Possible Side Effects

The drug's more common side effects include altered blood pressure, chest pain, headache, agitation, stomach upset, and urinary tract infection.

Which Nutrients Are Robbed

Taking this medicine may deplete your supply of, increase your need for, or interfere with the activity of:

- Potassium

Additional Ways This Drug May Upset Your Nutritional Balance

Ferric gluconate can cause low blood sugar (hypoglycemia), abdominal pain, heartburn, nausea, and vomiting, all of which can upset your eating habits and possibly interfere with good nutrition. It can also cause diarrhea, which can hamper nutrient absorption.

This drug can also trigger hyperkalemia, or too much potassium in the blood.

Restoring Your Nutritional Balance

Since ferric gluconate can cause potassium to either rise or fall, ask your physician to monitor your levels of this nutrient.

Consult with your physician before making any changes to your diet or supplemental regimen.

FLUCONAZOLE, ITRACONAZOLE, AND VORICONAZOLE

(floo-KOE-nuh-zole, i-tra-KOE-nuh-zole, vor-i-KOE-nuh-zole)

Brand Names: Fluconazole: Apo-Fluconazole, Diflucan
Itraconazole: Sporanox
Voriconazole: VFEND

About Fluconazole, Itraconazole, and Voriconazole

These three drugs, all of which end in "azole," are members of a group of synthetic antifungal medicines first used in the 1980s. The azoles were developed to supplement or replace older antifungal drugs that had serious side effects. These side effects made the drugs dangerous to use for extended periods of time or, in some cases, dangerous to use at all.

Fluconazole, itraconazole, and voriconazole fight a variety of fungi, including many species of *Candida* (yeastlike fungus). They destroy fungus cells by interfering with their ability to manufacture ergosterol, an important ingredient in their cell walls.

Fluconazole is used primarily to treat oral or vaginal *Candida* and certain ailments associated with AIDS.

Itraconazole is used to treat various fungal infections in patients with weakened immune systems, fungal infections of the nails, and other ailments.

Voriconazole, the last of the trio to be introduced in the United States, is used to treat various fungal infections, including infections caused by *Aspergillus fumigatus*, a fungus that can trigger wheezing, shortness of breath, fever, and bloody sputum.

Possible Side Effects

Fluconazole's more common side effects include headache, nausea, and abdominal pain. Itraconazole's more common side effects include nausea, rash, and water retention. Voriconazole's more common side effects include vision problems, nausea, vomiting, fever, and chills.

Which Nutrients Are Robbed

Taking these medicines may deplete your supply of, increase your need for, or interfere with the activity of:

Fluconazole and itraconazole: potassium
Voriconazole: magnesium and potassium

Additional Ways This Drug May Upset Your Nutritional Balance

Fluconazole can cause abdominal pain, changes in taste, nausea, and vomiting; itraconazole can cause abdominal pain, loss of appetite, and vomiting; and voriconazole can cause abdominal pain, nausea, and vomiting. These side effects can upset your eating habits and possibly interfere with good nutrition. All three drugs can also cause diarrhea, which can hamper nutrient absorption.

Restoring Your Nutritional Balance

To compensate for the nutrient loss caused by fluconazole, itraconazole, and voriconazole, speak to your physician about taking 100–300 mg potassium per day. And if you're taking voriconazole, ask about the feasibility of taking 500–1,000 mg magnesium per day, as well.

You can also eat foods that contain the depleted nutrients:

- Magnesium: Florida avocado, toasted wheat germ, almonds, shredded wheat cereal, pumpkin seeds
- Potassium: dried figs, California avocado, papaya, banana, dates

Consult with your physician before making any changes to your diet or supplemental regimen.

FLUCYTOSINE (floo-SYE-toe-seen)

Brand Names: Ancobon, Ancotil

About Flucytosine

In 1957, medical researchers were hoping that flucytosine would prove to be a new drug to treat cancer. Their hopes were dashed when they realized that it was ineffective against cancer; however, it was a fairly powerful antifungal medicine.

Fungi are plants that trigger moldlike or yeastlike infections in humans. We call these mycotic infections. ("Myco" is doctor-speak for things related to fungi.) Some fungi invade the skin or nails, while others make their way inside the body proper and take up residence in the liver, kidneys, lungs, or elsewhere.

Flucytosine doesn't attack fungal cells from the outside, the way other antifungal medicines do. Instead, it moves right into the cells, where it's converted into other substances that interfere with the ability of the fungus to manufacture DNA and RNA. Unable to pass on genetic information properly, the fungal cells falter.

Flucytosine is generally used as a partner treatment with amphotericin B or other drugs to treat certain fungal infections.

Possible Side Effects

The drug's side effects include headache, hallucinations, staggering and uncoordinated movement (ataxia), weakness, and stomach upset.

Which Nutrients Are Robbed

Taking this medicine may deplete your supply of, increase your need for, or interfere with the activity of:

- Calcium
- Potassium
- Magnesium
- Sodium

Additional Ways This Drug May Upset Your Nutritional Balance

Flucytosine can cause low blood sugar (hypoglycemia), nausea, vomiting, abdominal pain, and loss of appetite, all of which can upset your eating habits and possibly interfere with good nutrition. It can also cause diarrhea, which can hamper nutrient absorption.

Restoring Your Nutritional Balance

To compensate for the nutrient loss caused by this drug, speak to your physician about taking 1,200 mg calcium and 500–1,000 mg magnesium per day. And ask your physician to consider the potential effects of sodium depletion and to monitor your potassium status to ensure that it remains within the normal range.

You can also eat foods that contain the depleted nutrients:

- Calcium: milk, dried figs, Swiss cheese, yogurt, tofu
- Magnesium: Florida avocado, toasted wheat germ, almonds, shredded wheat cereal, pumpkin seeds

Consult with your physician before making any changes to your diet or supplemental regimen.

FLUDROCORTISONE (floo-droe-KOR-ti-sohn)

Brand Name: Florinef

About Fludrocortisone

Perched atop each kidney is a little gland called the adrenal gland. The adrenals are not very impressive looking, resembling little ski hats for the kidneys. But they're vital because they secrete the hormones cortisol, aldosterone, adrenaline, and other substances that help control the heart rate, blood pressure, blood sugar, and the levels of salt and potassium. These substances also help combat infections, manufacture carbohydrates, and perform many other functions.

If your adrenals are harmed—perhaps by an errant immune system, infection, or cancer—you may suffer from Addison's disease. With your adrenals unable to pump out sufficient quantities of the vital hormones, you may be hit with muscle weakness, fatigue, dizziness when standing up, darkened patches of skin, weight loss, dehydration, lack of appetite, vomiting, and diarrhea.

Symptoms of Addison's may be relatively mild, becoming a problem only when you're stressed. However, the disease can progress to cause very low blood pressure and severe weakness, significant abdominal pain and kidney failure. Untreated, Addison's disease can be fatal.

One of the problems caused by the deficiency of the hormone aldosterone is the retention of potassium and the loss of large amounts of sodium in the urine. The kidneys are no longer able to concentrate the urine, so you may urinate way too much and become severely dehydrated. The combination of dehydration and low sodium levels can lead to shock.

Fludrocortisone reverses this harmful process by forcing the body to reabsorb sodium before it's flushed out with the urine, and getting rid of excess potassium instead. This helps restore the sodium/potassium balance and maintain proper water balance.

Possible Side Effects

The drug's side effects include hypertension, congestive heart failure, convulsions, headache, and peptic ulcer.

Which Nutrients Are Robbed

Taking this medicine may deplete your supply of, increase your need for, or interfere with the activity of:

- Phosphorus
- Potassium

Additional Ways This Drug May Upset Your Nutritional Balance

Fludrocortisone can cause a peptic ulcer, which can upset your eating habits and possibly interfere with good nutrition.

Restoring Your Nutritional Balance

To compensate for the nutrient loss caused by this drug, speak to your physician about taking 700 mg phosphorus per day. And ask your physician to monitor your potassium status.

You can also eat foods that contain the depleted nutrient:

- Phosphorus: plain nonfat yogurt, lentils, salmon, milk, halibut

Consult with your physician before making any changes to your diet or supplemental regimen.

FLUNISOLIDE (floo-NISS-oh-lide)

Brand Names: AeroBid-M, Alti-Flunisolide, Apo-Flunisolide, Nasalide, Nasarel, Rhinalar

About Flunisolide

A lot of people buy medicines to get rid of their wheezy-sneezy-stuffy-nose-watery-eyes misery. They're likely suffering from what we call "hay fever" and what doctors call allergic rhinitis. This can be a regular problem that strikes seasonally when certain kinds of pollen are released, or a one-time occurrence due to exposure to some brand-new allergen.

Whatever the impetus, in some people the body reacts to the presence of harmless pollen, dust mites, animal dander, or other substances by pushing the panic button and setting off a full-fledged allergic response. Suddenly your nose is stuffed, runny, or itchy; your eyes are watery; your eyelids are inflamed; and you may start wheezing or have other symptoms.

Flunisolide, a corticosteroid that comes in the form of a nasal spray, fights the inflammation response that causes nasal symptoms. Flunisolide is also used to treat asthma.

Possible Side Effects

The drug's side effects include headache, dizziness, and a decreased sense of smell and taste.

Which Nutrients Are Robbed

Taking this medicine may deplete your supply of, increase your need for, or interfere with the activity of:

- Vitamin A
- Folic acid
- Vitamin B_6
- Vitamin C
- Vitamin D
- Vitamin K
- Calcium
- Magnesium
- Potassium
- Selenium
- Zinc
- Melatonin

Restoring Your Nutritional Balance

To compensate for the nutrient loss caused by this drug, speak to your physician about taking 5,000 IU vitamin A, 400–800 mcg folic acid, 50–100 mg vitamin B_6, 250–1,500 mg vitamin C, 400 IU vitamin D, 60–80 mcg vitamin K, 1,200 mg calcium, 500–1,000 mg magnesium, 100–300 mg potassium, 20–100 mcg of selenium, 50–200 mg zinc, and 1–3 mg melatonin per day.

You can also eat foods that contain the depleted nutrients:

- Vitamin A: beef liver, chicken liver, cheese pizza, whole milk, cheddar cheese
- Folic acid: beef liver, fortified breakfast cereals, spinach, great northern beans, asparagus
- Vitamin B_6: potato, banana, garbanzo beans, chicken breast, fortified oatmeal
- Vitamin C: papaya, guava, red pepper, cantaloupe, black currants
- Vitamin D: salmon, mackerel, sardines, eel, fortified milk
- Vitamin K: kale, broccoli, parsley, Swiss chard, spinach
- Calcium: milk, dried figs, Swiss cheese, yogurt, tofu
- Magnesium: Florida avocado, toasted wheat germ, almonds, shredded wheat cereal, pumpkin seeds
- Potassium: dried figs, California avocado, papaya, banana, dates
- Selenium: Brazil nuts, tuna, beef liver, turkey breast, spaghetti with meat sauce
- Zinc: oysters, beef shank, chicken, pork tenderloin, plain yogurt

Consult with your physician before making any changes to your diet or supplemental regimen.

FLUOROURACIL (flure-oh-YOOR-uh-sil)

Brand Names: Adrucil, Carac, Efudex, Fluoroplex

About Fluorouracil

Breast cancer is the second most common cancer to strike women (after skin cancer), diagnosed in over 215,000 women a year and killing about one in five of these women. Certain factors, such as age, family history of the disease, and alcoholic beverage consumption, are linked to breast cancer, but many women who develop the disease have no known risk factors.

The first symptom of breast cancer can be a lump in the breast, and often the woman herself discovers the lump. If the cancer has spread to nearby lymph nodes (the one in the nearest armpit is the most likely to be affected), the node may feel like it has hard little lumps in it. In some cases, the breast may be swollen, red, and warm, the skin may develop a texture like an orange peel, there may be a discharge from the nipple, or the nipple may invert.

After the cancer has been removed surgically, doctors typically prescribe radiation therapy or chemotherapy to track down and destroy any cancer cells that may have escaped the surgeon's scalpel—especially while they're still small and easier to kill. Doctors have had a great deal of experience with fluorouracil plus the drugs cyclophosphamide and methotrexate. Taken together, this trio is called CMF. Fluorouracil works by interfering with the manufacture and function of DNA and RNA, thus killing cancer and other rapidly multiplying cells. Cyclophosphamide prevents cancer cells from dividing, while methotrexate prevents them from manufacturing new DNA and reproducing.

Fluorouracil is also used to treat cancers of the rectum, colon, stomach, and pancreas. In topical form, it is used for certain skin cancers.

Possible Side Effects

The drug's more common side effects include loss of hair, anemia, stomach upset, fever, and rash.

Which Nutrients Are Robbed

Taking this medicine may deplete your supply of, increase your need for, or interfere with the activity of:

- Thiamin
- Vitamin B_6

Additional Ways This Drug May Upset Your Nutritional Balance

Fluorouracil can cause heartburn, nausea, vomiting, and loss of appetite, all of which can upset your eating habits and possibly interfere with good nutrition. It can also cause diarrhea, which can hamper nutrient absorption.

Restoring Your Nutritional Balance

To compensate for the nutrient loss caused by this drug, speak to your physician about taking 25–100 mg thiamin and 50–100 mg vitamin B_6 per day.

You can also eat foods that contain the depleted nutrients:

- Thiamin: braised liver, turkey heart, roasted chicken, gefilte fish, sardines
- Vitamin B_6: potato, banana, garbanzo beans, chicken breast, fortified oatmeal

Consult with your physician before making any changes to your diet or supplemental regimen.

FLUOXETINE (floo-OKS-e-teen)

Brand Names: Prozac, Sarafem

About Fluoxetine

Depression is an ancient affliction. In the Old Testament, Job lamented, "My soul is weary of my life." Hippocrates, the noted ancient Greek physician, called depression melancholia, which means "black bile," one of the four humors, or fluids, that he believed controlled health. In more modern times, depression has been seen as a weakness, then as an expression of inner conflict, and, today, as the result of unhappy circumstances or disturbances in brain chemistry.

Depression causes a variety of symptoms, including feelings of sadness, worthlessness, helplessness and hopelessness, difficulty in concentrating, trouble making decisions, loss of interest in hobbies, withdrawal from work, anxiety, and various physical complaints (such as headaches, loss of energy, lack of interest in sex, and so on).

For decades, doctors have used drugs to treat depression with a fair amount of success, although most of these drugs have serious side effects. And then, in the late 1980s, along came fluoxetine, commonly known as Prozac.

Almost as soon as it made its debut, Prozac was more than just another antidepressant. It seemed to do more than lift the mood. According to many who took it, Prozac increased energy and optimism and made it "feel good to be you." By the mid-1990s, Prozac was a household word, the second best-selling drug in the world, featured in *Newsweek* magazine, and the subject of a best-selling book.

Prozac was the first in a new family of drugs called the selective serotonin reuptake inhibitors (SSRIs), which work by increasing the levels of serotonin, a chemical messenger (neurotransmitter) in the brain. Serotonin is a "feel-good" neurotransmitter, delivering an "everything-is-great" message to the brain. Prozac and the other SSRIs keep serotonin from being reabsorbed after it completes its biochemical task. Instead, the serotonin hangs around longer, in effect delivering its "everything-is-great" message over and over again.

Prozac and the other SSRIs have effectively pushed the older antidepressants to the sidelines. Although not necessarily stronger than the older drugs, the SSRIs tend to have fewer toxic side effects.

Prozac is used to treat depression, obsessive-compulsive disorder, panic disorder, and bulimia nervosa.

Possible Side Effects

The drug's more common side effects include insomnia, headache, nausea, nervousness, anxiety, muscle weakness, and tremor.

Which Nutrients Are Robbed

Taking this medicine may deplete your supply of, increase your need for, or interfere with the activity of:

- Melatonin

Additional Ways This Drug May Upset Your Nutritional Balance

Fluoxetine can cause nausea, vomiting, diarrhea, loss of appetite, changes in taste, and stomach upset, all of which can upset your eating habits and possibly interfere with good nutrition.

Restoring Your Nutritional Balance

To compensate for the nutrient loss caused by this drug, speak to your physician about taking 1–3 mg melatonin per day.

Consult with your physician before making any changes to your diet or supplemental regimen.

FLUPHENAZINE (floo-FEN-uh-zeen)

Brand Names: Apo-Fluphenazine, Modecate, Moditen Enanthate, PMS-Fluphenazine Decanoate, Prolixin, Prolixin Decanoate, Prolixin Enanthate (DSC)

About Fluphenazine

Remember *Harvey*, the old movie starring Jimmy Stewart, who played a man who had an invisible friend (a rabbit, actually) that no one else could see? Some people have said that having schizophrenia is like living in that movie. You're absolutely sure that certain people are with you or talking to you. And certain things seem to be undeniably true, but you can't get others to believe you.

Schizophrenia is a worldwide problem that typically makes its first appearance in young adulthood. It seems to be due to a combination of genetic and environmental factors, but we can't say for certain which ones bring it on or why one person develops schizophrenia while his or her sibling does not.

Experts disagree as to whether schizophrenia is several distinct diseases or one ailment with different manifestations. But we can distinguish among those who have what is called disorganized schizophrenia, characterized by incoherence; paranoid schizophrenia, characterized by the feeling that people are out to get you or by delusions of grandeur; and catatonic schizophrenia, with its hallmark excitement and/or stupor.

Fluphenazine is one of the many drugs used to treat schizophrenia. This medicine apparently works by blocking receptors for the neurotransmitter dopamine and decreasing its activity in the brain.

Possible Side Effects

The drug's side effects include drowsiness, headache, fluctuations in blood pressure, rapid heartbeat, dizziness, and weight gain.

Which Nutrients Are Robbed

Taking this medicine may deplete your supply of, increase your need for, or interfere with the activity of:

- Riboflavin
- Coenzyme Q_{10}

Additional Ways This Drug May Upset Your Nutritional Balance

Fluphenazine can cause loss of appetite, which can upset your eating habits and possibly interfere with good nutrition.

Restoring Your Nutritional Balance

To compensate for the nutrient loss caused by this drug, speak to your physician about taking 25–100 mg riboflavin and 30–100 mg coenzyme Q_{10} per day.

You can also eat foods that contain the depleted nutrients:

- Riboflavin: dried sunflower seeds, orange juice, bulgur, spinach noodles, pine nuts
- Coenzyme Q_{10}: beef, chicken, trout, salmon, oranges, broccoli

Consult with your physician before making any changes to your diet or supplemental regimen.

FLURBIPROFEN (flure-BI-proe-fen)

Brand Names: Alti-Flurbiprofen, Ansaid, Apo-Flurbiprofen, Froben, Froben-SR, Novo-Flurprofen, Nu-Flurprofen, Ocufen

About Flurbiprofen

Osteoarthritis (OA) and rheumatoid arthritis (RA) are the two most common forms of arthritis. They both bedevil the joints, but they're very different diseases, with different causes and courses. Here are some of the differences:

OSTEOARTHRITIS	RHEUMATOID ARTHRITIS
Most prominent symptom: pain in the joint; swelling and inflammation are less prominent	Most prominent symptom: swelling and inflammation of the joints
Typically appears in one joint at a time	Often appears simultaneously in two "opposite" joints: that is, in both wrists or in both ankles
Usually strikes those age 40 and up; not common in children	Usually strikes those between the ages of 25 and 50, but will also strike children, causing juvenile rheumatoid arthritis
Doesn't spread beyond the afflicted joints	May go beyond the joints to trigger fatigue, weight loss, fever, and other potentially serious symptoms
Caused by a local breakdown in body cells and/or tissues	Caused by an errant immune system that attacks the joints and possibly other parts of the body

Although OA and RA are very different, the treatment regimen for both includes drugs that quell pain and inflammation, like flurbiprofen. That's because reducing inflammation can lessen the pain, and easing pain can make inflammation more bearable.

In addition to OA and RA, flurbiprofen may be used to treat inflammation of the eye following certain surgeries.

Possible Side Effects

The drug's more common side effects include eye irritation, headache, dizziness, stomach upset, ringing in the ears, and rash.

Which Nutrients Are Robbed

Taking this medicine may deplete your supply of, increase your need for, or interfere with the activity of:

- Folic acid

Additional Ways This Drug May Upset Your Nutritional Balance

Flurbiprofen can cause heartburn, indigestion, nausea, and vomiting, all of which can upset your eating habits and possibly interfere with good nutrition.

Restoring Your Nutritional Balance

To compensate for the nutrient loss caused by this drug, speak to your physician about taking 400–800 mcg folic acid per day.

You can also eat foods that contain the depleted nutrient:

* Folic acid: beef liver, fortified breakfast cereals, spinach, great northern beans, asparagus

Consult with your physician before making any changes to your diet or supplemental regimen.

FLUTICASONE (floo-TIK-uh-sohn)

Brand Names: Cutivate, Flonase, Flovent, Flovent Rotadisk

About Fluticasone

Asthma is a terrifying disease that literally leaves you gasping for breath. The muscles surrounding the airways (bronchial tubes) clamp down, making them smaller, while an outpouring of thick mucous clogs up these narrowed tubes. Depending on the severity of the attack, you may wheeze and feel a little out of breath, or you may go into respiratory failure, a life-threatening condition that demands immediate medical attention.

An asthma attack can be triggered by exposure to allergens, such as dust, feathers, pollen, cold air, certain foods, various drugs, animals, or plants. It may follow an upper respiratory tract infection or an exercise session and may be made worse by emotional stress or exposure to noxious fumes and other irritants.

Fortunately, many people have relatively mild asthma that can be managed with medicines such as fluticasone, a corticosteroid used in aerosol form to help prevent future attacks. It's also used to treat hay fever and certain skin inflammations.

Possible Side Effects

The drug's more common side effects include headache, fever, nausea, vomiting, upper respiratory infection, and throat irritation.

Which Nutrients Are Robbed

Taking this medicine may deplete your supply of, increase your need for, or interfere with the activity of:

- Vitamin A
- Folic acid
- Vitamin B$_6$
- Vitamin C
- Vitamin D
- Vitamin K
- Calcium
- Magnesium
- Potassium
- Selenium
- Zinc
- Melatonin

Additional Ways This Drug May Upset Your Nutritional Balance

Fluticasone can cause nausea and vomiting, both of which can upset your eating habits and possibly interfere with good nutrition.

Restoring Your Nutritional Balance

To compensate for the nutrient loss caused by this drug, speak to your physician about taking 5,000 IU vitamin A, 400–800 mcg folic acid, 50–100 mg vitamin B$_6$, 250–1,500 mg vitamin C, 400 IU vitamin D, 60–80 mcg vitamin K, 1,200 mg calcium, 500–1,000 mg magnesium, 100–300 mg potassium, 20–100 mcg selenium, 50–200 mg zinc, and 1–3 mg melatonin per day.

You can also eat foods that contain the depleted nutrients:

- Vitamin A: beef liver, chicken liver, cheese pizza, whole milk, cheddar cheese
- Folic acid: beef liver, fortified breakfast cereals, spinach, great northern beans, asparagus
- Vitamin B$_6$: potato, banana, garbanzo beans, chicken breast, fortified oatmeal
- Vitamin C: papaya, guava, red pepper, cantaloupe, black currants
- Vitamin D: salmon, mackerel, sardines, eel, fortified milk
- Vitamin K: kale, broccoli, parsley, Swiss chard, spinach
- Calcium: milk, dried figs, Swiss cheese, yogurt, tofu
- Magnesium: Florida avocado, toasted wheat germ, almonds, shredded wheat cereal, pumpkin seeds
- Potassium: dried figs, California avocado, papaya, banana, dates
- Selenium: Brazil nuts, tuna, beef liver, turkey breast, spaghetti with meat sauce
- Zinc: oysters, beef shank, chicken, pork tenderloin, plain yogurt

Consult with your physician before making any changes to your diet or supplemental regimen.

FLUVASTATIN (FLOO-va-stat-in)

Brand Names: Lescol, Lescol XL

About Fluvastatin

According to the Third Report of the National Cholesterol Education Program, this is what your "cholesterol numbers" mean:

Total Cholesterol
> Less than 200: Desirable
> 200–239: Borderline high
> 240 and up: High

HDL "Good" Cholesterol
> Less than 40: A major risk factor for heart disease
> 60 and up: Protective against heart disease

LDL "Bad" Cholesterol
> Less than 100: Optimal
> 100–129: Near optimal
> 130–159: Borderline high
> 160–189: High
> 190 and up: Very high

Diet and exercise can reduce the total cholesterol and LDL and raise the HDL. For some people, that's all it takes. Others—tens of millions of others, worldwide—may need additional help from cholesterol-lowering drugs.

One of the popular statin drugs, fluvastatin is used in conjunction with diet and exercise to reduce cholesterol levels and the risk of heart disease. It works by interfering with the body's ability to manufacture cholesterol. Unfortunately, it also interferes with the body's ability to synthesize coenzyme Q_{10}, which is crucial to heart health.

Possible Side Effects

The drug's more common side effects include headache, stomach upset, diarrhea, muscle pain, and insomnia.

Which Nutrients Are Robbed

Taking this medicine may deplete your supply of, increase your need for, or interfere with the activity of:

- Coenzyme Q_{10}

Additional Ways This Drug May Upset Your Nutritional Balance

Fluvastatin can cause a feeling of bloating, abdominal pain, and nausea, all of which can upset your eating habits and possibly interfere with good nutrition. It can also cause diarrhea, which can hamper nutrient absorption.

This drug may cause blood levels of vitamin A to rise.

Restoring Your Nutritional Balance

To compensate for the nutrient loss caused by this drug, speak to your physician about taking 30–100 mg coenzyme Q_{10} per day.

You can also eat foods that contain the depleted nutrient:

- Coenzyme Q_{10}: beef, chicken, trout, salmon, oranges, broccoli

Consult with your physician before making any changes to your diet or supplemental regimen.

FONDAPARINUX (fon-duh-PA-ri-nuks)

Brand Name: Arixtra

About Fondaparinux

Veins return "used" blood to the heart and sometimes, in the process, a blood clot (thrombus) forms and sticks to a vein's inside wall. The thrombus might remain in place, or it might dislodge and float through the bloodstream on its way back toward the heart. This free-floating kind of clot is called an embolus.

Damage to veins during surgery or prolonged bed rest after surgery can cause a blood clot to form, which is a real concern for surgeons who fix broken hips or insert hip or knee replacements. If a thrombus forms in one of the deeper veins in the leg (a condition called deep vein thrombosis), it may very well travel up through the heart and into the lungs, where it can lodge in an artery and cause a pulmonary embolism. This is a "lung attack," the death of lung tissue caused by a stoppage in the blood flow. The problem could be mild or deadly, depending on which artery in the lung is blocked.

But a thrombus can cause trouble even if it doesn't free itself and travel to the lungs. For example, it may block the flow of blood in a major leg vein, causing pain and swelling. If the clot is converted to scar tissue, the valves inside the veins may be damaged and unable to move blood back to the heart effectively. This can cause fluid accumulation in the ankle and on up to the thigh, depending on where the damaged valves are.

Fondaparinux is a newer drug used to prevent deep vein thrombosis in people who are undergoing hip surgery, knee replacement, or hip replacement. It works by interfering with one of the biochemical factors that causes blood to clot.

Possible Side Effects

The drug's more common side effects include anemia, fever, water retention, nausea, vomiting, and rash.

Which Nutrients Are Robbed

Taking this medicine may deplete your supply of, increase your need for, or interfere with the activity of:

- Potassium

Additional Ways This Drug May Upset Your Nutritional Balance

Fondaparinux can cause heartburn, bloating, nausea, and vomiting, all of which can upset your eating habits and possibly interfere with good nutrition. It can also cause diarrhea, which can hamper nutrient absorption.

Restoring Your Nutritional Balance

To compensate for the nutrient loss caused by this drug, speak to your physician about taking 100–300 mg potassium per day.

You can also eat foods that contain the depleted nutrient:

- Potassium: dried figs, California avocado, papaya, banana, dates

Consult with your physician before making any changes to your diet or supplemental regimen.

FOSCARNET (foss-KAR-net)

Brand Name: Foscavir

About Foscarnet

Herpes (technically herpes simplex) became big news in the 1980s, with newspaper headlines and magazine covers sounding the alarm of a "new epidemic." The problem never grew to the gigantic proportions some feared, but for the person who contracts it, herpes can be devastating.

Herpes, which can cause the appearance of small, painful, fluid-filled blisters inside the mouth and on the lips, eyes, and/or genitals, is caused by a virus that takes up residence inside nerve cells. Every so often this virus "wakes up" and begins reproducing itself, sending out legions of new viruses that cause tingling, eruptions, itching, and pain. The blisters pop, turning into sores and then scabs. An outbreak can also cause generalized aching and headache, fever, and a feeling of being sick.

Foscarnet is an antiviral medicine that combats viruses by interfering with their ability to manufacture and use DNA and RNA. The drug is used to treat herpes infections that do not respond to the drug acyclovir. It's also used to treat infections caused by a related virus called cytomegalovirus, or CMV for short.

Possible Side Effects

The drug's more common side effects include seizures, anemia, fever, headache, nausea, vomiting, and diarrhea.

Which Nutrients Are Robbed

Taking this medicine may deplete your supply of, increase your need for, or interfere with the activity of:

- Calcium
- Phosphorus
- Magnesium
- Potassium

Additional Ways This Drug May Upset Your Nutritional Balance

Foscarnet can cause nausea and vomiting, which can upset your eating habits and possibly interfere with good nutrition. It can also cause diarrhea, which can hamper nutrient absorption.

This drug can also trigger hyperphosphatemia, or too much phosphorus in the blood.

Restoring Your Nutritional Balance

To compensate for the nutrient loss caused by this drug, speak to your physician about taking 1,200 mg calcium, 500–1,000 mg magnesium, and 100–300 mg potassium per day. And ask your physician to monitor your phosphorus status.

You can also eat foods that contain the depleted nutrients:

- Calcium: milk, dried figs, Swiss cheese, yogurt, tofu
- Magnesium: Florida avocado, toasted wheat germ, almonds, shredded wheat cereal, pumpkin seeds
- Potassium: dried figs, California avocado, papaya, banana, dates

Consult with your physician before making any changes to your diet or supplemental regimen.

FOSINOPRIL (foe-SIN-oh-pril)

Brand Name: Monopril

About Fosinopril

The human heart is a mechanical marvel, a four-chambered pump that can keep a tremendous volume of fluid in continuous circulation for 80 years or longer. It's also a "smart" pump that's able to increase or decrease its output almost immediately in response to the body's need for oxygen and nutrients.

Blood enters the heart through the right atrium—the upper, smaller chamber on the right side of the heart. It quickly drops down into the right ventricle, which pumps it out to the lungs. There, the blood drops off the carbon dioxide it's been holding and takes up a new load of oxygen before returning to the heart. Reentering the heart through the left atrium—the small chamber on the top left side of the heart—the blood pauses briefly before dropping down into the left ventricle. This is the strongest of the four heart chambers, for it must pump blood not just to the next chamber or to the nearby lungs, but throughout the entire body, from scalp to toes.

Any damage to the left ventricle can be devastating, for the heart will no longer be able to do its job effectively. Unfortunately, after a heart attack, the heart can begin to remodel or rebuild certain tissues, a process that can weaken the left ventricle and contribute to heart failure.

Fosinopril helps slow damage to the left ventricle following a heart attack, which most likely is why it reduces the rate of future heart problems and death in people who have had heart attacks.

Fosinopril is used to prevent left ventricular dysfunction following a heart attack, as well as for elevated blood pressure and congestive heart failure.

Possible Side Effects

The drug's more common side effects include dizziness, cough, headache, weakness, musculoskeletal pain, and stomach upset.

Which Nutrients Are Robbed

Taking this medicine may deplete your supply of, increase your need for, or interfere with the activity of:

- Sodium
- Zinc

Additional Ways This Drug May Upset Your Nutritional Balance

Fosinopril can cause nausea and vomiting, which can upset your eating habits and possibly interfere with good nutrition. It can also cause diarrhea, which can hamper nutrient absorption.

This drug can also trigger hyperkalemia, or too much potassium in the blood.

Restoring Your Nutritional Balance

To compensate for the nutrient loss caused by this drug, speak to your physician about taking 50–200 mg zinc per day. And ask your physician to consider the potential effects of sodium depletion.

You can also eat foods that contain the depleted nutrient:

- Zinc: oysters, beef shank, chicken, pork tenderloin, plain yogurt

Consult with your physician before making any changes to your diet or supplemental regimen.

FOSPHENYTOIN (foss-FEN-i-toyn)

Brand Name: Cerebyx

About Fosphenytoin

A seizure can be a very mild, once-in-a-lifetime response to a very high fever, a lack of calcium in the blood, a drug, or some other problem.

But some seizures recur and the problem can grow. The most serious kind of seizure is called *status epilepticus*, a potentially fatal condition that requires immediate medical treatment. In status epilepticus, the "electrical storms" in your brain don't stop. Instead, they rage throughout large areas of your gray matter, triggering a generalized seizure affecting both halves of your brain that can last up to 15 minutes—a long time for a seizure. Or you may suffer from seizure after seizure, without becoming fully conscious between each episode.

The powerful muscle contractions triggered by a seizure, coupled with the uncontrolled jerking movements of the limbs, can lead to broken bones and other injuries. You may injure yourself when you lose consciousness and fall. And a prolonged electrical storm in your brain can cause brain damage.

Fosphenytoin is used to treat status epilepticus, as well as seizures that might strike during neurosurgery. It's also used when it's not advisable to use the drug's close chemical cousin, phenytoin. Fosphenytoin is a prodrug of phenytoin. This means that once inside the body, it's converted to phenytoin. As phenytoin, it helps stabilize nerve cell membranes and quiets seizure activity.

Possible Side Effects

The drug's side effects depend on the method of administration. Common side effects with IV administration include dizziness, excessive sleepiness, itching, and involuntary movement of the eye. Common side effects with intramuscular injection include dizziness, lack of coordination, nausea, vomiting, and muscle weakness.

Which Nutrients Are Robbed

Taking this medicine may deplete your supply of, increase your need for, or interfere with the activity of:

- Biotin
- Folic acid
- Vitamin K
- Calcium

- Thiamin
- Vitamin B$_{12}$
- Vitamin D
- Phosphorus
- Potassium

Additional Ways This Drug May Upset Your Nutritional Balance

Fosphenytoin can cause nausea and vomiting, which can upset your eating habits and possibly interfere with good nutrition.

Fosphenytoin can also trigger hyperkalemia, or too much potassium in the blood.

Restoring Your Nutritional Balance

To compensate for the nutrient loss caused by this drug, speak to your physician about taking 500–1,000 mcg biotin, 25–100 mg thiamin, 500–1,000 mcg vitamin B$_{12}$, 400 IU vitamin D, 60–80 mcg vitamin K, 1,200 mg calcium, and 700 mg phosphorus per day. And because fosphenytoin can cause potassium levels to either rise or fall, ask your physician to monitor your potassium status. Taking folic acid can increase the risk of seizures in some people, so discuss the use of this nutrient with your physician.

You can also eat foods that contain the depleted nutrients:

- Biotin: beef liver, soybeans, rice bran, peanut butter, barley
- Thiamin: braised liver, turkey heart, roasted chicken, gefilte fish, sardines
- Vitamin B$_{12}$: beef liver, rainbow trout, sockeye salmon, beef, haddock
- Vitamin D: salmon, mackerel, sardines, eel, fortified milk
- Vitamin K: kale, broccoli, parsley, Swiss chard, spinach
- Calcium: milk, dried figs, Swiss cheese, yogurt, tofu
- Phosphorus: plain nonfat yogurt, lentils, salmon, milk, halibut

Consult with your physician before making any changes to your diet or supplemental regimen.

FROVATRIPTAN (froe-vuh-TRIP-tan)

Brand Name: Frova

About Frovatriptan

We really don't know what causes migraine headaches. Arteries in the brain may widen and narrow inappropriately, the flow of blood through the brain may be altered, and pain receptors may be stimulated. Although all of these things happen and all are undoubtedly important pieces of the puzzle, we can't yet fit them together.

This much we do know: Migraines hurt, with the pain ranging from moderate to incapacitating, and movement, light, sounds, or smells often make the pain even worse.

But pain isn't the only problem. Migraine headaches may be preceded by an aura, which includes odd visual sensations (flashing lights, zigzagging lines) and, in some cases, difficulty with balance or speech. There may also be nausea and mood changes—who wouldn't be depressed if her head was pounding and movement or sound made her want to vomit?

There are several treatments for migraines. Some of these are effective, but none of them actually cures the underlying problem(s).

Frovatriptan is prescribed to prevent migraines, although no one knows exactly how it works. (This isn't surprising since we don't know exactly what it's supposed to fix.) However, we do know that the drug binds to certain receptor sites for specific nerves in the head, forcing key blood vessels to constrict and release fewer substances that may be encouraging the migraine.

Possible Side Effects

The drug's more common side effects include dizziness, fatigue, headache, flushing, and hot or cold sensations.

Which Nutrients Are Robbed

Taking this medicine may deplete your supply of, increase your need for, or interfere with the activity of:

- Calcium

Additional Ways This Drug May Upset Your Nutritional Balance

Frovatriptan can cause low blood sugar (hypoglycemia), abdominal pain, heartburn, and nausea, all of which can upset your eating habits and possibly interfere with good nutrition. It can also cause diarrhea, which can hamper nutrient absorption.

Restoring Your Nutritional Balance

To compensate for the nutrient loss caused by this drug, speak to your physician about taking 1,200 mg calcium per day.

You can also eat foods that contain the depleted nutrient:

• Calcium: milk, dried figs, Swiss cheese, yogurt, tofu

Consult with your physician before making any changes to your diet or supplemental regimen.

FUROSEMIDE (fyoor-OH-se-mide)

Brand Names: Apo-Furosemide, Furoside, Lasix, Lasix Special

About Furosemide

There are many reasons why you might find yourself with too much calcium in your bloodstream (a condition called hypercalcemia). It could be due to a problem with your bones, your body's storehouse for calcium. Certain tumors and thyroid problems can make your bones lose their grip on calcium, which then migrates into the bloodstream. Excess calcium in the blood can also be caused by taking certain drugs or large amounts of calcium and vitamin D supplements, or by long periods of immobilization.

When blood levels of calcium rise above normal, there may be muscle weakness, confusion, and lack of appetite. If calcium levels continue to increase, delirium, abnormal heart rhythms, coma, and even death can result.

For certain emergency cases, the treatment includes a salt-water solution plus furosemide, a diuretic that encourages the kidneys to send extra fluid to the bladder for excretion, taking calcium along with it. Furosemide is also used to release the excess fluid seen in congestive heart failure, elevated blood pressure, and certain cases of kidney or liver disease.

Possible Side Effects

The drug's side effects include dizziness, fever, restlessness, stomach upset, and muscle spasms.

Which Nutrients Are Robbed

Taking this medicine may deplete your supply of, increase your need for, or interfere with the activity of:

- Thiamin
- Vitamin B$_6$
- Vitamin C
- Calcium
- Chloride
- Magnesium
- Phosphorus
- Potassium
- Sodium
- Zinc

Additional Ways This Drug May Upset Your Nutritional Balance

Furosemide can cause nausea, vomiting, loss of appetite, and oral and gastric irritation, all of which can upset your eating habits and possibly interfere with good nutrition. It can also cause diarrhea, which can hamper nutrient absorption.

Restoring Your Nutritional Balance

To compensate for the nutrient loss caused by this drug, speak to your physician about taking 25–100 mg thiamin, 50–100 mg vitamin B$_6$, 250–1,500 mg vitamin C, 500–1,000 mg magnesium, 700 mg phosphorus, and 50–200 mg zinc per day. And ask your physician to consider the potential effects of sodium and chloride depletion, and whether you should be getting extra calcium via food or supplements.

A Note on Potassium: "Regular" diuretics lower potassium levels, while potassium-sparing diuretics do not—they may increase levels instead. It is not uncommon for doctors to prescribe two different diuretics. That's why you should speak to your physician about your potassium levels, and whether it is appropriate for you to take supplements or eat potassium-rich foods.

You can also eat foods that contain the depleted nutrients:

- Thiamin: braised liver, turkey heart, roasted chicken, gefilte fish, sardines
- Vitamin B$_6$: potato, banana, garbanzo beans, chicken breast, fortified oatmeal
- Vitamin C: papaya, guava, red pepper, cantaloupe, black currants
- Magnesium: Florida avocado, toasted wheat germ, almonds, shredded wheat cereal, pumpkin seeds
- Phosphorus: plain nonfat yogurt, lentils, salmon, milk, halibut
- Zinc: oysters, beef shank, chicken, pork tenderloin, plain yogurt

Consult with your physician before making any changes to your diet or supplemental regimen.

GATIFLOXACIN (ga-ti-FLOKS-uh-sin)

Brand Name: Tequin

About Gatifloxacin

The air you inhale moves through your nose or mouth and into your main airway, called the windpipe or trachea. As the air travels downward into the chest, the trachea branches into two smaller airways called *bronchi*, each of which leads directly into a lung. There the bronchi split into smaller and smaller branches, eventually becoming millions of tiny airways called bronchioles, some of which are only half a millimeter wide.

Naturally, you want to keep airways of all sizes as wide open as possible so air can move easily in and out of your lungs. But the airflow can be disrupted by a chronic inflammation of the bronchi (bronchitis), in which the smaller branches of the bronchial tree secrete excessive amounts of mucous, become inflamed, and go into spasm. The problem can be made worse by invading bacteria, resulting in difficulty breathing and a long-standing, sputum-producing cough.

Gatifloxacin is one of the antibiotics used for chronic bronchitis worsened by the invasion of bacteria. The drug works by preventing bacteria from manufacturing new DNA as part of their replication process.

Gatifloxacin is also used to treat gonorrhea and certain infections of the urinary tract and rectum.

Possible Side Effects

The drug's more common side effects include vaginitis, diarrhea, headache, and dizziness.

Which Nutrients Are Robbed

Taking this medicine may deplete your supply of, increase your need for, or interfere with the activity of:

- Biotin
- Inositol
- Thiamin
- Riboflavin
- Niacin
- Vitamin B_6
- Vitamin B_{12}
- Vitamin K
- Zinc
- *Bifidobacterium bifidum*
- *Lactobacillus acidophilus*

Additional Ways This Drug May Upset Your Nutritional Balance

Gatifloxacin can cause low blood sugar (hypoglycemia) and nausea, which can upset your eating habits and possibly interfere with good nutrition. It can also cause diarrhea, which can hamper nutrient absorption.

Restoring Your Nutritional Balance

To compensate for the nutrient loss caused by this drug, speak to your physician about taking 500–1,000 mcg biotin, 250–1,000 mg inositol, 25–100 mg thiamin, 25–100 mg riboflavin, 50–100 mg niacin, 50–100 mg vitamin B_6, 500–1,000 mcg vitamin B_{12}, 60–80 mcg vitamin K, 50–200 mg zinc, 15 billion live *Bifidobacterium bifidum* organisms, and 15 billion live *Lactobacillus acidophilus* organisms per day.

You can also eat foods that contain the depleted nutrients:

- Biotin: beef liver, soybeans, rice bran, peanut butter, barley
- Inositol: cantaloupe, oranges, green beans, grapefruit juice, limes
- Thiamin: braised liver, turkey heart, roasted chicken, gefilte fish, sardines
- Riboflavin: dried sunflower seeds, orange juice, bulgur, spinach noodles, pine nuts
- Niacin: chicken breast, beef liver, mackerel, barley, bulgur
- Vitamin B_6: potato, banana, garbanzo beans, chicken breast, fortified oatmeal
- Vitamin B_{12}: beef liver, rainbow trout, sockeye salmon, beef, haddock
- Vitamin K: kale, broccoli, parsley, Swiss chard, spinach
- Zinc: oysters, beef shank, chicken, pork tenderloin, plain yogurt
- *Bifidobacterium bifidum*: Jerusalem artichokes, asparagus, garlic, and onions may stimulate the growth or activity of this probiotic
- *Lactobacillus acidophilus*: yogurt containing live lactobacillus cultures, kefir, acidophilus milk

Consult with your physician before making any changes to your diet or supplemental regimen.

GEMFIBROZIL (jem-FYE-broe-zil)

Brand Names: Apo-Gemfibrozil, Gen-Fibro, Lopid, Nu-Gemfibrozil

About Gemfibrozil

There's the "total" cholesterol, the "good" cholesterol, the "bad" cholesterol, and the "no-one-ever-gave-it-a-nickname" cholesterol.

The total cholesterol is the number your doctor typically tells you about after your annual exam, perhaps frowning if it's above 200 and smiling if it's below 200. The total cholesterol is sort of a summation of the levels of cholesterol and fat in your blood.

The good cholesterol is the HDL, or high density lipoprotein. Made up of protein, cholesterol, and a little bit of fat, HDL carries cholesterol out of body tissues and to the liver for processing and removal.

The bad cholesterol is the LDL, or low density lipoprotein. Made up of a large amount of cholesterol, plus protein and fats, LDL's job is to take cholesterol to various body cells. Unfortunately, it also carries cholesterol to the artery walls, where the cholesterol tends to stick and cause atherosclerosis (hardening the arteries).

The no-one-ever-gave-it-a-nickname cholesterol is VLDL, or very low density lipoprotein. Full of fats, plus smaller amounts of cholesterol and protein, it carries fat from the liver to the body cells.

You can think of total cholesterol as something that can trigger heart disease if found in excess, and of LDL and VLDL as little buses that transport cholesterol and fat around the body. You want to keep your cholesterol, LDL, and VLDL down to safe levels.

On the other hand, you want to have plenty of HDL, which serves as a sort of garbage truck for cholesterol, picking it up and taking it to the liver for deposition and removal.

Gemfibrozil helps control excess cholesterol. It seems to work by slowing the liver's release of VLDL. It also lowers LDL somewhat, and pushes up the HDL.

Gemfibrozil is usually prescribed for those with high cholesterol and high blood fat levels.

Possible Side Effects

The drug's more common side effects include stomach upset, fatigue, vertigo, and eczema.

Which Nutrients Are Robbed

Taking this medicine may deplete your supply of, increase your need for, or interfere with the activity of:

- Vitamin E
- Potassium
- Coenzyme Q_{10}

Additional Ways This Drug May Upset Your Nutritional Balance

Gemfibrozil can cause heartburn, abdominal pain, nausea, and vomiting, all of which can upset your eating habits and possibly interfere with good nutrition. It can also cause diarrhea, which can hamper nutrient absorption.

Restoring Your Nutritional Balance

To compensate for the nutrient loss caused by this drug, speak to your physician about taking 400 IU vitamin E, 30–100 mg coenzyme Q_{10}, and 100–300 mg potassium per day.

You can also eat foods that contain the depleted nutrients:

- Vitamin E: wheat germ oil, almonds, safflower oil, corn oil, soybean oil
- Coenzyme Q_{10}: beef, chicken, trout, salmon, oranges, broccoli
- Potassium: dried figs, California avocado, papaya, banana, dates

Consult with your physician before making any changes to your diet or supplemental regimen.

GEMTUZUMAB OZOGAMICIN (gem-TOO-ze-mab oh-zoe-GAM-i-sin)

Brand Name: Mylotarg

About Gemtuzumab Ozogamicin

Chemotherapy drugs have added years to the lives of countless cancer patients. But their serious side effects have sometimes made patients wonder if going through the treatment was worth it.

Pharmaceutical companies are currently testing new cancer drugs that are more powerful and better able to zero in on the cancer cells, while leaving the healthy ones alone. One of the newer approaches adopts the action of the immune system's antibodies.

Antibodies are biological weapons designed to seek out and destroy specific bacteria, viruses, and other invaders. The antibodies distinguish between friend and foe by looking for particular features on the invading cell.

Gemtuzumab ozogamicin uses the same strategy by combining an antibody with an antitumor drug. It specifically looks for the CD33 antibody that's found on cancerous white blood cells in over 80 percent of those who have acute myeloid leukemia. The antibody binds to the cancerous cell, which allows the antitumor drug to enter the cell, bind to its DNA, and destroy it.

Gemtuzumab ozogamicin is used to treat acute myeloid leukemia in senior citizens who have not been helped by chemotherapy or who have suffered a remission.

Possible Side Effects

The drug's more common side effects include lowered or elevated blood pressure, fever, chills, and headache.

Which Nutrients Are Robbed

Taking this medicine may deplete your supply of, increase your need for, or interfere with the activity of:

- Magnesium
- Potassium

Additional Ways This Drug May Upset Your Nutritional Balance

Gemtuzumab ozogamicin can cause nausea, vomiting, loss of appetite, and abdominal pain, all of which can upset your eating habits and possibly interfere with good nutrition. It can also cause diarrhea, which can hamper nutrient absorption.

Restoring Your Nutritional Balance

To compensate for the nutrient loss caused by this drug, speak to your physician about taking 500–1,000 mg magnesium and 100–300 mg potassium per day.

You can also eat foods that contain the depleted nutrients:

- Magnesium: Florida avocado, toasted wheat germ, almonds, shredded wheat cereal, pumpkin seeds
- Potassium: dried figs, California avocado, papaya, banana, dates

Consult with your physician before making any changes to your diet or supplemental regimen.

GENTAMICIN (jen-tuh-MYE-sin)

Brand Names: Garamycin, G-Mycin, Jenamicin

About Gentamicin

Because the bones are well protected by the skin and the immune system, they don't often become infected. But when they do, the bone marrow may swell and press against the blood vessels in the bone. If the blood flow in those vessels either slows appreciably or stops, parts of the bone may die.

Bones can become infected via an invading organism in the blood or when an infection in nearby tissues moves into them. Joint replacement surgery may also be the culprit: Bacteria or fungi in nearby areas can be swept into the bone as holes are drilled and artificial parts are attached. Symptoms of a bone infection include pain, swelling, discomfort with movement, fatigue, and fever, among other things.

Gentamicin is used to treat bone infections and severe bacterial infections that won't respond to other antibiotics. If treated promptly, a bone infection can be eliminated. If not, it can become chronic, spread to adjacent soft tissue, and cause pus to drain through openings in the skin.

Possible Side Effects

Gentamicin's more common side effects include vertigo, unstable gait, and hearing and kidney damage.

Which Nutrients Are Robbed

Taking this medicine may deplete your supply of, increase your need for, or interfere with the activity of:

- Biotin
- Inositol
- Thiamin
- Riboflavin
- Niacin
- Vitamin B_6
- Vitamin B_{12}
- Vitamin K
- Calcium
- Magnesium
- Potassium
- Sodium
- *Bifidobacterium bifidum*
- *Lactobacillus acidophilus*

Restoring Your Nutritional Balance

To compensate for the nutrient loss caused by this drug, speak to your physician about taking 500–1,000 mcg biotin, 250–1,000 mg inositol, 25–100

mg thiamin, 25–100 mg riboflavin, 50–100 mg niacin, 50–100 mg vitamin B_6, 500–1,000 mcg vitamin B_{12}, 60–80 mcg vitamin K, 1,200 mg calcium, 500–1,000 mg magnesium, 100–300 mg potassium, 15 billion live *Bifidobacterium bifidum* organisms, and 15 billion live *Lactobacillus acidophilus* organisms per day. And ask your physician to consider the potential effects of sodium depletion.

You can also eat foods that contain the depleted nutrients:

- Biotin: beef liver, soybeans, rice bran, peanut butter, barley
- Inositol: cantaloupe, oranges, green beans, grapefruit juice, limes
- Thiamin: braised liver, turkey heart, roasted chicken, gefilte fish, sardines
- Riboflavin: dried sunflower seeds, orange juice, bulgur, spinach noodles, pine nuts
- Niacin: chicken breast, beef liver, mackerel, barley, bulgur
- Vitamin B_6: potato, banana, garbanzo beans, chicken breast, fortified oatmeal
- Vitamin B_{12}: beef liver, rainbow trout, sockeye salmon, beef, haddock
- Vitamin K: kale, broccoli, parsley, Swiss chard, spinach
- Calcium: milk, dried figs, Swiss cheese, yogurt, tofu
- Magnesium: Florida avocado, toasted wheat germ, almonds, shredded wheat cereal, pumpkin seeds
- Potassium: dried figs, California avocado, papaya, banana, dates
- *Bifidobacterium bifidum*: Jerusalem artichokes, asparagus, garlic, and onions may stimulate the growth or activity of this probiotic
- *Lactobacillus acidophilus*: yogurt containing live lactobacillus cultures, kefir, acidophilus milk

Consult with your physician before making any changes to your diet or supplemental regimen.

GLYBURIDE, GLIMEPIRIDE, GLIPIZIDE (GLYE-byoor-ide, GLYE-me-per-ride, GLIP-i-zide)

Brand Names: Glyburide: Albert Glyburide, Apo-Glyburide, DiaBeta, Euglucon, Gen-Glybe, Glynase, Med-Glybe, Micronase, Novo-Glyburide, Nu-Glyburide
Glimepiride: Amaryl
Glipizide: Glucotrol, Glucotrol XL

About Glyburide, Glimepiride, and Glipizide

These three drugs are the "new and improved," second-generation versions of the sulfonylureas, drugs that have long been used to treat type 2 diabetes by encouraging the pancreas to produce more of the hormone insulin.

Millions of Americans have developed insulin resistance, which means that certain body cells don't respond well to insulin's request to "open up" and accept blood sugar for fuel or storage. To understand how insulin works, imagine being locked in a room without any food. The only way you can get food is through the local grocery store's delivery service. Luckily, the delivery boy has the key to your room and a plentiful supply of food. But when he comes to deliver the food, he can't make the key work because the big lock on your door has become rusty. No matter how hard he tries, the delivery boy just can't seem to turn the lock and open the door. Once in a while, he gets lucky, but even then he can open the door only enough to shove a few groceries inside. But you can't get everything that you need. Eventually you starve to death because you simply can't get enough food.

Something similar happens with type 2 diabetes. The blood sugar is delivered, but the delivery boy (insulin) has trouble opening the "locks" on the cell membranes, so he can't get sufficient glucose into the cells.

These three drugs—glyburide, glipizide, and glimepiride—help the body open those rusty locks by stimulating the production of additional insulin. With extra men on the job, insulin may be able to spring the rusty locks and deliver the goods.

Glyburide, glipizide, and glimepiride are all used to treat type 2 diabetes. One may be chosen over the others depending on how long it keeps working in the body, the side effects it's likely to trigger, and your specific needs.

Possible Side Effects

Glyburide's side effects include headache, dizziness, and hepatitis. Glipizide's side effects include rash and sensitivity to light. Glimepiride's more common side effects include headache, dizziness, and nausea.

Which Nutrients Are Robbed

Taking these medicines may deplete your supply of, increase your need for, or interfere with the activity of:

- Sodium
- Coenzyme Q_{10}

Additional Ways These Drugs May Upset Your Nutritional Balance

Glimepiride can cause low blood sugar (hypoglycemia) and nausea. Glipizide can cause hypoglycemia, loss of appetite, heartburn, nausea, and vomiting. Glyburide can cause hypoglycemia, heartburn, loss of appetite, and nausea. All of these side effects can upset your eating habits and possibly interfere with good nutrition.

Both glipizide and glyburide can also cause diarrhea, which can hamper nutrient absorption.

Restoring Your Nutritional Balance

To compensate for the nutrient loss caused by these drugs, speak to your physician about taking 30–100 mg coenzyme Q_{10} per day. And ask your physician to consider the potential effects of sodium depletion.

You can also eat foods that contain the depleted nutrient:

- Coenzyme Q_{10}: beef, chicken, trout, salmon, oranges, broccoli

Consult with your physician before making any changes to your diet or supplemental regimen.

GLYBURIDE PLUS METFORMIN (GLYE-byoor-ide, met-FOR-min)

Brand Name: Glucovance

About Glyburide plus Metformin

Imagine that the sanitation trucks in your city aren't very good at emptying the trash cans, so the waste piles up and sits on the street for a long time. The city could respond by acquiring and sending out more trash trucks. Although these new trucks might not be any better than the old ones, just the fact that there are more of them will mean that more trash can be cleared away.

Using glyburide to treat type 2 diabetes is like putting more trucks on the job. With type 2 diabetes, the insulin that ferries the body's fuel (glucose) into the cells can't do its job as well as it should, for the cells have become resistant to it. Glyburide helps overcome this problem by stimulating the pancreas to produce larger amounts of insulin in order to get more glucose into the cells. More insulin, just like more trucks, helps ensure that the job gets done.

Metformin is also used to treat diabetes but has other means of attack. It appears to help remove excess glucose from the blood and simultaneously slow the release of more glucose.

To learn more about these drugs, read the separate entries on glyburide and metformin on pages 295 and 360.

Possible Side Effects

Glyburide's side effects include headache, dizziness, and hepatitis. Metformin's side effects include diarrhea, nausea, bloating, and an unpleasant taste in the mouth.

Which Nutrients Are Robbed

Taking this medicine may deplete your supply of, increase your need for, or interfere with the activity of:

- Folic acid
- Vitamin B_{12}
- Sodium
- Coenzyme Q_{10}

Additional Ways These Drugs May Upset Your Nutritional Balance

Glyburide can cause low blood sugar (hypoglycemia), nausea, heartburn, and loss of appetite. Metformin can trigger nausea, vomiting, indigestion, abdominal discomfort, heartburn, and changes in taste. All of these side effects can upset your eating habits and possibly interfere with good nutrition. Both glyburide and metformin can also cause diarrhea, which can hamper nutrient absorption.

Restoring Your Nutritional Balance

To compensate for the nutrient loss caused by this drug, speak to your physician about taking 400–800 mcg folic acid, 500–1,000 mcg vitamin B_{12}, and 30–100 mg coenzyme Q_{10} per day. And ask your physician to consider the potential effects of sodium depletion.

You can also eat foods that contain the depleted nutrients:

- Folic acid: beef liver, fortified breakfast cereals, spinach, great northern beans, asparagus
- Vitamin B_{12}: beef liver, rainbow trout, sockeye salmon, beef, haddock
- Coenzyme Q_{10}: beef, chicken, trout, salmon, oranges, broccoli

Consult with your physician before making any changes to your diet or supplemental regimen.

GRISEOFULVIN (gri-see-oh-FUL-vin)

Brand Names: Fulvicin, Grifulvin V, Grisactin, Gris-PEG

About Griseofulvin

We've all seen those commercials showing some poor guy taking off his shoes in the locker room and sadly examining his itching, burning feet. He's suffering from what doctors call *tinea pedis,* better known as athlete's foot. A common problem caused by fungi found in communal showers or other areas where people walk barefoot, athlete's foot causes redness, cracking of the skin, and fluid-filled blisters, in addition to the itching and burning.

Griseofulvin, a derivative of penicillin, is used to treat severe cases of athlete's foot. Although we don't know exactly how this medicine works, we do know that it finds its way into newly forming skin and prevents fungal infections from taking hold. So instead of destroying old infections, as some antifungal medications do, griseofulvin helps prevent new ones. Because it can take anywhere from a few weeks to a few months for old, infected skin, nails, or hair to be shed and replaced, it takes at least that long for griseofulvin to produce results.

Possible Side Effects

The drug's side effects include rash, skin eruptions (urticaria), confusion, and menstrual irregularities.

Which Nutrients Are Robbed

Taking this medicine may deplete your supply of, increase your need for, or interfere with the activity of:

- Vitamin K

Additional Ways This Drug May Upset Your Nutritional Balance

Griseofulvin can cause nausea and vomiting, which can upset your eating habits and possibly interfere with good nutrition. It can also cause diarrhea, which can hamper nutrient absorption.

Restoring Your Nutritional Balance

To compensate for the nutrient loss caused by this drug, speak to your physician about taking 60–80 mcg vitamin K per day.

You can also eat foods that contain the depleted nutrient:

• Vitamin K: kale, broccoli, parsley, Swiss chard, spinach

Consult with your physician before making any changes to your diet or supplemental regimen.

HALOPERIDOL (hal-oh-PER-i-dole)

Brand Names: Haldol, Haldol Decanoate, Peridol, Novo-Peridol

About Haloperidol

Tourette's syndrome is a baffling disease. For unknown reasons, a person may begin to display muscular tics. But not just simple tics that vanish with time, like tightening a cheek muscle. Instead, the tic is a complex pattern of movements that may include rolling the head from side to side, opening and closing the mouth, and stretching the neck. Next might come vocal tics: snorting, humming, and/or barking, which can progress to cursing. Unexplained and unmotivated hitting, kicking, and other inappropriate behavior may also develop. This inappropriate behavior makes it difficult for those with Tourette's to function in society, which may explain why children with Tourette's have a hard time learning, while adults can become aggressive and self-destructive.

Clonidine and other drugs typically are prescribed for milder cases of Tourette's, but in more severe cases, an antipsychotic drug called haloperidol may be used. Haloperidol affects the way the neurotransmitter dopamine is handled in the central nervous system, which may be the way this drug combats the tics of Tourette's.

In addition to Tourette's, haloperidol is used to treat schizophrenia and may be prescribed for children with severe behavioral problems.

Possible Side Effects

The drug's side effects include anxiety, agitation, irregular heartbeat, and blurred vision.

Which Nutrients Are Robbed

Taking this medicine may deplete your supply of, increase your need for, or interfere with the activity of:

- Sodium
- Coenzyme Q_{10}

Additional Ways These Drugs May Upset Your Nutritional Balance

Haloperidol can cause low blood sugar (hypoglycemia), nausea, vomiting, and loss of appetite, all of which can upset your eating habits and possibly interfere with good nutrition. It can also cause diarrhea, which can hamper nutrient absorption.

Restoring Your Nutritional Balance

To compensate for the nutrient loss caused by this drug, speak to your physician about taking 30–100 mg coenzyme Q_{10} per day. And ask your physician to consider the potential effects of sodium depletion.

You can also eat foods that contain the depleted nutrient:

- Coenzyme Q_{10}: beef, chicken, trout, salmon, oranges, broccoli

Consult with your physician before making any changes to your diet or supplemental regimen.

HEPARIN (HEP-uh-rin)

Brand Names: Calcilean, Calciparine, Hepalean, Hep-Lock, Liquaemin

About Heparin

Coagulation—stopping the bleeding—is a complex process involving platelets and clotting factors. This built-in, step-by-step procedure literally turns liquid into solid and can be a lifesaver when you cut yourself. Yet it can also threaten your life if your blood "solidifies" at the wrong time and produces a blood clot that triggers a heart attack, stroke, or other problem. A blood clot can also cause the sudden blockage of the pulmonary artery. If that happens, blood flow to an area of the lung will be slowed or stopped and lung tissue may die.

Unwanted blood clots can form for various reasons, one of which is inactivity. Sitting for hours during a very long airplane ride raises the odds of developing a blood clot. Surgery is another cause of blood clots, especially in older people, as is kidney dialysis.

To help prevent such blood clots, doctors may prescribe heparin. Although the drug doesn't stop the clotting process directly, it does spur the activity of one of the body's natural anticlotting substances, antithrombin III. Normally, antithrombin III works rather slowly, but heparin puts it into high gear, causing it to work about 1,000 times faster.

Possible Side Effects

The drug's side effects include unexplained bruising, a persistent erection, blood in the urine, and bleeding from the gums.

Which Nutrients Are Robbed

Taking this medicine may deplete your supply of, increase your need for, or interfere with the activity of:

- Vitamin D
- Calcium

Additional Ways This Drug May Upset Your Nutritional Balance

Heparin can cause nausea and vomiting, which can upset your eating habits and possibly interfere with good nutrition.

This drug can also trigger hyperkalemia, or too much potassium in the blood.

Restoring Your Nutritional Balance

To compensate for the nutrient loss caused by this drug, speak to your physician about taking 400 IU vitamin D and 1,200 mg calcium per day.

You can also eat foods that contain the depleted nutrients:

- Vitamin D: salmon, mackerel, sardines, eel, fortified milk
- Calcium: milk, dried figs, Swiss cheese, yogurt, tofu

Consult with your physician before making any changes to your diet or supplemental regimen.

HYDRALAZINE, HYDRALAZINE PLUS HYDROCHLOROTHIAZIDE (hye-DRAL-uh-zeen, hye-droe-klor-oh-THYE-uh-zide)

Brand Names: Hydralazine: Apo-Hydral, Apresoline, Novo-Hylazin
Hydralazine plus hydrochlorothiazide: Apresazide

About Hydralazine, Hydralazine plus Hydrochlorothiazide

Hydralazine, which widens the smaller arteries known as arterioles, is used to treat moderate or severe hypertension, as well as congestive heart failure.

High blood pressure is, in some ways, like heavy traffic: too many cars trying to move down a road that's only so wide. But imagine what would happen if the road suddenly widened, adding two or three extra lanes. The congestion would clear, cars would travel faster, and the pressure exerted by heavy traffic would ease. Hydralazine works in a similar manner, getting the arteries to widen a bit, which makes arterial roadways easier to travel and lowers the blood pressure.

In many cases, physicians find that they produce better results for their patients by combining two kinds of blood pressure medication, sometimes within the same pill. That's the case with hydralazine plus hydrochlorothiazide. While hydralazine "opens" the arteries, hydrochlorothiazide (a diuretic) helps the body excrete fluid. Going back to our traffic analogy, we can say that hydralazine makes the roadway wider, while hydrochlorothiazide diverts some of the traffic off the road. More lanes plus fewer cars equals a lot less congestion. (For more information, see the entry on hydrochlorothiazide on page 304.)

Possible Side Effects

Hydralazine's side effects include rapid heartbeat, rash, and impotence. Hydrochlorothiazide's more common side effects include low blood pressure and skin sensitivity to light.

Which Nutrients Are Robbed

Taking these medicines may deplete your supply of, increase your need for, or interfere with the activity of:

Hydralazine: vitamin B_6, magnesium, potassium, zinc, coenzyme Q_{10}
Hydralazine plus hydrochlorothiazide: vitamin B_6, magnesium, phosphorus, potassium, sodium, zinc, coenzyme Q_{10}

Additional Ways These Drugs May Upset Your Nutritional Balance

Hydralazine can cause loss of appetite, nausea, and vomiting, while hydrochlorothiazide can cause loss of appetite. These side effects can upset your eating habits and possibly interfere with good nutrition. Hydralazine can also cause diarrhea, which can hamper nutrient absorption.

Restoring Your Nutritional Balance

To compensate for the nutrient loss caused by these drugs, speak to your physician about taking 50–100 mg vitamin B_6, 500–1,000 mg magnesium, 700 mg phosphorus, 50–200 mg zinc, and 30–100 mg coenzyme Q_{10} per day. And ask your physician to consider the potential effects of sodium depletion.

A Note on Potassium: "Regular" diuretics lower potassium levels, while potassium-sparing diuretics do not—they may increase levels instead. It is not uncommon for doctors to prescribe two different diuretics. That's why you should speak to your physician about your potassium levels, and whether it is appropriate for you to take supplements or eat potassium-rich foods.

You can also eat foods that contain the depleted nutrients:

- Vitamin B_6: potato, banana, garbanzo beans, chicken breast, fortified oatmeal
- Magnesium: Florida avocado, toasted wheat germ, almonds, shredded wheat cereal, pumpkin seeds
- Phosphorus: plain nonfat yogurt, lentils, salmon, milk, halibut
- Zinc: oysters, beef shank, chicken, pork tenderloin, plain yogurt
- Coenzyme Q_{10}: beef, chicken, trout, salmon, oranges, broccoli

Consult with your physician before making any changes to your diet or supplemental regimen.

HYDROCHLOROTHIAZIDE, HYDROCHLOROTHIAZIDE PLUS SPIRONOLACTONE, HYDROCHLOROTHIAZIDE PLUS TRIAMTERENE (hye-droe-klor-oh-THYE-uh-zide, speer-on-oh-LAK-tohn, trye-AM-ter-een)

Brand Names: Hydrochlorothiazide: Apo-Hydro, Diuchlor H, Esidrix, Hydrochlor, Hydro-D, Microzide, Neo-Codema, Oretic, Urozide
Hydrochlorothiazide plus spironolactone: Aldactazide, Novo-Spirozine, Spirozide

Hydrochlorothiazide plus triamterene: Apo-Triazide, Dyazide, Maxzide, Novo-triamzide

About Hydrochlorothiazide and Its Companions

A simple way to reduce elevated blood pressure (hypertension) is to flush some of the fluid out of the body—that's something like relieving the pressure in an overinflated tire by letting some of the air out. Unfortunately, we don't have little valves that we can open to release excess fluid. Instead, doctors prescribe drugs called diuretics that encourage the body to send extra fluid to the bladder for excretion. This translates to a reduction in blood volume, which, in turn, cuts down on the heart's workload and lowers blood pressure.

Hydrochlorothiazide is one of the thiazide diuretics, a group of medicines that help the body release fluid by interfering with the reabsorption of sodium and chloride in the kidneys. Besides treating high blood pressure, hydrochlorothiazide is used to ease the fluid buildup seen in congestive heart failure and to treat a kidney problem called *nephritic syndrome.* This disease, which can be caused by a bacterial, viral, or parasitic infection, damages the kidneys, causing fluid retention, blood in the urine, and elevated blood pressure.

Since hydrochlorothiazide can flush too much potassium out of the body along with the extra fluid, it's sometimes combined with spironolactone or triamterene, two potassium-sparing diuretics that help the body hold on to this important mineral.

Possible Side Effects

Hydrochlorothiazide's more common side effects include low blood pressure and sensitivity to light. Spironolactone's side effects include drowsiness, impotence, and enlargement of the breasts in males (*gynecomastia*). Triamterene's side effects include excessively high potassium levels and kidney stones.

Which Nutrients Are Robbed

Taking these medicines may deplete your supply of, increase your need for, or interfere with the activity of:

- *Hydrochlorothiazide:* vitamin D, calcium, magnesium, phosphorus, potassium, sodium, zinc, coenzyme Q_{10}
- *Hydrochlorothiazide plus spironolactone:* magnesium, phosphorus, sodium, zinc, coenzyme Q_{10}
- *Hydrochlorothiazide plus triamterene:* folic acid, vitamin B_6, calcium, magnesium, sodium, zinc, coenzyme Q_{10}

Additional Ways These Drugs May Upset Your Nutritional Balance

Hydrochlorothiazide can cause loss of appetite, while spironolactone can trigger loss of appetite, nausea, and vomiting. These side effects can upset your eating habits and possibly interfere with good nutrition. Spironolactone can cause diarrhea, which may interfere with nutrient absorption.

Both spironolactone and triamterene can cause hyperkalemia, or too much potassium in the blood.

Restoring Your Nutritional Balance

To compensate for the nutrient loss caused by *hydrochlorothiazide*, speak to your physician about taking 400 IU vitamin D, 1,200 mg calcium, 500–1,000 mg magnesium, 700 mg phosphorus, 50–200 mg zinc, and 30–100 mg coenzyme Q_{10} per day. And ask your physician to consider the potential effects of sodium depletion.

To compensate for the nutrient loss caused by *hydrochlorothiazide plus spironolactone*, speak to your physician about taking 500–1,000 mg magnesium, 700 mg phosphorus, 50–200 mg zinc, and 30–100 mg coenzyme Q_{10} per day. And ask your physician to consider the potential effects of sodium depletion.

To compensate for the nutrient loss caused by *hydrochlorothiazide plus triamterene,* speak to your physician about taking 400–800 mcg folic acid, 50–100 mg vitamin B_6, 1,200 mg calcium, 500–1,000 mg magnesium, 50–200 mg zinc, and 30–100 mg coenzyme Q_{10} per day. And ask your physician to consider the potential effects of sodium depletion.

A Note on Potassium: "Regular" diuretics lower potassium levels, while potassium-sparing diuretics do not—they may increase levels instead. It is not uncommon for doctors to prescribe two different diuretics. That's why you should speak to your physician about your potassium levels, and whether it is appropriate for you to take supplements or eat potassium-rich foods.

You can also eat foods that contain the depleted nutrients:

- Folic acid: beef liver, fortified breakfast cereals, spinach, great northern beans, asparagus
- Vitamin B_6: potato, banana, garbanzo beans, chicken breast, fortified oatmeal
- Vitamin D: salmon, mackerel, sardines, eel, fortified milk
- Calcium: milk, dried figs, Swiss cheese, yogurt, tofu
- Magnesium: Florida avocado, toasted wheat germ, almonds, shredded wheat cereal, pumpkin seeds
- Phosphorus: plain nonfat yogurt, lentils, salmon, milk, halibut

- Zinc: oysters, beef shank, chicken, pork tenderloin, plain yogurt
- Coenzyme Q_{10}: beef, chicken, trout, salmon, oranges, broccoli

Consult with your physician before making any changes to your diet or supplemental regimen.

HYDROCODONE PLUS ACETAMINOPHEN (hye-droe-KOE-dohn, uh-seet-uh-MIN-oh-fen)

Brand Names: Anexsia, Anodynos-DHC, Bancap HC, Co-Gesic, Dolacet, DuoCet, Hydrocet, Hydrogesic, Hy-Phen, Lorcet, Lorcet-HD, Lorcet Plus, Lortab, Margesic H, Medipain 5, Norco, Stagesic, T-Gesic, Vapocet, Vicodin, Vicodin ES, Vicodin HP, Zydone

About Hydrocodone plus Acetaminophen

Hydrocodone is an opioid painkiller that works like morphine on the central nervous system. That is, it works by imitating the body's own endorphins.

Endorphins, which are also known as endogenous opioid peptides, are naturally occurring, very powerful painkillers. They work by plugging into specific receptor sites in the nervous system and triggering a "relief" message. Hydrocodone and other morphine-like drugs also plug themselves into these receptors, but trigger weaker "relief" messages. Fortunately, these lesser responses are often good enough. Hydrocodone is typically combined with acetaminophen or another painkiller.

Acetaminophen takes a completely different approach to quelling pain. It slows the production of the prostaglandins that "encourage" pain. (For more on acetaminophen, see the entry on page 90.) The combination of hydrocodone plus acetaminophen is often used to treat moderate to severe pain.

Possible Side Effects

The side effects of hydrocodone plus acetaminophen include low blood pressure, a slow heartbeat, decreased urination, and weakness.

Which Nutrients Are Robbed

Taking this medicine may deplete your supply of, increase your need for, or interfere with the activity of:

- Glutathione

Additional Ways This Drug May Upset Your Nutritional Balance

Hydrocodone and acetaminophen can cause nausea and vomiting, which can upset your eating habits and possibly interfere with good nutrition.

Restoring Your Nutritional Balance

To compensate for the nutrient loss caused by this drug, speak to your physician about taking 800–2,000 mg n-acetyl cysteine (a precursor to glutathione) per day.

Consult with your physician before making any changes to your diet or supplemental regimen.

HYDROCODONE PLUS ASPIRIN (hye-droe-KOE-dohn, ASS-pir-in)

Brand Names: Alor 5/500, Azdone, Damason-P, Lortab ASA, Panasal 5/500

About Hydrocodone plus Aspirin

About 100 years ago, the great physician Sir William Osler said that morphine was "God's own medicine." And indeed, it is a powerful painkiller that's still the gold standard when measuring the effects of other powerful painkillers.

Unfortunately, morphine has side effects—such as drowsiness, dizziness, and nausea—that make it impractical for treating all but the most serious cases of pain. Instead, weaker drugs are often preferred, such as hydrocodone, which travels to the opiate receptors in the central nervous system, "plugs in," and relieves pain. It also suppresses coughs.

The combination of hydrocodone plus aspirin is used to treat moderate to moderately severe pain. Whereas hydrocodone has morphine-like actions that quell pain, aspirin works to inhibit pain and relieve inflammation by interfering with the production of prostaglandins.

Possible Side Effects

The more common side effects seen with the combination of hydrocodone plus aspirin include dizziness, sedation, fatigue, and weakness.

Which Nutrients Are Robbed

Taking this medicine may deplete your supply of, increase your need for, or interfere with the activity of:

- Folic acid
- Vitamin C
- Iron
- Potassium
- Sodium

Additional Ways This Drug May Upset Your Nutritional Balance

Hydrocodone and aspirin can cause vomiting, which can upset your eating habits and possibly interfere with good nutrition.

Aspirin can also trigger hyperkalemia, or too much potassium in the blood.

Restoring Your Nutritional Balance

To compensate for the nutrient loss caused by this drug, speak to your physician about taking 400–800 mcg folic acid and 250–1,500 mg vitamin C per day. And ask your physician to consider the potential effects of iron and sodium depletion and to monitor your potassium status.

You can also eat foods that contain the depleted nutrients:

- Folic acid: beef liver, fortified breakfast cereals, spinach, great northern beans, asparagus
- Vitamin C: papaya, guava, red pepper, cantaloupe, black currants

Consult with your physician before making any changes to your diet or supplemental regimen.

HYDROCORTISONE (hye-droe-KOR-ti-sohn)

Brand Names: A-Hydrocort, Allercort, Bactine, Cortamed, Cortef, Cortril, Emo-Cort, Hydrocortone, Solu-Cortef

About Hydrocortisone

A glucocorticosteroid is a steroid hormone that influences the metabolism of fat, protein, and carbohydrate; encourages the manufacture of RNA and protein in the liver; and "puts a damper" on the inflammation process. Several different glucocorticosteroids are used to treat a variety of diseases, especially those involving inflammation.

Hydrocortisone, the original glucocorticosteroid that you can rub on your skin, was introduced back in 1952. It works by constricting nearby blood vessels, lowering the amount of histamine secreted by immune system cells, and otherwise reducing inflammation and its symptoms. This makes it helpful in treating skin problems that are caused by allergies and immune system reactions.

Hydrocortisone is also used to treat adrenal crisis, which is also known as acute adrenocortical insufficiency. This problem strikes when the adrenal glands cannot make sufficient amounts of the steroid hormone cortisol. When levels of this vital substance fall below normal, you can suffer from abdominal pain, fever, diarrhea, nausea, vomiting, confusion, and low blood pressure. Several things can cause this condition, including: surgery, infection, or another stress; surgical removal of the adrenal glands; and destruction of the pituitary gland, which "gives instructions" to the adrenals.

Hydrocortisone is used to manage acute adrenocortical insufficiency, certain skin conditions, and ulcerative colitis.

Possible Side Effects

The drug's more common side effects include insomnia, nervousness, and increased appetite.

Which Nutrients Are Robbed

Taking this medicine may deplete your supply of, increase your need for, or interfere with the activity of:

- Vitamin A
- Vitamin B$_6$
- Folic acid
- Vitamin C
- Vitamin D
- Calcium
- Magnesium
- Potassium
- Selenium
- Zinc

Additional Ways This Drug May Upset Your Nutritional Balance

Hydrocortisone can cause indigestion, which can upset your eating habits and possibly interfere with good nutrition.

Restoring Your Nutritional Balance

To compensate for the nutrient loss caused by this drug, speak to your physician about taking 5,000 IU vitamin A, 50–100 mg vitamin B$_6$, 400–800 mcg folic acid, 250–1,500 mg vitamin C, 400 IU vitamin D, 1,200 mg calcium, 500–1,000 mg magnesium, 100–300 mg potassium, 20–100 mcg selenium, and 50–200 mg zinc per day.

You can also eat foods that contain the depleted nutrients:

- Vitamin A: beef liver, chicken liver, cheese pizza, whole milk, cheddar cheese
- Vitamin B$_6$: potato, banana, garbanzo beans, chicken breast, fortified oatmeal
- Folic acid: beef liver, fortified breakfast cereals, spinach, great northern beans, asparagus
- Vitamin C: papaya, guava, red pepper, cantaloupe, black currants
- Vitamin D: salmon, mackerel, sardines, eel, fortified milk
- Calcium: milk, dried figs, Swiss cheese, yogurt, tofu
- Magnesium: Florida avocado, toasted wheat germ, almonds, shredded wheat cereal, pumpkin seeds
- Potassium: dried figs, California avocado, papaya, banana, dates
- Selenium: Brazil nuts, tuna, beef liver, turkey breast, spaghetti with meat sauce
- Zinc: oysters, beef shank, chicken, pork tenderloin, plain yogurt

Consult with your physician before making any changes to your diet or supplemental regimen.

IBUPROFEN (eye-byoo-PROE-fen)

Brand Names: Actiprofen, Advil, Advil Migraine Liqui-Gels, Apo-Ibuprofen, Bayer Select Pain Relief Formula, Children's Advil Oral Suspension, Children's Motrin Oral Suspension, Dynafed IB, Genpril, Haltran, IBU, Ibuprin, Ibuprohm, Junior Strength Motrin, Menadol, Midol IB, Motrin, Motrin IB, Motrin Migraine Pain, Novo-Profen, Nu-Ibuprofen, Nuprin, Saleto-200, Saleto-400, Saleto-600, Saleto-800

About Ibuprofen

In 1984, ibuprofen was approved for sale over-the-counter. Sold under a variety of brand names, it quickly became and remains a popular remedy for pain and inflammation.

Ibuprofen is used to treat a variety of conditions causing pain and/or inflammation, including juvenile rheumatoid arthritis, dysmenorrhea, gout, ankylosing spondylitis, and acute migraine headache. It's also helpful in reducing fever.

The drug works by interfering with substances called COX (cyclooxygenase), which produce, among other things, the prostaglandins that play a role in inflammation. Inflammation is one of the body's defenses: When the body is wounded or invaded, it fights back by sending more blood to the affected area and bringing in more immune system cells. These are the body's army: macrophages that engulf and destroy invaders, neutrophils that engage the enemy in hand-to-hand combat, antibodies that learn how to target specific invaders, and others. The whole purpose is to clean up the mess caused by an injury or, if germs have invaded, to destroy the enemy.

The inflammation process is helpful, but it can be painful. And sometimes it goes on too long or occurs without a good reason. Ibuprofen helps reduce inflammation indirectly, by hindering the production of the prostaglandins that serve as the "bugle call" for the whole process. In real-life terms, this would be like destroying your enemy's telephones and radios so the opposing general can't give his troops the order to advance.

Possible Side Effects

The drug's more common side effects include headache, fluid retention, rash, and nervousness.

Which Nutrients Are Robbed

Taking this medicine may deplete your supply of, increase your need for, or interfere with the activity of:

• Folic acid

Additional Ways This Drug May Upset Your Nutritional Balance

Ibuprofen can cause nausea, vomiting, peptic ulcer, heartburn, and indigestion, all of which can upset your eating habits and possibly interfere with good nutrition.

Restoring Your Nutritional Balance

To compensate for the nutrient loss caused by this drug, speak to your physician about taking 400–800 mcg folic acid per day.

You can also eat foods that contain the depleted nutrient:

• Folic acid: beef liver, fortified breakfast cereals, spinach, great northern beans, asparagus

Consult with your physician before making any changes to your diet or supplemental regimen.

IMATINIB (i-MAT-in-ib)

Brand Name: Gleevec

About Imatinib

In chronic myeloid leukemia (CML), the bone marrow produces cancerous white blood cells that, instead of defending the body against invaders, eventually fill up much of the available space in the bone marrow and crowd out other developing blood cells. In time, these cancerous white blood cells spill over into the bloodstream.

In the early stages, CML may produce fatigue, weakness, weight loss, or other symptoms—or may not trigger any symptoms at all. But as the disease advances, a blast crisis will inevitably develop.

During a blast crisis, the bone marrow produces large numbers of immature white blood cells, but not enough red blood cells and platelets. It's as if a silverware factory were to spew out tremendous quantities of poorly made forks, while making only a few spoons and knives. Not only is it harder to eat with an inferior-quality fork, foods that require a spoon or a knife become very difficult to handle. Similarly, the immature white blood cells can't do a good job of defending the body against either common or extraordinary germs. In addition, a lack of red blood cells causes anemia, and without platelets there can be bruising and excessive bleeding.

Imatinib is one of the drugs used to treat chronic myeloid leukemia when it has evolved to the point of a blast crisis. Although its actions are not fully understood, we do know that imatinib interferes with an enzyme produced by the abnormal chromosome that's associated with CML. Without this enzyme, it's harder for the colony of cancerous white blood cells to grow.

Possible Side Effects

The drug's more common side effects include fluid retention, headache, fever, and rash.

Which Nutrients Are Robbed

Taking this medicine may deplete your supply of, increase your need for, or interfere with the activity of:

- Potassium

Additional Ways This Drug May Upset Your Nutritional Balance

Imatinib can cause abdominal pain, loss of appetite, nausea, and vomiting, all of which can upset your eating habits and possibly interfere with good nutrition. It can also cause diarrhea, which can hamper nutrient absorption.

Restoring Your Nutritional Balance

To compensate for the nutrient loss caused by this drug, speak to your physician about taking 100–300 mg potassium per day.

You can also eat foods that contain the depleted nutrient:

- Potassium: dried figs, California avocado, papaya, banana, dates

Consult with your physician before making any changes to your diet or supplemental regimen.

IMIPRAMINE (im-IP-ruh-meen)

Brand Names: Apo-Imipramine, Impril, Janimine, Novo-Pramine, PMS-Imipramine, Tofranil, Tofranil-PM

About Imipramine

Parents look forward to the day when young children can go the entire night without wetting their diapers—or the bed. Luckily, most children quickly learn to recognize the signs of a full bladder, wake up at night when it's time to urinate, and make that long trek to the bathroom. But some children progress more slowly. By the age of 4, some 30 percent are still wetting the bed, and two years later, 10 percent are still hoping to wake up in the morning to find dry sheets. At the age of 12, some 3 percent of youngsters continue to wet the bed, and the problem can persist up to the age of 18 in a very small number of people.

Bedwetting—technically enuresis—may be caused by the slow maturation of nerves in the urinary tract, an infection in the tract, a narrowing of the tube that carries urine from the bladder to the outside of the body, or psychological problems.

As the numbers suggest, most children grow out of the bedwetting problem on their own. They can also use helpful techniques, such as abstaining from liquids for a couple of hours before going to bed, using bedwetting alarms, keeping a log of wet and dry nights, and so on. If these approaches don't work, imipramine may be prescribed.

Imipramine is an antidepressant that also relaxes the bladder, while tightening up the sphincter, the bladder's "exit door."

In addition to treating bedwetting, imipramine may be used for depression, chronic pain, panic disorder and attention deficit hyperactivity disorder (ADHD).

Possible Side Effects

The drug's side effects include rapid heartbeat, congestive heart failure, changes in libido, and fatigue.

Which Nutrients Are Robbed

Taking this medicine may deplete your supply of, increase your need for, or interfere with the activity of:

- Riboflavin
- Coenzyme Q_{10}
- Sodium

Additional Ways This Drug May Upset Your Nutritional Balance

Imipramine can cause nausea, vomiting, changes in taste, and loss of appetite, all of which can upset your eating habits and possibly interfere with good nutrition. It can also cause diarrhea, which can hamper nutrient absorption.

Restoring Your Nutritional Balance

To compensate for the nutrient loss caused by this drug, speak to your physician about taking 25–100 mg riboflavin and 30–100 mg coenzyme Q_{10} per day. And ask your physician to consider the potential effects of sodium depletion.

You can also eat foods that contain the depleted nutrients:

- Riboflavin: dried sunflower seeds, orange juice, bulgur, spinach noodles, pine nuts
- Coenzyme Q_{10}: beef, chicken, trout, salmon, oranges, broccoli

Consult with your physician before making any changes to your diet or supplemental regimen.

INAMRINONE (in-AM-ri-nohn)

Brand Name: Inamrinone

About Inamrinone

The heart is on a very demanding schedule: it must contract 60 times a minute or more for about 77 years (on average), squeezing out a full "serving" of blood with each contraction. The typical heart performs its job perfectly decade after decade, until the end of life. But in about 1 percent of us, the heart can't meet its rigid work schedule because it doesn't pump well enough to keep adequate amounts of blood pulsing through the arteries and veins. Insufficient amounts of oxygen and nutrients are delivered to the various cells, and waste products begin to accumulate. As a result, the muscles tire, the kidneys don't work well, and fluid backs up into the bloodstream and maybe even the lungs.

Inamrinone is one of the drugs doctors prescribe for heart failure if other drugs don't work. It works by increasing the cardiac output, or the amount of blood squirted out of the heart every minute. It also helps open up the blood vessels, making it easier for the heart to push the blood through.

Possible Side Effects

The drug's more common side effects include irregular heartbeat, low blood pressure, and nausea.

Which Nutrients Are Robbed

Taking this medicine may deplete your supply of, increase your need for, or interfere with the activity of:

- Potassium

Additional Ways This Drug May Upset Your Nutritional Balance

Inamrinone can cause nausea, which can upset your eating habits and possibly interfere with good nutrition.

Restoring Your Nutritional Balance

To compensate for the nutrient loss caused by this drug, speak to your physician about taking 100–300 mg potassium per day.

You can also eat foods that contain the depleted nutrient:

- Potassium: dried figs, California avocado, papaya, banana, dates

Consult with your physician before making any changes to your diet or supplemental regimen.

INDAPAMIDE (in-DAP-uh-mide)

Brand Names: Apo-Indapadmide, Gen-Indapamide, Lozide, Lozol, Novo-Indapamide, Nu-Indapamide

About Indapamide

There are several ways of treating elevated blood pressure. One approach, which has been in use since the mid-1900s, is to reduce the blood volume. You can think of high blood pressure as very heavy traffic, bumper-to-bumper cars packed on a busy highway. Everybody's trying to get down the same road at once, exerting a great deal of pressure on the highway. Now imagine that a bunch of those cars take a quick and early exit. The road is still the same size, with the same capacity, but there is a lot less pressure on the system. Traffic unblocks, everybody is able to accelerate, and the problem disappears.

Physicians take a similar approach with elevated blood pressure, relieving the pressure on the blood vessel "highways" by disposing of some of the fluid in the blood. They do this through the use of diuretics such as indapamide, which stimulate the body to excrete more water, resulting in lower blood volume and lower blood pressure.

Indapamide is used to treat elevated blood pressure, congestive heart failure, and other problems involving excess fluid in the body.

Possible Side Effects

The drug's more common side effects include nausea, vomiting, heart palpitations, dizziness, anxiety, and depression.

Which Nutrients Are Robbed

Taking this medicine may deplete your supply of, increase your need for, or interfere with the activity of:

- Magnesium
- Phosphorus
- Potassium
- Sodium
- Zinc
- Coenzyme Q_{10}

Additional Ways This Drug May Upset Your Nutritional Balance

Indapamide can cause loss of appetite, nausea, vomiting, abdominal pain, and bloating, all of which can upset your eating habits and possibly interfere with good nutrition. It can also cause diarrhea, which can hamper nutrient absorption.

This drug can also trigger hypercalcemia, or too much calcium in the blood.

Restoring Your Nutritional Balance

To compensate for the nutrient loss caused by this drug, speak to your physician about taking 500–1,000 mg magnesium, 700 mg phosphorus, 50–200 mg zinc, and 30–100 mg coenzyme Q_{10} per day. And ask your physician to consider the potential effects of sodium depletion.

A Note on Potassium: "Regular" diuretics lower potassium levels, while potassium-sparing diuretics do not—they may increase levels instead. It is not uncommon for doctors to prescribe two different diuretics. That's why you should speak to your physician about your potassium levels, and whether it is appropriate for you to take supplements or eat potassium-rich foods.

You can also eat foods that contain the depleted nutrients:

- Magnesium: Florida avocado, toasted wheat germ, almonds, shredded wheat cereal, pumpkin seeds
- Phosphorus: plain nonfat yogurt, lentils, salmon, milk, halibut
- Zinc: oysters, beef shank, chicken, pork tenderloin, plain yogurt
- Coenzyme Q_{10}: beef, chicken, trout, salmon, oranges, broccoli

Consult with your physician before making any changes to your diet or supplemental regimen.

INDOMETHACIN (in-doe-METH-uh-sin)

Brand Names: Apo-Indomethacin, Indocid, Indocid SR, Indochron E-R, Indocin, Indocin I.V., Indocin SR, Novo-Methacin, Nu-Indo, Pro-Indo

About Indomethacin

Like other nonsteroidal anti-inflammatory drugs (NSAIDs), indomethacin is useful in treating a variety of diseases that cause pain and/or inflammation.

One of the diseases for which it's used is ankylosing spondylitis, an arthritis-like condition that attacks the spine. The problem often begins with waxing and waning periods of back pain. Early morning stiffness is a common symptom. Over time, bony "bridges" form from one vertebra to the next, locking them to each other and turning the once-flexible spine into a rigid rod. If you've ever seen a person with a straight back that is bent forward at the waist (as if he's doing an imitation of Groucho Marx), you've witnessed the results of ankylosing spondylitis.

And that's not all. Ankylosing spondylitis can also cause anemia, fatigue, loss of appetite, difficulty breathing, damage to the heart valves, and compressed nerves.

There is no cure for ankylosing spondylitis, but indomethacin can help relieve the pain and inflammation it causes. This, in turn, makes it easier to get through the day and to do the stretching and strengthening exercises that can help maintain spine flexibility and strength.

Possible Side Effects

Indomethacin's side effects include headache, ulcers, dizziness, fatigue, and depression.

Which Nutrients Are Robbed

Taking this medicine may deplete your supply of, increase your need for, or interfere with the activity of:

- Folic acid
- Iron

Additional Ways This Drug May Upset Your Nutritional Balance

Indomethacin can cause low blood sugar (hypoglycemia), nausea, abdominal distress, and heartburn, all of which can upset your eating habits and possibly interfere with good nutrition. It can also cause diarrhea, which can hamper nutrient absorption.

This drug can also trigger hyperkalemia, or too much potassium in the blood.

Restoring Your Nutritional Balance

To compensate for the nutrient loss caused by this drug, speak to your physician about taking 400–800 mcg folic acid per day. And ask your physician to consider the potential effects of iron depletion.

You can also eat foods that contain the depleted nutrient:

- Folic acid: beef liver, fortified breakfast cereals, spinach, great northern beans, asparagus

Consult with your physician before making any changes to your diet or supplemental regimen.

INTERFERON ALFA-2A (in-ter-FEER-on AL-fa too ay)

Brand Name: Roferon-A

About Interferon Alfa-2a

Inside the marrow of your bones are stem cells that give birth to white blood cells, or leukocytes (which comes from *leukos* and *kytos*, the Greek words for "white" and "cell"). A crucial part of the body's immune system, the leukocytes come in several different varieties.

But when something goes wrong with their "birthing" process, the leukocytes can become cancerous, multiplying at a dangerous rate and interfering with or replacing other cells in the bone marrow that should have matured into healthy blood cells. The cancerous leukocytes may also spread to the liver, spleen, brain, and other parts of the body.

This type of cancer is called leukemia, and it can take different forms. One of these is *hairy cell leukemia*, so-named because the affected cells have little hairlike projections. Hairy cell leukemia is uncommon and slow-growing. The disease produces an enlarged spleen, typically strikes in middle age, and favors men over women.

Interferon Alpha-2a is used to combat hairy cell leukemia. This drug is a biologic response modifier, a medication that works by changing the ways that cancer cells interact with the body on both the metabolic and immune levels.

Interferon Alpha-2a is also used to treat Kaposi's sarcoma (a type of cancer associated with AIDS), hepatitis C, and chronic myelogenous leukemia. In this form of leukemia, large numbers of immature white blood cells are produced, leading to fatigue, weakness, lack of appetite, weight loss, bruising, and bleeding.

Possible Side Effects

The drug's more common side effects include fatigue, headache, and psychiatric disturbances, such as depression and suicidal thoughts.

Which Nutrients Are Robbed

Taking these medicines may deplete your supply of, increase your need for, or interfere with the activity of:

- Calcium
- Sodium

Additional Ways This Drug May Upset Your Nutritional Balance

Interferon Alfa-2a can cause abdominal pain, loss of appetite, changes in taste, nausea, and vomiting, all of which can upset your eating habits and possibly interfere with good nutrition. It can also cause diarrhea, which can hamper nutrient absorption.

Interferon Alfa-2a can also trigger hyperphosphatemia, or too much phosphorus in the blood.

Restoring Your Nutritional Balance

To compensate for the nutrient loss caused by this drug, speak to your physician about taking 1,200 mg calcium per day. And ask your physician to consider the potential effects of sodium depletion.

You can also eat foods that contain the depleted nutrient:

- Calcium: milk, dried figs, Swiss cheese, yogurt, tofu

Consult with your physician before making any changes to your diet or supplemental regimen.

INTERFERON ALFA-2B (in-ter-FEER-on AL-fa too bee)

Brand Name: Intron A

About Interferon Alfa-2b

Hepatitis is an inflammation of the liver that stems from both viral and nonviral sources. The viral kind is typically caused by hepatitis virus A, B, C, D, or E, although it may also develop from yellow fever, infectious mononucleosis, or other ailments. Nonviral hepatitis can stem from excessive alcohol consumption or the use of certain drugs, among other things.

In hepatitis A or C, the symptoms may come and go and be barely noticeable. The B and E forms are more severe. When symptoms do strike, they can include nausea, vomiting, fever, and poor appetite. As the bloodstream fills with pigment manufactured by the liver, the skin and the whites of the eyes may become yellowish and the urine may darken (a condition called jaundice). With hepatitis B, there may also be hives and joint pain.

In many people, an attack of hepatitis resolves itself, and little or no treatment is needed. But for others, the inflammation of the liver continues for at least six months, a condition called chronic hepatitis. Its symptoms include fatigue, a low-grade fever, abdominal discomfort, and a general feeling of malaise. The spleen may enlarge, and spiderlike blood vessels may become visible in the skin. In some people, the disease grows progressively worse, causing severe liver damage.

Interferon Alfa-2b is one of the drugs used to treat chronic hepatitis B and C, as well as certain forms of cancer. The drug is a biological response modifier, which means that it augments the immune system's behavior.

Possible Side Effects

The drug's more common side effects include fatigue, headache, and fever.

Which Nutrients Are Robbed

Taking these medicines may deplete your supply of, increase your need for, or interfere with the activity of:

• Calcium

Additional Ways This Drug May Upset Your Nutritional Balance

Interferon Alfa-2b can cause abdominal pain, loss of appetite, changes in taste, nausea, and vomiting, all of which can upset your eating habits and possibly interfere with good nutrition. It can also cause diarrhea, which can hamper nutrient absorption.

Restoring Your Nutritional Balance

To compensate for the nutrient loss caused by this drug, speak to your physician about taking 1,200 mg calcium per day.

You can also eat foods that contain the depleted nutrient:

• Calcium: milk, dried figs, Swiss cheese, yogurt, tofu

Consult with your physician before making any changes to your diet or supplemental regimen.

ISONIAZID (eye-soe-NYE-uh-zid)

Brand Names: Isotamine, Laniazid Oral, Nydrazid Injection, PMS-Isoniazid

About Isoniazid

Certain types of germs called mycobacteria, which can cause serious infections such as tuberculosis (TB), are very difficult to get rid of once they've invaded the body. That's because antibiotics, which target rapidly growing organisms, don't work well against these slow-growers, which can become dormant, or hibernate. They can also hide inside immune system cells called macrophages, where many drugs can't reach them, and they are very good at developing resistance to drugs in general. So it's not surprising to find that it usually takes a couple of drugs to kill mycobacteria. In fact, doctors usually give patients with TB a "cocktail" of several different drugs all at once, hoping to destroy all strains of the bacteria before a resistant one can emerge.

Isoniazid is one of these antimycobacterial drugs. It's actually a pro-drug, which means that it has to be activated by another substance in the body before it can begin killing the mycobacteria. Besides being used to treat active tuberculosis infections, isoniazid is also given to prevent TB in those who may have been exposed to it or who have positive skin tests.

Possible Side Effects

The drug's more common side effects include loss of appetite, dark urine, stomach pain, and weakness.

Which Nutrients Are Robbed

Taking this medicine may deplete your supply of, increase your need for, or interfere with the activity of:

- Folic acid
- Niacin
- Vitamin B_6
- Vitamin B_{12}
- Vitamin D
- Calcium
- Phosphorus

Additional Ways This Drug May Upset Your Nutritional Balance

Isoniazid can cause loss of appetite, nausea, vomiting, and stomach pain, all of which can upset your eating habits and possibly interfere with good nutrition.

Restoring Your Nutritional Balance

To compensate for the nutrient loss caused by this drug, speak to your physician about taking 400–800 mcg folic acid, 50–100 mg niacin, 50–100 mg vitamin B_6, 500–1,000 mcg vitamin B_{12}, 400 IU vitamin D, 1,200 mg calcium, and 700 mg phosphorus per day.

You can also eat foods that contain the depleted nutrients:

* Folic acid: beef liver, fortified breakfast cereals, spinach, great northern beans, asparagus
* Niacin: chicken breast, beef liver, mackerel, barley, bulgur
* Vitamin B_6: potato, banana, garbanzo beans, chicken breast, fortified oatmeal
* Vitamin B_{12}: beef liver, rainbow trout, sockeye salmon, beef, haddock
* Vitamin D: salmon, mackerel, sardines, eel, fortified milk
* Calcium: milk, dried figs, Swiss cheese, yogurt, tofu
* Phosphorus: plain nonfat yogurt, lentils, salmon, milk, halibut

Consult with your physician before making any changes to your diet or supplemental regimen.

KANAMYCIN (kan-uh-MYE-sin)

Brand Name: Kantrex

About Kanamycin

Kanamycin is an antibiotic used to treat pneumonia caused by *Klebsiella pneumoniae* bacteria. Normally, the *K. pneumoniae* and other bacteria are kept from infecting your lower respiratory tract by your immune system, your cough reflex, and little hairs that line your airways and propel mucus upward. But if your natural defenses have been weakened, you're hit by a particularly strong strain of bacteria, or too many bacteria invade all at once, you may develop pneumonia.

Pneumonia can cause fever, breathing difficulties, and a cough, perhaps with sputum. You may sweat, feel chilled and fatigued, have headaches and abdominal pain, and experience other symptoms. Your doctor may also find that your heart is beating too rapidly, that he or she can hear odd noises when you breathe (called rales), and that tapping on your chest produces a dull sound.

Pneumonia is a major cause of death in the United States, which is why physicians often treat it quickly and aggressively. Kanamycin, which burrows into bacteria and prevents them from synthesizing new proteins, is one of the antibiotics that may be used. It's not typically a first-choice medication, for there are newer, less toxic drugs available, so it's generally reserved for bacterial strains that are resistant to other drugs.

Possible Side Effects

The drug's side effects include potentially significant damage to the ears and kidneys.

Which Nutrients Are Robbed

Taking this medicine may deplete your supply of, increase your need for, or interfere with the activity of:

- Biotin
- Inositol
- Thiamin
- Riboflavin
- Niacin
- Vitamin B_6
- Vitamin B_{12}
- Vitamin K
- Calcium
- Magnesium
- Potassium
- *Bifidobacterium bifidum*
- *Lactobacillus acidophilus*

Restoring Your Nutritional Balance

To compensate for the nutrient loss caused by this drug, speak to your physician about taking 500–1,000 mcg biotin, 250–1,000 mg inositol, 25–100 mg thiamin, 25–100 mg riboflavin, 50–100 mg niacin, 50–100 mg vitamin B_6, 500–1,000 mcg vitamin B_{12}, 60–80 mcg vitamin K, 1,200 mg calcium, 500–1,000 mg magnesium, 100–300 mg potassium, 15 billion live *Bifidobacterium bifidum* organisms, and 15 billion live *Lactobacillus acidophilus* organisms per day.

You can also eat foods that contain the depleted nutrients:

- Biotin: beef liver, soybeans, rice bran, peanut butter, barley
- Inositol: cantaloupe, oranges, green beans, grapefruit juice, limes
- Thiamin: braised liver, turkey heart, roasted chicken, gefilte fish, sardines
- Riboflavin: dried sunflower seeds, orange juice, bulgur, spinach noodles, pine nuts
- Niacin: chicken breast, beef liver, mackerel, barley, bulgur
- Vitamin B_6: potato, banana, garbanzo beans, chicken breast, fortified oatmeal

- Vitamin B$_{12}$: beef liver, rainbow trout, sockeye salmon, beef, haddock
- Vitamin K: kale, broccoli, parsley, Swiss chard, spinach
- Calcium: milk, dried figs, Swiss cheese, yogurt, tofu
- Magnesium: Florida avocado, toasted wheat germ, almonds, shredded wheat cereal, pumpkin seeds
- Potassium: dried figs, California avocado, papaya, banana, dates
- *Bifidobacterium bifidum*: Jerusalem artichokes, asparagus, garlic, and onions may stimulate the growth or activity of this probiotic
- *Lactobacillus acidophilus*: yogurt containing live lactobacillus cultures, kefir, acidophilus milk

Consult with your physician before making any changes to your diet or supplemental regimen.

KETOPROFEN (kee-toe-PROE-fen)

Brand Names: Actron, Apo-Keto, Apo-Keto-E, Novo-Keto-EC, Nu-Ketoprofen, Nu-Ketoprofen-E, Orafen, Orudis, Orudis KT, Oruvail, PMS-Ketoprofen, Rhodis, Rhodis-EC

About Ketoprofen

Here's a quick look at rheumatoid arthritis (RA), by the numbers.

- 1: That's the percentage of people worldwide who have rheumatoid arthritis.
- 2: That's the number of "opposite" joints typically attacked at once. Other forms of arthritis may strike just one knee joint, one elbow joint, or one finger joint at a time, but rheumatoid arthritis typically strikes in twos: both elbows, both ankles, or both wrists simultaneously.
- 10: That's the percentage of those with RA who are likely to be permanently disabled by the disease.
- 25 to 50: That's the age at which rheumatoid arthritis usually appears, although it can strike at any age.
- 75: That's the percentage of people who can enjoy reasonably good relief from their symptoms, given the right treatment.

One final number: two. That's the number of ways that ketoprofen helps relieve the symptoms of rheumatoid arthritis. First, it helps to relieve pain. Second, it helps to reduce the swelling that can cause pain and contribute to deformity in the joints. Ketoprofen isn't a cure for RA, but it can make living with the disease much more bearable. The drug is also used to treat osteoarthritis and dysmenorrhea.

Possible Side Effects

The drug's more common side effects include headache and stomach upset.

Which Nutrients Are Robbed

Taking this medicine may deplete your supply of, increase your need for, or interfere with the activity of:

- Folic acid

Additional Ways This Drug May Upset Your Nutritional Balance

Ketoprofen can cause nausea, vomiting, and abdominal distress, all of which can upset your eating habits and possibly interfere with good nutrition. It can also cause diarrhea, which can hamper nutrient absorption.

Restoring Your Nutritional Balance

To compensate for the nutrient loss caused by this drug, speak to your physician about taking 400–800 mcg folic acid per day.

You can also eat foods that contain the depleted nutrient:

- Folic acid: beef liver, fortified breakfast cereals, spinach, great northern beans, asparagus

Consult with your physician before making any changes to your diet or supplemental regimen.

KETOROLAC (kee-toe-ROLE-ak)

Brand Names: Acular, Toradol

About Ketorolac

Ketorolac is a multipurpose pain reliever with some ability to relieve inflammation. It's often used for moderately severe acute pain—the kind that arises in response to an injury, inflammation, or surgery. In other words, there's a clear reason for the pain, which fades away when the underlying problem clears up.

Some recent studies have shown ketorolac's versatility. In 2003, an article appearing in the *American Journal of Obstetrics and Gynecology* reported that ketorolac "is efficacious in reducing postoperative pain and narcotics usage after Cesarean section."[2] A study appearing in the *Journal of Urology* in 2004 reported that "ketorolac is a safe and effective supplement to opioid-based analgesia for pain control after partial nephrectomy."[3] (Nephro- is the Greek root for "kidney," and -ectomy means "to remove surgically," so a partial nephrectomy means taking out part of the kidney.) The high pain levels that are normally seen after this surgery usually require treatment with opioid drugs. But when the people in this study were given ketorolac, they were able to get off opioids sooner. Not only that, they enjoyed a better and less painful recovery.

There's a serious risk of becoming physically or psychologically dependent on opioid drugs, so doctors prefer to limit their use as much as possible. For many people, ketorolac can be a safe and effective substitute for opioids. The drug is also used for eye problems such as allergic conjunctivitis.

Possible Side Effects

Ketorolac's more common side effects include headache and gastrointestinal pain. When it's used for the eyes, the more common side effects include burning and stinging of the eyes.

Which Nutrients Are Robbed

Taking this medicine may deplete your supply of, increase your need for, or interfere with the activity of:

• Folic acid

Additional Ways This Drug May Upset Your Nutritional Balance

Ketorolac can cause gastrointestinal pain, a feeling of fullness, nausea, and vomiting, all of which can upset your eating habits and possibly interfere with good nutrition. It can also cause diarrhea, which can hamper nutrient absorption.

Restoring Your Nutritional Balance

To compensate for the nutrient loss caused by this drug, speak to your physician about taking 400–800 mcg folic acid per day.

You can also eat foods that contain the depleted nutrient:

- Folic acid: beef liver, fortified breakfast cereals, spinach, great northern beans, asparagus

Consult with your physician before making any changes to your diet or supplemental regimen.

LABETALOL (lah-BET-uh-lole)

Brand Names: Normodyne, Tradnate

About Labetalol

Labetalol exerts a "Whoa, Nelly!" action on the certain parts of the body.

The brain is constantly sending messages to all parts of the body, instructing it to work faster or slower, do more or less, pump harder or more gently, and so on. But sometimes these messages have ill effects. For example, if you have elevated blood pressure, you probably don't want your heart to work any harder than necessary, because that can drive your blood pressure up even further.

Drugs called beta-blockers work by heading these messages off at the pass, thereby preventing the heart from overworking. They're called beta-blockers because they do their job at special areas in the body called beta receptors.

Here's one way to understand what beta-blockers do: Suppose some crazed jockeys jump onto the backs of a pack of horses and start whipping the animals over and over, forcing them to run much too fast for much too long. Sooner or later, the horses will simply keel over and die.

Now imagine the beta-blockers as nice, relaxed cowboys who ride those horses at a slow to medium (but steady) pace. Instead of being forced to race at an exhausting pace, the horses move along at a comfortable trot, arriving at their destination without overdoing it. It's as if the gentle cowboys have pushed aside the crazy jockeys and cried "Whoa, Nelly!" to the overworked, galloping horses. This is something like the effect of beta-blockers on the heart.

Labetalol is one of the "Whoa, Nelly!" beta-blockers that's used to treat mild to severe hypertension. In extreme cases, it may be given intravenously.

Possible Side Effects

The drug's more common side effects include dizziness and nausea.

Which Nutrients Are Robbed

Taking this medicine may deplete your supply of, increase your need for, or interfere with the activity of:

- Coenzyme Q_{10}
- Melatonin

Additional Ways This Drug May Upset Your Nutritional Balance

Labetalol can cause low blood sugar (hypoglycemia), changes in taste, nausea, and vomiting, all of which can upset your eating habits and possibly interfere with good nutrition.

Restoring Your Nutritional Balance

To compensate for the nutrient loss caused by this drug, speak to your physician about taking 30–100 mg coenzyme Q_{10} and 1–3 mg melatonin per day.

You can also eat foods that contain the depleted nutrient:

- Coenzyme Q_{10}: beef, chicken, trout, salmon, oranges, broccoli

Consult with your physician before making any changes to your diet or supplemental regimen.

LAMIVUDINE (lah-MI-vyoo-deen)

Brand Names: Epivir, Epivir HBV

About Lamivudine

Viruses burrow into and take over body cells, turning them into little factories that churn out copies of the virus. Hidden inside body cells, viruses are tough to kill—especially since you don't want to kill the host cell in the process. Antibacterial and antifungal drugs can't do the job, but drugs called reverse transcriptase inhibitors can. Here's how:

A virus penetrates a body cell (a "slave cell") and reveals its nucleic acids, which the slave cell uses as a template for making DNA and RNA for new viruses. Reverse transcriptase inhibitors insert themselves into the new viral DNA chains. Their unauthorized presence halts the building of the new DNA chains, and the new virus dies before it is born.

Lamivudine is a reverse transcriptase inhibitor used to manage HIV infections and treat chronic hepatitis B.

Possible Side Effects

The drug's more common side effects include headache, fatigue, and musculoskeletal pain.

Which Nutrients Are Robbed

Taking this medicine may deplete your supply of, increase your need for, or interfere with the activity of:

- Vitamin B_{12}
- Zinc
- Copper
- Carnitine

Additional Ways This Drug May Upset Your Nutritional Balance

Lamivudine can cause nausea, vomiting, loss of appetite, abdominal pain, and heartburn, all of which can upset your eating habits and possibly interfere with good nutrition. It can also cause diarrhea, which can hamper nutrient absorption.

Restoring Your Nutritional Balance

To compensate for the nutrient loss caused by this drug, speak to your physician about taking 500–1,000 mcg vitamin B_{12}, 2 mcg copper, 50–200 mg zinc, and 250–1,000 mg carnitine per day.

You can also eat foods that contain the depleted nutrients:

- Vitamin B_{12}: beef liver, rainbow trout, sockeye salmon, beef, haddock
- Copper: beef liver, almonds, raw mushrooms, hazelnuts, lentils
- Zinc: oysters, beef shank, chicken, pork tenderloin, plain yogurt
- Carnitine: ground beef, pork, Canadian bacon, whole milk, cod

Consult with your physician before making any changes to your diet or supplemental regimen.

LANSOPRAZOLE (lan-SOE-prah-zole)

Brand Name: Prevacid

About Lansoprazole

The stomach secretes high-powered acid to break down the food that you eat. This is absolutely necessary for proper digestion, but not such a good thing when the acid eats away at your stomach lining or flows back up into your esophagus, burning the sensitive tissue and causing pain.

There are a couple of strategies for handling problems due to excess stomach acid. One is to take antacids to neutralize acid that is already present. Another is to prevent overproduction of acid in the first place, which is the approach taken by a group of medicines called the proton pump inhibitors.

Proton pumps are portions of specialized cells in the stomach that produce acid. When their action is inhibited, production of stomach acid drops markedly.

Lansoprazole, a proton pump inhibitor, is used to treat gastroesophageal reflux disease (GERD), better known as heartburn. It is also used to treat certain kinds of gastric and duodenal ulcers, inflammation of the lining of the esophagus (esophagitis), and Zollinger-Ellison syndrome, a condition that stimulates the body to pump out tremendous amounts of acid.

As lansoprazole begins to work, abdominal pain and irritation begin to lessen, and X rays will most likely show that any existing duodenal ulcers are healing.

Possible Side Effects

The drug's more common side effects include constipation and abdominal pain.

Which Nutrients Are Robbed

Taking this medicine may deplete your supply of, increase your need for, or interfere with the activity of:

- Beta-carotene
- Thiamin
- Folic acid
- Vitamin B_{12}
- Iron
- Zinc

Additional Ways This Drug May Upset Your Nutritional Balance

Lansoprazole can cause abdominal pain and nausea, which can upset your eating habits and possibly interfere with good nutrition. It can also cause diarrhea, which can hamper nutrient absorption.

Restoring Your Nutritional Balance

To compensate for the nutrient loss caused by this drug, speak to your physician about taking 25,000 IU beta-carotene, 25–100 mg thiamin, 400–800 mcg folic acid, 500–1,000 mcg vitamin B_{12}, and 50–200 mg zinc per day. And ask your doctor to consider the potential effects of iron depletion.

You can also eat foods that contain the depleted nutrients:

- Beta-carotene: carrot, spinach, mango, cantaloupe, apricot nectar
- Thiamin: braised liver, turkey heart, roasted chicken, gefilte fish, sardines
- Folic acid: beef liver, fortified breakfast cereals, spinach, great northern beans, asparagus
- Vitamin B_{12}: beef liver, rainbow trout, sockeye salmon, beef, haddock
- Zinc: oysters, beef shank, chicken, pork tenderloin, plain yogurt

Consult with your physician before making any changes to your diet or supplemental regimen.

LEFLUNOMIDE (le-FLOO-noe-mide)

Brand Name: Arava

About Leflunomide

Leflunomide is a newer immunosuppressive drug used to treat rheumatoid arthritis. It apparently helps slow the proliferation of T-cells and autoantibodies (specialized weapons made by the body that attack body tissues).

When an invader or other foreign entity is found in the body, macrophages and other immune system cells ingest it and then present pieces of it to the T-cells. It's like giving a picture of a "most wanted" criminal to police officers. The T-cells then patrol the bloodstream and lymph system, seeking out the suspect (and its clones) and destroying them. Other immune system cells called B-cells also learn to recognize these "bad guys," but instead of trying to destroy them in hand-to-hand combat, they make special weapons called *antibodies* that find and destroy the enemy.

The immune system is supposed to distinguish between the body's own tissues and invaders. But sometimes the immune system gets confused and thinks that healthy body tissue is an invader. That's what happens in rheumatoid arthritis, when the body attacks the joints and their supporting tissues. Antibodies become autoantibodies that destroy body tissue.

Leflunomide helps relieve the symptoms of rheumatoid arthritis by stifling an errant immune system, reducing pain and inflammation, and slowing damage to the afflicted joints.

Possible Side Effects

The drug's side effects include respiratory tract infections, back pain, hair loss, headache, and eczema.

Which Nutrients Are Robbed

Taking this medicine may deplete your supply of, increase your need for, or interfere with the activity of:

- Potassium

Additional Ways This Drug May Upset Your Nutritional Balance

Leflunomide can cause nausea, loss of appetite, and vomiting, all of which can upset your eating habits and possibly interfere with good nutrition. It can also cause diarrhea, which can hamper nutrient absorption.

Restoring Your Nutritional Balance

To compensate for the nutrient loss caused by this drug, speak to your physician about taking 100–300 mg potassium per day.

You can also eat foods that contain the depleted nutrient:

- Potassium: dried figs, California avocado, papaya, banana, dates

Consult with your physician before making any changes to your diet or supplemental regimen.

LEVALBUTEROL (lee-val-BYOO-ter-ole)

Brand Name: Xopenex

About Levalbuterol

Asthma makes breathing difficult for about 18 million Americans. There are many triggers for the disease, including viral infections, cigarette smoke, pollen, dust mite particles, and even cold air. Whatever the precipitating cause, the airways narrow, swell, and fill with mucus, leaving less—sometimes very little—room for air to flow in and out.

Airways narrow when the muscles wrapped around them contract—in this case, contract inappropriately. With asthma, this narrowing is just part of the problem, for inflammation sets in and excess mucus clings to the airway walls, narrowing the passageways even more.

Of course, these airway muscles don't contract on their own. The breathing tubes are studded with various receptors. When the appropriate substances plug into the right receptors, the airway muscles either contract or relax. Levalbuterol help combat asthma by inserting itself into the appropriate receptors and giving the air tubes the order to relax and open wider. As a result, there's more room in the airways and breathing is easier.

Possible Side Effects

The drug's more common side effects include rapid heartbeat, viral infections, and nasal inflammation.

Which Nutrients Are Robbed

Taking this medicine may deplete your supply of, increase your need for, or interfere with the activity of:

- Potassium

Additional Ways This Drug May Upset Your Nutritional Balance

Levalbuterol can cause a feeling of fullness, heartburn, and nausea, all of which can upset your eating habits and possibly interfere with good nutrition.

Restoring Your Nutritional Balance

To compensate for the nutrient loss caused by this drug, speak to your physician about taking 100–300 mg potassium per day.

You can also eat foods that contain the depleted nutrient:

- Potassium: dried figs, California avocado, papaya, banana, dates

Consult with your physician before making any changes to your diet or supplemental regimen.

LEVODOPA, LEVODOPA PLUS CARBIDOPA (lee-voe-DOE-pah, kar-bi-DOE-pah)

Brand Names: Levodopa: Dopar, Larodopa
Levodopa plus Carbidopa: Sinemet, Sinemet CR, Lodosyn

About Levodopa, Levodopa plus Carbidopa

Parkinson's disease is a devastating condition that slowly but surely leaves its victims with tremors of the hands, arms, legs, face, and jaw; a slow, shuffling gait; rigid muscles; and impaired balance. The muscles tremble when they're not being used, and there may be difficulty speaking, swallowing, or initiating muscle movement, along with a lack of facial expression and other problems.

The disease destroys cells in a part of the brain responsible for controlling movement, coordination, and balance. In order to perform these functions, these brain cells must produce a chemical called dopamine. When Parkinson's strikes, the cells begin to degenerate and make less dopamine, resulting in the characteristic impairments in movement.

Levodopa helps slow the progression of Parkinson's by supplying the missing dopamine to the brain cells. Once it gets inside the brain, levodopa is converted to dopamine, allowing the brain to restore smooth muscle movement that is easier to initiate, coordinate, and control. (I like to think of levodopa as *lev*itating of *dopa*mine levels.)

Levodopa may be used alone or mixed with carbidopa, which makes levodopa more powerful and helps reduce its side effects.

Possible Side Effects

Levodopa's side effects include chest pain, confusion, and nightmares. Side effects seen with levodopa plus carbidopa include irregular heartbeat, dizziness, and increased libido.

Which Nutrients Are Robbed

Taking this medicine may deplete your supply of, increase your need for, or interfere with the activity of:

- Potassium
- SAMe

Additional Ways This Drug May Upset Your Nutritional Balance

Levodopa and carbidopa can cause loss of appetite, nausea, vomiting, gastrointestinal bleeding, changes in taste, and heartburn, all of which can upset your eating habits and possibly interfere with good nutrition. It can also cause diarrhea, which can hamper nutrient absorption.

Restoring Your Nutritional Balance

To compensate for the nutrient loss caused by this drug, speak to your physician about taking 100–300 mg potassium and 200–400 mg SAMe per day.

You can also eat foods that contain the depleted nutrient:

- Potassium: dried figs, California avocado, papaya, banana, dates

Consult with your physician before making any changes to your diet or supplemental regimen.

LEVOFLOXACIN (lee-voe-FLOKS-uh-sin)

Brand Names: Levaquin, Quixin

About Levofloxacin

The *maxillary sinus* is one of four groups of sinuses (hollow areas) in the facial bones. The sinuses help reduce the weight of the bones while keeping them strong.

The sinuses are lined with membranes, which produce a sticky substance (mucus) that traps dirt and other particles in a form that can easily be expelled from the body. The sinuses have tiny slots through which excess mucus, trapped bacteria, and other foreign particles can drain.

Unfortunately, these small hollows can become infected and inflamed, sometimes as the result of an upper respiratory infection. When that happens, the tiny slots through which the sinuses drain their excess mucus and trapped dirt can become blocked. Unexpelled matter then backs up within the sinuses, causing pain, tenderness, headache, and possibly a fever. In severe cases, a sinus infection can spread to the bone or the brain.

Levofloxacin is one of the antibiotics used to treat infection of the maxillary sinus (maxillary sinusitis). The drug works by preventing the invading bacteria from forming new DNA and replicating.

In addition to maxillary sinusitis, levofloxacin is used to treat chronic bronchitis, pneumonia, and skin and urinary tract infections caused by bacteria. It's also used for bacterial conjunctivitis (inflammation of the inner surface of the eyelids).

Possible Side Effects

The drug's more common side effects include dizziness, headache, insomnia, and fever.

Which Nutrients Are Robbed

Taking this medicine may deplete your supply of, increase your need for, or interfere with the activity of:

- Biotin
- Inositol
- Thiamin
- Riboflavin
- Niacin
- Vitamin B_6
- Vitamin B_{12}
- Vitamin K
- Zinc
- *Bifidobacterium bifidum*
- *Lactobacillus acidophilus*

Additional Ways This Drug May Upset Your Nutritional Balance

Levofloxacin can cause nausea and vomiting, which can upset your eating habits and possibly interfere with good nutrition. It can also cause diarrhea, which can hamper nutrient absorption.

Restoring Your Nutritional Balance

To compensate for the nutrient loss caused by this drug, speak to your physician about taking 500–1,000 mcg biotin, 250–1,000 mg inositol, 25–100 mg thiamin, 25–100 mg riboflavin, 50–100 mg niacin, 50–100 mg vitamin B_6, 500–1,000 mcg vitamin B_{12}, 60–80 mcg vitamin K, 50–200 mg zinc, 15 billion live *Bifidobacterium bifidum* organisms, and 15 billion live *Lactobacillus acidophilus* organisms per day.

You can also eat foods that contain the depleted nutrients:

- Biotin: beef liver, soybeans, rice bran, peanut butter, barley
- Inositol: cantaloupe, oranges, green beans, grapefruit juice, limes
- Thiamin: braised liver, turkey heart, roasted chicken, gefilte fish, sardines
- Riboflavin: dried sunflower seeds, orange juice, bulgur, spinach noodles, pine nuts
- Niacin: chicken breast, beef liver, mackerel, barley, bulgur
- Vitamin B_6: potato, banana, garbanzo beans, chicken breast, fortified oatmeal
- Vitamin B_{12}: beef liver, rainbow trout, sockeye salmon, beef, haddock
- Vitamin K: kale, broccoli, parsley, Swiss chard, spinach

- Zinc: oysters, beef shank, chicken, pork tenderloin, plain yogurt
- *Bifidobacterium bifidum*: Jerusalem artichokes, asparagus, garlic, and onions may stimulate the growth or activity of this probiotic
- *Lactobacillus acidophilus*: yogurt containing live lactobacillus cultures, kefir, acidophilus milk

Consult with your physician before making any changes to your diet or supplemental regimen.

LEVONORGESTREL (LEE-voe-nor-jes-trel)

Brand Names: Norplant Implant, Plan B

About Levonorgestrel

The morning-after pill offers emergency, after-the-act contraception. Within 72 hours after a single episode of unprotected sex or contraception failure, a woman who wants to prevent pregnancy may be given two doses of levonorgestrel, one 12 hours after the first.

Levonorgestrel is a progestin, a synthetic version of the hormone progesterone. It works by delaying or preventing ovulation and/or altering the lining of the uterus to make it very difficult for the embryo to implant itself. Using this medicine is *not* an effective way to terminate an existing pregnancy.

Besides serving as a morning-after pill, levonorgestrel provides long-term contraception. It can be put into an intrauterine device (IUD) and implanted in the uterus to provide contraception. It's also the hormone used in the Norplant system, in which small capsules inserted into a woman's body slowly release levonorgestrel to prevent pregnancy. These capsules can remain in the body for up to five years.

Possible Side Effects

The drug's more common side effects include elevated blood pressure, depression, abdominal pain, and upper respiratory tract infection.

Which Nutrients Are Robbed

Taking this medicine may deplete your supply of, increase your need for, or interfere with the activity of:

- Folic acid
- Riboflavin
- Vitamin B_6
- Vitamin B_{12}
- Vitamin C
- Magnesium
- Zinc

Additional Ways This Drug May Upset Your Nutritional Balance

Depending on which form you take, levonorgestrel can cause nausea, vomiting, and abdominal pain, which can upset your eating habits and possibly interfere with good nutrition. It can also cause diarrhea, which can hamper nutrient absorption.

Restoring Your Nutritional Balance

To compensate for the nutrient loss caused by this drug, speak to your physician about taking 400–800 mcg folic acid, 25–100 mg riboflavin, 50–100 mg vitamin B_6, 500–1,000 mcg vitamin B_{12}, 250–1,500 mg vitamin C, 500–1,000 mg magnesium, and 50–200 mg zinc per day.

You can also eat foods that contain the depleted nutrients:

- Folic acid: beef liver, fortified breakfast cereals, spinach, great northern beans, asparagus
- Riboflavin: dried sunflower seeds, orange juice, bulgur, spinach noodles, pine nuts
- Vitamin B_6: potato, banana, garbanzo beans, chicken breast, fortified oatmeal
- Vitamin B_{12}: beef liver, rainbow trout, sockeye salmon, beef, haddock
- Vitamin C: papaya, guava, red pepper, cantaloupe, black currants
- Magnesium: Florida avocado, toasted wheat germ, almonds, shredded wheat cereal, pumpkin seeds
- Zinc: oysters, beef shank, chicken, pork tenderloin, plain yogurt

Consult with your physician before making any changes to your diet or supplemental regimen.

LINEZOLID (li-NEZ-oh-lid)

Brand Name: Zyvox

About Linezolid

If you're unlucky enough to be hospitalized and your bad luck streak continues, you may find yourself one of many who develop a nosocomial infection. "Nosocomial" isn't the name of some exotic bacteria; it's doctor-speak for an infection that was acquired in the hospital. Unfortunately, these infections can sometimes be very serious, because the germs that manage to survive in the antiseptic hospital environment are usually very hearty, very dangerous, and very difficult to destroy.

One of the drugs used to treat certain nosocomial infections is linezolid, a newer type of synthetic antimicrobial. It works by preventing the germs from manufacturing protein, a necessary step for reproducing. Linezolid is also used to treat infections caused by a number of different streptococci and staphylococci, as well as infections caused by organisms resistant to other drugs.

Possible Side Effects

The drug's more common side effects include elevated blood pressure, headache, fever, diarrhea, and rash.

Which Nutrients Are Robbed

Taking this medicine may deplete your supply of, increase your need for, or interfere with the activity of:

- Biotin
- Inositol
- Thiamin
- Riboflavin
- Niacin
- Vitamin B$_6$
- Vitamin B$_{12}$
- Vitamin K
- *Bifidobacterium bifidum*
- *Lactobacillus acidophilus*

Additional Ways This Drug May Upset Your Nutritional Balance

Linezolid can cause nausea, vomiting, and changes in taste, all of which can upset your eating habits and possibly interfere with good nutrition. It can also cause diarrhea, which can hamper nutrient absorption.

Restoring Your Nutritional Balance

To compensate for the nutrient loss caused by this drug, speak to your physician about taking 500–1,000 mcg biotin, 250–1,000 mg inositol, 25–100

mg thiamin, 25–100 mg riboflavin, 50–100 mg niacin, 50–100 mg vitamin B_6, 500–1,000 mcg vitamin B_{12}, 60–80 mcg vitamin K, 15 billion live *Bifidobacterium bifidum* organisms, and 15 billion live *Lactobacillus acidophilus* organisms per day.

You can also eat foods that contain the depleted nutrients:

- Biotin: beef liver, soybeans, rice bran, peanut butter, barley
- Inositol: cantaloupe, oranges, green beans, grapefruit juice, limes
- Thiamin: braised liver, turkey heart, roasted chicken, gefilte fish, sardines
- Riboflavin: dried sunflower seeds, orange juice, bulgur, spinach noodles, pine nuts
- Niacin: chicken breast, beef liver, mackerel, barley, bulgur
- Vitamin B_6: potato, banana, garbanzo beans, chicken breast, fortified oatmeal
- Vitamin B_{12}: beef liver, rainbow trout, sockeye salmon, beef, haddock
- Vitamin K: kale, broccoli, parsley, Swiss chard, spinach
- *Bifidobacterium bifidum*: Jerusalem artichokes, asparagus, garlic, and onions may stimulate the growth or activity of this probiotic
- *Lactobacillus acidophilus*: yogurt containing live lactobacillus cultures, kefir, acidophilus milk

Consult with your physician before making any changes to your diet or supplemental regimen.

LISINOPRIL (lyse-IN-oh-pril)

Brand Names: Apo-Lisinopril, Prinivil, Zestril

About Lisinopril

A lot can go wrong with the human heart. It can suffer from a heart attack, be assaulted by elevated blood pressure, or "fade away" due to congestive heart failure. It can also be assaulted by bacteria, hit with inflammation, or hamstrung by birth defects.

You'd think that each problem would need a different solution, but some drugs, like lisinopril, can attack several problems at once. Lisinopril can widen certain blood vessels, making it easier for the heart to force blood though, and can help rid the body of excess fluid. Both of these actions reduce the heart's workload and help lower elevated blood pressure. And lisinopril can slow the remodeling (or remaking) of certain parts of the heart following a heart attack, a process that can weaken the heart in the long run. (The body's efforts to solve immediate problems by "patching things over" can sometimes lead to long-term difficulties.)

The drug can help you survive the critical hours and days following a heart attack, while staving off the long-term threats of hypertension and heart failure.

Possible Side Effects

Lisinopril's more common side effects include headache, dizziness, chest pain, and cough.

Which Nutrients Are Robbed

Taking this medicine may deplete your supply of, increase your need for, or interfere with the activity of:

• Zinc

Additional Ways This Drug May Upset Your Nutritional Balance

Lisinopril can cause nausea, vomiting, and abdominal pain, all of which can upset your eating habits and possibly interfere with good nutrition. It can also cause diarrhea, which can hamper nutrient absorption.

The drug can also cause hyperkalemia, or too much potassium in the blood.

Restoring Your Nutritional Balance

To compensate for the nutrient loss caused by this drug, speak to your physician about taking 50–200 mg zinc per day.

You can also eat foods that contain the depleted nutrient:

• Zinc: oysters, beef shank, chicken, pork tenderloin, plain yogurt

Consult with your physician before making any changes to your diet or supplemental regimen.

LITHIUM (LITH-ee-um)

Brand Names: Carbolith, Duralith, Eskalith, Lithane, Lithobid, Lithonate

About Lithium

Episodes of mania usually develop over a couple of days. At first you feel full of energy and exuberance: The world looks great! As the episode progresses, your energy levels soar even higher. You can work or play for hours, you need little sleep, and your head is full of great ideas. Unfortunately, you probably flit from one thought or plan to the next, rarely focusing on one long enough to see it through. You may also become irritated at the slowness of those around you and angry at those who say there's something wrong with you. You may believe that you are more powerful, smarter, or richer than you really are.

Manic episodes like this are typically a part of bipolar disease (formerly known as manic-depression), which is characterized by episodes of mania alternating with episodes of depression. Bipolar disease, ranging from mild to severe, afflicts almost 2 percent of Americans.

Lithium is an antimanic or mood-stabilizing drug that helps prevent mood swings in perhaps three-quarters of people with bipolar disease. Although lithium has long been used to treat mania and bipolar disease, the drug is a puzzle. Its antimania benefits were discovered by accident, and to this day we don't know exactly how it works. But lithium *is* helpful in calming and preventing the manic phase of bipolar disease. It's also used to treat mania in senior citizens.

Possible Side Effects

Side effects include muscle weakness, tremors, fatigue, loss of appetite, nausea, and diarrhea.

Which Nutrients Are Robbed

Taking this medicine may deplete your supply of, increase your need for, or interfere with the activity of:

- Inositol

Additional Ways This Drug May Upset Your Nutritional Balance

Lithium can cause loss of appetite, changes in taste, nausea, and vomiting, which can upset your eating habits and possibly interfere with good nutrition. It can also cause diarrhea, which can hamper nutrient absorption.

Restoring Your Nutritional Balance

To compensate for the nutrient loss caused by this drug, speak to your physician about taking 250–1,000 mg inositol per day.

You can also eat foods that contain the depleted nutrient:

• Inositol: cantaloupe, oranges, green beans, grapefruit juice, limes

Consult with your physician before making any changes to your diet or supplemental regimen.

LOMEFLOXACIN (loe-me-FLOKS-uh-sin)

Brand Name: Maxaquin

About Lomefloxacin

The kidneys, which are placed to the right and left of the spine in the lower-middle portion of the back, continually filter waste products out of the blood and mix them with water to produce urine. The ureter is a tube that leads from each kidney to the bladder, which serves as the holding tank for the urine. When the bladder fills to a certain point, it signals the brain that it's time to urinate. Then the muscular bladder walls squeeze the urine into the urethra, the final piece of tubing in the urinary system, which carries the fluid out of the body.

Ideally, there are no bacteria or other germs in the bladder. And although there may be some in the urethra, there shouldn't be enough to cause problems. Unfortunately, infectious organisms do get into the urinary system, often by crawling up through the urethra, which is open and exposed to the outside environment. Germs can also enter the urinary system by getting into the blood, then traveling to the kidneys.

If an infection settles in the kidneys or the ureters, which are higher up in the body, it's called an upper urinary tract infection. If it settles is in the bladder or urethra, it's called a lower urinary tract infection.

Lomefloxacin is one of the antibiotics used to treat either type of urinary tract infection caused by *Escherichia coli* (*E. coli*) and certain other bacteria. It's well absorbed from the intestines and may have to be taken only once a day.

Possible Side Effects

The drug's side effects include dizziness, photosensitivity, and headache.

Which Nutrients Are Robbed

Taking this medicine may deplete your supply of, increase your need for, or interfere with the activity of:

- Biotin
- Inositol
- Thiamin
- Riboflavin
- Niacin
- Vitamin B_6

- Vitamin B_{12}
- Vitamin K
- Zinc
- *Bifidobacterium bifidum*
- *Lactobacillus acidophilus*

Additional Ways This Drug May Upset Your Nutritional Balance

Lomefloxacin can cause low blood sugar (hypoglycemia) and nausea, which can upset your eating habits and possibly interfere with good nutrition.

Restoring Your Nutritional Balance

To compensate for the nutrient loss caused by this drug, speak to your physician about taking 500–1,000 mcg biotin, 250–1,000 mg inositol, 25–100 mg thiamin, 25–100 mg riboflavin, 50–100 mg niacin, 50–100 mg vitamin B_6, 500–1,000 mcg vitamin B_{12}, 60–80 mcg vitamin K, 50–200 mg zinc, 15 billion live *Bifidobacterium bifidum* organisms, and 15 billion live *Lactobacillus acidophilus* organisms per day.

You can also eat foods that contain the depleted nutrients:

- Biotin: beef liver, soybeans, rice bran, peanut butter, barley
- Inositol: cantaloupe, oranges, green beans, grapefruit juice, limes
- Thiamin: braised liver, turkey heart, roasted chicken, gefilte fish, sardines
- Riboflavin: dried sunflower seeds, orange juice, bulgur, spinach noodles, pine nuts
- Niacin: chicken breast, beef liver, mackerel, barley, bulgur
- Vitamin B_6: potato, banana, garbanzo beans, chicken breast, fortified oatmeal
- Vitamin B_{12}: beef liver, rainbow trout, sockeye salmon, beef, haddock
- Vitamin K: kale, broccoli, parsley, Swiss chard, spinach
- Zinc: oysters, beef shank, chicken, pork tenderloin, plain yogurt
- *Bifidobacterium bifidum*: Jerusalem artichokes, asparagus, garlic, and onions may stimulate the growth or activity of this probiotic
- *Lactobacillus acidophilus*: yogurt containing live lactobacillus cultures, kefir, acidophilus milk

Consult with your physician before making any changes to your diet or supplemental regimen.

LOVASTATIN (LOE-vuh-stat-in)

Brand Names: Apo-Lovastatin, Altocor, Mevacor

About Lovastatin

Cholesterol is absolutely necessary to good health. It is a crucial ingredient used in the manufacture of cell membranes, adrenal and sex hormones, and many other things. But it also scares the bejeezus out of the millions of Americans whose levels are too high, because a high level of blood cholesterol is a major risk factor for heart attacks and strokes.

Why do cholesterol levels skyrocket in certain people? There are several reasons, including:

- *Age.* Cholesterol levels rise with age, although this may be at least partially due to decreased levels of exercise and increased weight.
- *Diet.* Too many calories in the diet, as well as too much saturated fat or cholesterol, is associated with elevated cholesterol levels.
- *Gender.* Before menopause, women typically have lower cholesterol levels than do men of the same age. After menopause, however, a woman's cholesterol levels rise, and so does her risk of heart disease.
- *Heredity.* In some people, the metabolic machinery is very efficient at making cholesterol, so they just naturally have high cholesterol levels.
- *Other diseases.* Liver disease, thyroid disease, and other ailments can lead to increased levels of blood cholesterol.
- *Physical activity.* More precisely, the *lack* of physical activity is linked to lower levels of HDL "good" cholesterol.
- *Weight.* Elevated LDL has also been linked to overweight and obesity.

You can't do anything about your gender or heredity, but many people have successfully lowered their cholesterol levels by changing their diet, increasing their exercise levels, and/or losing weight.

If these nondrug approaches don't work for you, your physician may prescribe a "statin" drug, such as lovastatin. Since their introduction in the 1980s, the statins have become tremendously popular and are successful in reducing cholesterol levels. These drugs work by interfering with a substance called HMG-CoA reductase, which the body uses to make cholesterol.

Lovastatin is used along with dietary therapy to reduce total cholesterol and LDL cholesterol, as well as to prevent or slow the progression of coronary artery disease.

Possible Side Effects

The drug's side effects include blurred vision, muscle cramps, joint pain, and a potentially fatal muscle disease called rhabdomyolysis.

Which Nutrients Are Robbed

Taking this medicine may deplete your supply of, increase your need for, or interfere with the activity of:

- Coenzyme Q_{10}

Additional Ways This Drug May Upset Your Nutritional Balance

Lovastatin can cause abdominal pain, bloating, heartburn, and nausea, all of which can upset your eating habits and possibly interfere with good nutrition. It can also cause diarrhea, which can hamper nutrient absorption.

This drug may cause blood levels of vitamin A to rise.

Restoring Your Nutritional Balance

To compensate for the nutrient loss caused by this drug, speak to your physician about taking 30–100 mg coenzyme Q_{10} per day.

You can also eat foods that contain the depleted nutrient:

- Coenzyme Q_{10}: beef, chicken, trout, salmon, oranges, broccoli

Consult with your physician before making any changes to your diet or supplemental regimen.

MAGNESIUM HYDROXIDE (mag-NEE-zee-um hye-DROKS-ide)

Brand Names: Phillips' Milk of Magnesia, Phillips' Chewable

About Magnesium Hydroxide

Phillips' Milk of Magnesia—in the recognizable blue bottle—is a familiar antidote for constipation. If you move your bowels two or fewer times per week, or if you have to strain and have terrible difficulty moving them, you are likely suffering from constipation.

Any number of things can cause constipation, including drugs, poor diet or bowel habits, irritable bowel syndrome, endocrine problems, even nerve damage. That's why it's important to have a physician rule out any underlying problems.

In many of us, the problem is triggered by lack of fiber and/or fluid in the diet. We need the appropriate amount of fluid in our stool to keep it soft, and fiber help draws that fluid in. If we're lacking either fluid or fiber, the stool can become hard and difficult to pass. Magensium hydroxide is an osmotic laxative, which means that it encourages the movement of fluid into the colon. This helps to soften the stool and stimulate the bowels to contract in the rhythmic movements (peristalsis) that push the stool out of the body.

Possible Side Effects

The drug's side effects include low blood pressure, abdominal cramps, and muscle weakness.

Which Nutrients Are Robbed

Taking this medicine may deplete your supply of, increase your need for, or interfere with the activity of:

- Folic acid
- Iron
- Vitamin D
- Phosphorus
- Calcium
- Zinc

Additional Ways This Drug May Upset Your Nutritional Balance

Magnesium hydroxide can cause diarrhea, which can hamper nutrient absorption.

This drug can also trigger hypermagnesemia, or too much magnesium in the blood.

Restoring Your Nutritional Balance

To compensate for the nutrient loss caused by this drug, speak to your physician about taking 400–800 mcg folic acid, 400 IU vitamin D, 1,200 mg calcium, 700 mg phosphorus, and 50–200 mg zinc per day. And ask your physician to consider the potential effects of iron depletion.

You can also eat foods that contain the depleted nutrients:

- Folic acid: beef liver, fortified breakfast cereals, spinach, great northern beans, asparagus

- Vitamin D: salmon, mackerel, sardines, eel, fortified milk
- Calcium: milk, dried figs, Swiss cheese, yogurt, tofu
- Phosphorus: plain nonfat yogurt, lentils, salmon, milk, halibut
- Zinc: oysters, beef shank, chicken, pork tenderloin, plain yogurt

Consult with your physician before making any changes to your diet or supplemental regimen.

MAGNESIUM OXIDE (mag-NEE-zee-um OKS-ide)

Brand Names: Mag-Ox 400, Mag-Gel 600, Uro-Mag

About Magnesium Oxide

There are only a few ounces of magnesium in your body, over half of which is stored in your bones and teeth. Only a small amount circulates in the bloodstream, but it is absolutely essential for good health, because magnesium is a necessary ingredient in more than 300 biochemical reactions. Utilized by every single cell in your body, magnesium plays an important part in energy metabolism, manufacture of genetic material, maintenance of normal muscle and nerve function, regulation of heart rhythm, and preservation of bones.

When you run short of magnesium—a condition called hypomagnesemia—you may suffer from weakness, anxiety, lack of appetite, poor coordination, and muscle spasms. If the deficiency becomes severe or continues for too long, you can develop elevated blood pressure, abnormal heart rhythms, swollen gums, and other problems.

Magnesium oxide is one of the supplements physicians use to replenish magnesium stores; 250 to 500 milligrams two to four times a day may be prescribed to treat chronic hypomagnesemia.

Possible Side Effects

The drug's side effects include low blood pressure, depression, breathing difficulty, and coma.

Which Nutrients Are Robbed

Taking this medicine may deplete your supply of, increase your need for, or interfere with the activity of:

- Calcium
- Potassium
- Phosphorus

Additional Ways This Drug May Upset Your Nutritional Balance

Magnesium oxide can cause nausea and vomiting, which can upset your eating habits and possibly interfere with good nutrition. It can also cause diarrhea, which can hamper nutrient absorption.

This drug can also trigger hypermagnesemia, or too much magnesium in the blood.

Restoring Your Nutritional Balance

To compensate for the nutrient loss caused by this drug, speak to your physician about taking 1,200 mg calcium, 700 mg phosphorus, and 100–300 mg potassium per day.

You can also eat foods that contain the depleted nutrients:

- Calcium: milk, dried figs, Swiss cheese, yogurt, tofu
- Phosphorus: plain nonfat yogurt, lentils, salmon, milk, halibut
- Potassium: dried figs, California avocado, papaya, banana, dates

Consult with your physician before making any changes to your diet or supplemental regimen.

MAGNESIUM SULFATE (mag-NEE-zee-um SUL-fate)

Brand Name: Epsom Salts

About Magnesium Sulfate

A lack of sufficient magnesium in the blood is called hypomagnesemia, a condition that can cause vomiting, weakness, muscle tremors, fatigue, and loss of appetite. Hypomagnesemia can be caused by a lack of magnesium in the diet, trouble with magnesium absorption, chronic diarrhea, or overconsumption of alcohol. Large amounts of magnesium can be lost through the urine due to high levels of certain hormones, diuretics, the drug amphotericin B, and other medications.

The treatment of hypomagnesemia consists of curing the underlying problems, if any, and replacing the missing magnesium. Magnesium sulfate, which can be injected into the muscles or veins, is used for this purpose, as well as to treat seizures related to eclampsia, constipation, and irregular heartbeat.

Possible Side Effects

The drug's side effects include flushing and drowsiness.

Which Nutrients Are Robbed

Taking this medicine may deplete your supply of, increase your need for, or interfere with the activity of:

- Calcium   • Phosphorus

Additional Ways This Drug May Upset Your Nutritional Balance

Magnesium sulfate can cause diarrhea, which can hamper nutrient absorption.

Restoring Your Nutritional Balance

To compensate for the nutrient loss caused by this drug, speak to your physician about taking 1,200 mg calcium and 700 mg phosphorus per day.

You can also eat foods that contain the depleted nutrients:

- Calcium: milk, dried figs, Swiss cheese, yogurt, tofu
- Phosphorus: plain nonfat yogurt, lentils, salmon, milk, halibut

Consult with your physician before making any changes to your diet or supplemental regimen.

MANNITOL (MAN-i-tole)

Brand Names: Osmitrol, Resectisol Irrigation Solution

About Mannitol

Mannitol is a diuretic used to treat, among other things, pressure in the brain caused by the buildup of excessive amounts of fluid. This problem can arise following a head injury, when fluid leaks out of the brain tissue and into the spaces between the brain and skull. The bony skull can't expand to accommodate the increased amounts of fluid, and this fluid pushes on the brain.

Mannitol is also used to treat acute liver failure, a potentially deadly disease that is often due to acetaminophen toxicity but that can also result from viral hepatitis, reactions to drugs, poisonous mushrooms, and cancer. The drug is also used to treat certain cases of kidney failure or pressure within the eyeball, and eliminate various toxic substances via the urine.

Possible Side Effects

Mannitol's side effects include heart failure, blurred vision, allergic reactions, and dizziness.

Which Nutrients Are Robbed

Taking this medicine may deplete your supply of, increase your need for, or interfere with the activity of:

- Potassium

Additional Ways This Drug May Upset Your Nutritional Balance

Mannitol can cause nausea and vomiting, all of which can upset your eating habits and possibly interfere with good nutrition.

Restoring Your Nutritional Balance

A Note on Potassium: "Regular" diuretics lower potassium levels, while potassium-sparing diuretics do not—they may increase levels instead. It is not uncommon for doctors to prescribe two different diuretics. That's why you should speak to your physician about your potassium levels, and whether it is appropriate for you to take supplements or eat potassium-rich foods.

Consult with your physician before making any changes to your diet or supplemental regimen.

MECLOFENAMATE (me-kloe-fen-AM-ate)

Brand Name: Meclomen

About Meclofenamate

Estimates of the number of people who suffer from one type of arthritis or another vary, but it's safe to say that:

- Over 20 million Americans suffer from osteoarthritis.
- More than 2 million have rheumatoid arthritis.
- About 1 million adults are afflicted with psoriatic arthritis.
- 300,000 struggle with ankylosing spondylitis.
- Close to 300,000 youngsters have juvenile rheumatoid arthritis.
- Over 3 million suffer from fibromyalgia.

All of these forms of arthritis can lead to inflammation—that heat, redness, and pain that bedevils afflicted joints.

The treatments for the different kinds of inflammatory arthritis vary, but they all work to reduce inflammation. Drugs like meclofenamate do so by interfering with the synthesis of prostaglandins, hormone-like substances that serve as ringleaders for the inflammatory brawls that can turn once-quiet, smoothly working joints into physiologic disaster areas. Eliminating inflammation may not solve the underlying problem, but it does reduce pain and may allow you to use your joint again.

Meclofenamate may be prescribed as part of the treatment for various forms of inflammatory arthritis or other disorders that cause inflammation and mild to moderate pain. It's also used for painful menstrual periods.

Possible Side Effects

The drug's more common side effects include dizziness, skin rash, and abdominal cramps.

Which Nutrients Are Robbed

Taking this medicine may deplete your supply of, increase your need for, or interfere with the activity of:

- Folic acid

Additional Ways This Drug May Upset Your Nutritional Balance

Meclofenamate can cause heartburn, indigestion, nausea, and vomiting, all of which can upset your eating habits and possibly interfere with good nutrition.

Restoring Your Nutritional Balance

To compensate for the nutrient loss caused by this drug, speak to your physician about taking 400–800 mcg folic acid per day.

You can also eat foods that contain the depleted nutrient:

- Folic acid: beef liver, fortified breakfast cereals, spinach, great northern beans, asparagus

Consult with your physician before making any changes to your diet or supplemental regimen.

MEFENAMIC ACID (me-fe-NAM-ik ASS-id)

Brand Name: Ponstel

About Mefenamic Acid

Doctors commonly prescribe nonsteroidal anti-inflammatory drugs (NSAIDs) to treat mild to moderate pain and/or inflammation, the kind seen in osteoarthritis, rheumatoid arthritis, ankylosing spondylitis, certain types of eye surgery, migraine headaches, and other problems. While the various NSAIDs are similar, each has specific properties that can make one better suited than others to handle certain problems. Mefenamic acid appears to have the edge when it comes to the treatment of dysmenorrhea (painful menstrual periods) and menorrhagia (unusually long periods with heavy bleeding).

Although we don't know what accounts for the pain in 75 percent of the women with painful periods, a good suspect is the prostaglandins. These are hormone-like substances that reduce the flow of blood to the uterus, cause it to contract, and make the nerve endings more likely to send pain messages to the brain. Mefenamic acid appears to interfere with substances called COX (cyclooxygenase), which serve as "parents" of the prostaglandins. This slows the production of prostaglandins and reduces pain.

Mefenamic acid also helps ease the symptoms of menorrhagia, and although the way it works is not completely clear, it often reduces unusually heavy bleeding.

Possible Side Effects

The drug's more common side effects include headache, flatulence, and dizziness.

Which Nutrients Are Robbed

Taking this medicine may deplete your supply of, increase your need for, or interfere with the activity of:

- Folic acid

Additional Ways This Drug May Upset Your Nutritional Balance

Mefenamic acid can cause heartburn, indigestion, nausea, vomiting, and abdominal cramping or pain, all of which can upset your eating habits and possibly interfere with good nutrition. It can also cause diarrhea, which can hamper nutrient absorption.

Restoring Your Nutritional Balance

To compensate for the nutrient loss caused by this drug, speak to your physician about taking 400–800 mcg folic acid per day.

You can also eat foods that contain the depleted nutrient:

- Folic acid: beef liver, fortified breakfast cereals, spinach, great northern beans, asparagus

Consult with your physician before making any changes to your diet or supplemental regimen.

MELOXICAM (mel-OKS-i-kam)

Brand Name: Mobic

About Meloxicam

The pain of osteoarthritis affects over 20 million Americans. We have a variety of medicines to ease that pain, most notably the nonsteroidal anti-inflammatories (NSAIDs), a group that includes aspirin and ibuprofen. However, a lesser-known NSAID, meloxicam, may be just as effective at relieving pain as the other NSAIDs, while slightly less likely to cause stomach ulcers. Recently approved in the United States as a treatment for osteoarthritis, meloxicam is a popular treatment overseas for painful joint conditions. Not everyone responds to this drug, but those who do enjoy a reduction in pain and an increase in mobility in their arthritic joints.

Possible Side Effects

The drug's more common side effects include headache, flu-like symptoms, and edema (an unusual accumulation of fluid in one or more parts of the body).

Which Nutrients Are Robbed

Taking this medicine may deplete your supply of, increase your need for, or interfere with the activity of:

- Folic acid

Additional Ways This Drug May Upset Your Nutritional Balance

Meloxicam can cause heartburn, bloating, nausea, and abdominal pain, all of which can upset your eating habits and possibly interfere with good nutrition. It can also cause diarrhea, which can hamper nutrient absorption.

Restoring Your Nutritional Balance

To compensate for the nutrient loss caused by this drug, speak to your physician about taking 400–800 mcg folic acid per day.

You can also eat foods that contain the depleted nutrient:

- Folic acid: beef liver, fortified breakfast cereals, spinach, great northern beans, asparagus

Consult with your physician before making any changes to your diet or supplemental regimen.

MESALAMINE (me-SAL-uh-meen)

Brand Names: Asacol Oral, Canasa, Pentasa Oral, Rowasa Rectal

About Mesalamine

Ulcerative colitis, which can strike at any age, produces inflammation and ulcers in the large intestine (colon) and triggers abdominal cramps, bloody diarrhea, and fever. In severe cases, a victim may have up to 20 bowel movements a day.

Crohn's disease, a related ailment, is a chronic inflammation of the intestinal wall, causing abdominal pain and cramps, diarrhea, fever, weight loss, and lack of appetite. Symptoms of Crohn's can afflict just about any part of the digestive tract, from the place where the food enters the body, to the place where it exits.

Mesalamine is an anti-inflammatory used for inflammatory bowel diseases such as ulcerative colitis and Crohn's disease. It acts locally in the bowel, instead of tracking down inflammation elsewhere in the body. It doesn't work for everybody, but for some it brings relief from abdominal pain and diarrhea within a few days or weeks.

Possible Side Effects

Side effects include headache, nausea, inflammation of the pancreas, back pain, and weakness.

Which Nutrients Are Robbed

Taking this medicine may deplete your supply of, increase your need for, or interfere with the activity of:

- Folic acid

Additional Ways This Drug May Upset Your Nutritional Balance

Mesalamine can cause nausea and vomiting, which can upset your eating habits and possibly interfere with good nutrition.

Restoring Your Nutritional Balance

To compensate for the nutrient loss caused by this drug, speak to your physician about taking 400–800 mcg folic acid per day.

You can also eat foods that contain the depleted nutrient:

- Folic acid: beef liver, fortified breakfast cereals, spinach, great northern beans, asparagus

Consult with your physician before making any changes to your diet or supplemental regimen.

MESORIDAZINE (mez-oh-RID-uh-zeen)

Brand Names: Serentil, Serentil Concentrate

About Mesoridazine

Schizophrenia typically strikes young men and women in their late teens to mid-20s. Although these people may be quite normal in the early part of their lives, over a period of a few weeks or years, their ability to work, interact with others, and care for themselves gradually declines. The symptoms can be divided into three groups, and those with schizophrenia may suffer symptoms from any or all of these groups.

- *Positive symptoms*: hearing voices, believing that people are following them or spying on them, thinking that certain words in a book or newspaper are messages to them, insisting that thoughts are being put into their heads by other people or things, or that others can hear or read their thoughts
- *Negative symptoms*: "flattening" of emotions, making little or no eye contact when speaking to others, finding little or no joy in previously enjoyable activities, lack of interest in social relationships
- *Cognitive impairment*: inability to concentrate, problems remembering, difficulty planning and organizing, inability to follow a story in a novel or on a TV show

No one really knows what causes schizophrenia; the best bet to date is that it stems from a combination of genetic and environmental factors. The overall risk of developing schizophrenia is 1 percent but if a parent or sibling has the disease, the risk jumps to 10 percent. And if a person's identical twin develops the problem, the risk shoots up to 50 percent.

Mesoridazine is one of the older antipsychotic drugs used to treat schizophrenia, and is no longer a first-line choice. It's typically prescribed for people who have not responded to other medications.

Possible Side Effects

The drug's side effects include rapid heartbeat, slurred speech, and involuntary movements or the lips, tongue, arms, or legs.

Which Nutrients Are Robbed

Taking this medicine may deplete your supply of, increase your need for, or interfere with the activity of:

- Riboflavin
- Coenzyme Q_{10}

Additional Ways This Drug May Upset Your Nutritional Balance

Mesoridazine can cause stomach pain, nausea, and vomiting, all of which can upset your eating habits and possibly interfere with good nutrition.

Restoring Your Nutritional Balance

To compensate for the nutrient loss caused by this drug, speak to your physician about taking 25–100 mg riboflavin and 30–100 mg coenzyme Q_{10} per day. You can also eat foods that contain the depleted nutrients:

- Riboflavin: dried sunflower seeds, orange juice, bulgur, spinach noodles, pine nuts
- Coenzyme Q_{10}: beef, chicken, trout, salmon, oranges, broccoli

Consult with your physician before making any changes to your diet or supplemental regimen.

METFORMIN, METFORMIN PLUS ROSIGLITAZONE
(met-FOR-min, roe-si-GLI-tuh-zohn)

Brand Names: Metformin: Glucophage, Glucophage XR
Metformin plus rosiglitazone: Apo-Metformin, Avandamet, Glycon, Gen-Metformin, Nu-Metformin, Novo-Metformin

About Metformin, Metformin plus Rosiglitazone

Diabetes is bad news for the body. But luckily, during the past several decades, more effective medicines have been developed to combat this disease. There are now five different groups of medicines that can be taken orally.

Metformin, which belongs to the group called the biguanides, is used to control blood glucose levels in those with type 2 diabetes. Although it's not completely clear how these drugs work, metformin appears to:

- Help clear blood sugar (glucose) from the blood
- Slow the production of new glucose in the liver
- Reduce the absorption of glucose from the gastrointestinal tract

It's very common for physicians to give patients two different drugs to combat diabetes, and metformin may be combined with the medication rosiglitazone. Rosiglitazone combats diabetes in several ways, chief of which is to reduce insulin resistance. Insulin resistance arises when the cells responsible for storing excess blood sugar refuse to "open up" when insulin comes knocking at the door. Rosiglitazone acts like a key, helping insulin open the door, so it can deposit the excess glucose inside the cell and clear it from the blood.

Possible Side Effects

Metformin's more common side effects include nausea, diarrhea, flatulence, and weakness. The more common side effects seen with metformin plus rosiglitazone include upper respiratory tract infection and diarrhea.

Which Nutrients Are Robbed

Taking this medicine may deplete your supply of, increase your need for, or interfere with the activity of:

- Folic acid   - Vitamin B_{12}

Additional Ways These Drugs May Upset Your Nutritional Balance

Metformin can cause low blood sugar (hypoglycemia), nausea, vomiting, indigestion, abdominal discomfort and distention, heartburn, and changes in taste, all of which can upset your eating habits and possibly interfere with good nutrition. It can also cause diarrhea, which can hamper nutrient absorption.

Metformin plus rosiglitazone can interfere with good nutrition by causing hypoglycemia and diarrhea.

Restoring Your Nutritional Balance

To compensate for the nutrient loss caused by this drug, speak to your physician about taking 400–800 mcg folic acid and 500–1,000 mcg vitamin B_{12} per day.

You can also eat foods that contain the depleted nutrients:

- Folic acid: beef liver, fortified breakfast cereals, spinach, great northern beans, asparagus
- Vitamin B_{12}: beef liver, rainbow trout, sockeye salmon, beef, haddock

Consult with your physician before making any changes to your diet or supplemental regimen.

METHAZOLAMIDE (meth-uh-ZOE-luh-mide)

Brand Names: Glauctabs, MZM, Neptazine

About Methazolamide

Your eyes are all wet.

You know about the fluid on the outer surface of the eye, and you know about tears. But there's also fluid inside your eyes, in between your pupils and corneas. This fluid is made by the ciliary bodies behind the iris, and drains into passageways located between the iris and the cornea.

In those with glaucoma, these drains become blocked and fluid starts to build up. Yet it continues to be manufactured, causing more and more fluid to be pushed into a confined space. The pressure within your eyeball increases, eventually becoming more than the optic nerve can handle, and your vision suffers. As the optic nerve is compressed, blind spots may develop along with a loss of peripheral vision, and eventually you will become blind.

This is what happens when glaucoma comes on gradually, as it often does. But it can also hit hard and fast, triggering a headache, eye pain, blurred vision, nausea, vomiting, and loss of vision in just a few hours if the problem isn't handled immediately.

Methazolamide is used in the treatment of both types of glaucoma. It works by decreasing the secretion of fluid from the ciliary bodies.

Possible Side Effects

The drug's side effects include depression, bone marrow depression, fatigue, and trembling.

Which Nutrients Are Robbed

Taking this medicine may deplete your supply of, increase your need for, or interfere with the activity of:

- Potassium

Additional Ways This Drug May Upset Your Nutritional Balance

Methazolamide can cause loss of appetite, changes in taste, nausea, and vomiting, all of which can upset your eating habits and possibly interfere with good nutrition. It can also cause diarrhea, which can hamper nutrient absorption.

Restoring Your Nutritional Balance

A Note on Potassium: "Regular" diuretics lower potassium levels, while potassium-sparing diuretics do not—they may increase levels instead. It is not uncommon for doctors to prescribe two different diuretics. That's why you should speak to your physician about your potassium levels, and whether it is appropriate for you to take supplements or eat potassium-rich foods.

Consult with your physician before making any changes to your diet or supplemental regimen.

METHOCARBAMOL PLUS ASPIRIN (meth-oh-KAR-buh-mole, ASS-pir-in)

Brand Name: Robaxisal

About Methocarbamol and Aspirin

You're probably all too familiar with the pain of a muscle spasm, whether it strikes in your calf when you're exercising or in the arch of your foot while you're lying in bed. Most muscle spasms are harmless problems caused by strain or trauma, but they can be serious problems if they're triggered by a spinal cord injury, cerebral palsy, or perhaps tetanus, a disease caused by the *Clostridium tetani* bacteria. When these bacterial spores enter the body, they produce a toxin that can cause the jaw to lock (which is why tetanus is sometimes called lockjaw). The toxin can also trigger difficulty swallowing, headache, and muscle spasms of the arms, legs, and neck.

Methocarbamol helps relieve muscle spasms linked to painful musculoskeletal ailments like tetanus. The drug, which is used in conjunction with physical therapy, works by depressing certain signals in the central nervous system.

Combining methocarbamol with aspirin helps relieve the pain associated with spasms.

Possible Side Effects

Methocarbamol's side effects include flushing of the face, light-headedness, fever, and kidney impairment, while aspirin's side effects include insomnia, rapid heartbeat, anemia, stomach ulcers, and liver damage.

Which Nutrients Are Robbed

Taking this medicine may deplete your supply of, increase your need for, or interfere with the activity of:

- Folic acid
- Vitamin C
- Iron
- Potassium
- Sodium

Additional Ways This Drug May Upset Your Nutritional Balance

Methocarbamol can cause nausea, vomiting, and changes in taste, while aspirin can cause heartburn, nausea, and vomiting. These side effects can upset your eating habits and possibly interfere with good nutrition.

Aspirin can also trigger hyperkalemia, or too much potassium in the blood.

Restoring Your Nutritional Balance

To compensate for the nutrient loss caused by this drug, speak to your physician about taking 400–800 mcg folic acid and 250–1,500 mg vitamin C per day. And ask your physician to consider the potential effects of iron and sodium depletion and to monitor your potassium status.

You can also eat foods that contain the depleted nutrients:

- Folic acid: beef liver, fortified breakfast cereals, spinach, great northern beans, asparagus
- Vitamin C: papaya, guava, red pepper, cantaloupe, black currants

Consult with your physician before making any changes to your diet or supplemental regimen.

METHOTREXATE (meth-oh-TREKS-ate)

Brand Names: Folex, Folex PFS, Methotrexate LPF, Rheumatrex

About Methotrexate

You might not think that cancer, rheumatoid arthritis, and psoriasis would have anything in common. After all, what does unregulated and unwarranted cell growth have to do with immune system problems or inflammation? But there is a connection: All three diseases can be treated with a powerful drug called methotrexate.

Methotrexate suppresses the immune system, which makes it helpful in treating rheumatoid arthritis, a disease in which the immune system attacks body tissues. Methotrexate is also structurally similar to folic acid, allowing it to interfere with the metabolism of that vitamin in rapidly reproducing cells, thus hindering their production of DNA, RNA, and protein. This results in the death of cells with a rapid turnover, a prime feature of cancer and psoriasis (in which the skin cells grow too fast, leaving flakes, bumps, and raised areas on the skin).

These combined properties make methotrexate useful for treating breast, lung, neck, and other forms of cancer, as well as rheumatoid arthritis and psoriasis.

Possible Side Effects

The drug's more common side effects include reddening of the skin, gingivitis, and kidney failure.

Which Nutrients Are Robbed

Taking this medicine may deplete your supply of, increase your need for, or interfere with the activity of:

- Folic acid
- Vitamin B_{12}
- Beta-carotene
- Calcium

Additional Ways This Drug May Upset Your Nutritional Balance

Methotrexate can cause nausea, vomiting, and loss of appetite, all of which can upset your eating habits and possibly interfere with good nutrition. It can also cause diarrhea, which can hamper nutrient absorption.

Restoring Your Nutritional Balance

To compensate for the nutrient loss caused by this drug, speak to your physician about taking 500–1,000 mcg vitamin B_{12}, 25,000 IU beta-carotene, and 1,200 mg calcium per day. Taking folic acid can interfere with methotrexate's action, so ask your physician to consider the potential effects of folic acid depletion.

Calcium citrate may lower the levels of methotrexate in your blood, so ask your physician which form of calcium is best for you.

You can also eat foods that contain the depleted nutrients:

- Vitamin B_{12}: beef liver, rainbow trout, sockeye salmon, beef, haddock
- Beta-carotene: carrot, spinach, mango, cantaloupe, apricot nectar
- Calcium: milk, dried figs, Swiss cheese, yogurt, tofu

Consult with your physician before making any changes to your diet or supplemental regimen.

METHSUXIMIDE (meth-SUKS-i-mide)

Brand Name: Celotin

About Methsuximide

This drug is a "pinch hitter," used to treat petit mal seizures when ethosuximide or other drugs are not helping.

Petit mal seizures are "quiet" seizures that often begin early in life. During an attack, the child is typically unaware of what is happening to him or around him. He may stare, his eyelids may flutter, and his facial muscles twitch. In a matter of seconds—usually just a few, but sometimes up to thirty—it's all over. The attack is brief and disappears without a trace; the victim might not even know that anything happened.

In addition to treating petit mal seizures, methsuximide has been tested as a treatment for partial seizures. A partial seizure can be simple, affecting only a small part of the brain and causing jerking in an arm or a leg. Or it can be complex. Complex partial seizures are "larger" seizures that may begin with staring and loss of awareness, then build to random movements of the limbs, an inability to understand what others are saying, and other symptoms. In some cases, the partial complex seizure may grow as the unexpected, uncontrolled "electrical firing" spreads to other parts of the brain, leading to loss of consciousness, frothing at the mouth, jerking of the limbs, and other symptoms.

The drug's mechanism of action is not fully understood; it may work by altering the way calcium is handled in the brain and changing the brain's metabolic rate.

Possible Side Effects

The drug's side effects include sore throat, fever, swollen glands, and itching.

Which Nutrients Are Robbed

Taking this medicine may deplete your supply of, increase your need for, or interfere with the activity of:

- Folic acid
- Vitamin K
- Vitamin D
- Calcium

Restoring Your Nutritional Balance

To compensate for the nutrient loss caused by this drug, speak to your physician about taking 400–800 mcg folic acid, 400 IU vitamin D, 60–80 mcg vitamin K, and 1,200 mg calcium per day.

You can also eat foods that contain the depleted nutrients:

- Folic acid: beef liver, fortified breakfast cereals, spinach, great northern beans, asparagus
- Vitamin D: salmon, mackerel, sardines, eel, fortified milk
- Vitamin K: kale, broccoli, parsley, Swiss chard, spinach
- Calcium: milk, dried figs, Swiss cheese, yogurt, tofu

Consult with your physician before making any changes to your diet or supplemental regimen.

METHYLDOPA (meth-il-DOE-pah)

Brand Names: Aldomet, Amodopa, Apo-Methyldopa, Dopamet, Novomedopa, Nu-Medopa

About Methyldopa

To get an idea of how high blood pressure (hypertension) medications work, imagine thousands of fans at a rock concert pushing their way down a corridor to get into the stadium and see their hero. These wall-to-wall bodies create a lot of pressure in that hallway. To reduce future pressure, you could allow fewer people in the hallway. To reduce the pressure right now, you could open some doors and kick some of the people out, or magically widen the hallway so that people could move about more easily.

Doctors take similar approaches to lowering blood pressure. They have drugs that slow the heart's output of blood (that's like letting fewer people into the hallway), diuretics that reduce the blood volume (similar to letting some of the people out of the hallway), and drugs that reduce the resistance of the blood vessels to the flow of blood (that's like making the hallway wider).

Methyldopa takes the third approach, treating mild to moderately severe hypertension by widening the blood vessels. It also slightly reduces the heart rate, which means that less blood is forced through the body's "hallways" at any given time. Both of these approaches result in a reduction in blood pressure.

Possible Side Effects

The drug's side effects include sedation, impotence, an unusually slow heartbeat, diarrhea, and fever.

Which Nutrients Are Robbed

Taking this medicine may deplete your supply of, increase your need for, or interfere with the activity of:

- Vitamin B_{12} • Coenzyme Q_{10}

Restoring Your Nutritional Balance

To compensate for the nutrient loss caused by this drug, speak to your physician about taking 500–1,000 mcg vitamin B_{12} and 30–100 mg coenzyme Q_{10} per day.

You can also eat foods that contain the depleted nutrients:

- Vitamin B_{12}: beef liver, rainbow trout, sockeye salmon, beef, haddock
- Coenzyme Q_{10}: beef, chicken, trout, salmon, oranges, broccoli

Consult with your physician before making any changes to your diet or supplemental regimen.

METHYLDOPA PLUS HYDROCHLOROTHIAZIDE (meth-il-DOE-pah, hye-droe-klor-oh-THYE-uh-zide)

Brand Names: Aldoril, Aldoril-15, Aldoril-25, Apo-Methazide, Novo-Doparil, PMS-Dopazide

About Methyldopa plus Hydrochlorothiazide

Suppose you wanted to send an e-mail message of great importance. Before you could get on-line, you would need to enter the correct password. Methyldopa reduces high blood pressure (hypertension) by acting like a password. It does this by inserting itself into special receptor sites in the brain that cause the brain to send instructions to the blood vessels to open up a bit wider. This opening of the blood vessels reduces their resistance to the flow of blood which, in turn, reduces the blood pressure.

Methyldopa may be combined with other drugs, such as hydrochlorothiazide, a diuretic that forces the body to release more fluid than usual via the urine. Reducing the amount of fluid in the blood makes it easier for the heart to pump the blood through the blood vessels, and lowers blood pressure.

Possible Side Effects

Methyldopa's side effects include sedation, impotence, an unusually slow heart rate, diarrhea, and fever. Hydrochlorothiazide's side effects include low blood pressure, photosensitivity, allergic reactions, and elevated calcium levels.

Which Nutrients Are Robbed

Taking this medicine may deplete your supply of, increase your need for, or interfere with the activity of:

- Vitamin B_6
- Magnesium
- Phosphorus
- Potassium
- Sodium
- Zinc
- Coenzyme Q_{10}

Additional Ways This Drug May Upset Your Nutritional Balance

Hydrochlorothiazide can cause loss of appetite, which can upset your eating habits and possibly interfere with good nutrition.

Restoring Your Nutritional Balance

To compensate for the nutrient loss caused by this drug, speak to your physician about taking 50–100 mg vitamin B_6, 500–1,000 mg magnesium, 700 mg phosphorus, 50–200 mg zinc, and 30–100 mg coenzyme Q_{10} per day. And ask your physician to consider the potential effects of sodium depletion.

A Note on Potassium: "Regular" diuretics lower potassium levels, while potassium-sparing diuretics do not—they may increase levels instead. It is not uncommon for doctors to prescribe two different diuretics. That's why you should speak to your physician about your potassium levels, and whether it is appropriate for you to take supplements or eat potassium-rich foods.

You can also eat foods that contain the depleted nutrients:

- Vitamin B_6: potato, banana, garbanzo beans, chicken breast, fortified oatmeal
- Magnesium: Florida avocado, toasted wheat germ, almonds, shredded wheat cereal, pumpkin seeds

- Phosphorus: plain nonfat yogurt, lentils, salmon, milk, halibut
- Zinc: oysters, beef shank, chicken, pork tenderloin, plain yogurt
- Coenzyme Q_{10}: beef, chicken, trout, salmon, oranges, broccoli

Consult with your physician before making any changes to your diet or supplemental regimen.

METHYLPREDNISOLONE (meth-il-pred-NIS-oh-lohn)

Brand Names: A-MethaPred, DepMedalone 40, DepMedalone 80, Depoject 40, Depoject 80, Depo-Medrol, Depopred, Depo-Predate, Duralone-40, Duralone-80, Med-Jec-40, Medralone 80, Medrol, Meprolone, Methacort 40, Methacort 80, Methylcotolone, Predacorten, Predacorten 80, Solu-Medrol

About Methylprednisolone

You might think that each drug is designed with a specific disease or two in mind—like Celebrex for arthritis, Nexium for heartburn, or Prozac for depression. But many, many drugs can be used to treat several different diseases because they have a common feature that a drug can attack. Methylprednisolone, for example, helps reduce inflammation, a condition that is common to all of these diseases:

- Alcoholic hepatitis: inflammation and death of liver tissue linked to excessive alcohol consumption
- Goodpasture's syndrome: a lung disease that triggers difficulty breathing and cough
- Inflammatory bowel disease: an intestinal condition that may take the form of ulcerative colitis and Crohn's disease
- Multiple sclerosis: a neurologic disease that causes weakness, poor vision, urinary incontinence, and other problems
- Pauci-immune glomerulonephritis: a kidney ailment that causes fever, weight loss, and malaise
- Polyarteritis nodosa: an inflammatory disease of the blood vessels that may cause fever, weight loss, pain, and other problems

Methylprednisolone can be used alone or in conjunction with other drugs to treat all these conditions.

Possible Side Effects

The drug's side effects include irregular heartbeat, insomnia, elevated blood fats, and muscle weakness.

Which Nutrients Are Robbed

Taking this medicine may deplete your supply of, increase your need for, or interfere with the activity of:

- Vitamin A
- Vitamin B$_6$
- Folic acid
- Vitamin C
- Vitamin D
- Vitamin K
- Calcium
- Magnesium
- Phosphorus
- Potassium
- Selenium
- Zinc

Additional Ways This Drug May Upset Your Nutritional Balance

Methylprednisolone can cause indigestion, nausea, vomiting, and abdominal distension, all of which can upset your eating habits and possibly interfere with good nutrition.

Restoring Your Nutritional Balance

To compensate for the nutrient loss caused by this drug, speak to your physician about taking 5,000 IU vitamin A, 50–100 mg vitamin B$_6$, 400–800 mcg folic acid, 250–1,500 mg vitamin C, 400 IU vitamin D, 60–80 mcg vitamin K, 1,200 mg calcium, 500–1,000 mg magnesium, 700 mg phosphorus, 100–300 mg potassium, 20–100 mcg selenium, and 50–200 mg zinc per day.

You can also eat foods that contain the depleted nutrients:

- Vitamin A: beef liver, chicken liver, cheese pizza, whole milk, cheddar cheese
- Vitamin B$_6$: potato, banana, garbanzo beans, chicken breast, fortified oatmeal
- Folic acid: beef liver, fortified breakfast cereals, spinach, great northern beans, asparagus
- Vitamin C: papaya, guava, red pepper, cantaloupe, black currants
- Vitamin D: salmon, mackerel, sardines, eel, fortified milk
- Vitamin K: kale, broccoli, parsley, Swiss chard, spinach
- Calcium: milk, dried figs, Swiss cheese, yogurt, tofu
- Magnesium: Florida avocado, toasted wheat germ, almonds, shredded wheat cereal, pumpkin seeds

- Phosphorus: plain nonfat yogurt, lentils, salmon, milk, halibut
- Potassium: dried figs, California avocado, papaya, banana, dates
- Selenium: Brazil nuts, tuna, beef liver, turkey breast, spaghetti with meat sauce
- Zinc: oysters, beef shank, chicken, pork tenderloin, plain yogurt

Consult with your physician before making any changes to your diet or supplemental regimen.

METOCLOPRAMIDE (met-oh-KLOE-prah-mide)

Brand Names: Apo-Metoclop, Reglan, Nu-Metoclopramide, PMS-Metoclopramide

About Metoclopramide

You can think of metoclopramide as a stop-and-go drug. On the stop side, it helps reduce the urge to vomit, which in doctor-speak makes it an antiemetic. ("Emesis" is the Greek word for "vomiting.") Metoclopramide is given along with certain types of chemotherapy or radiation treatments, during labor or delivery, and in the case of emergency surgery, when there is no time to wait for the stomach to empty out.

On the go side, metoclopramide helps improve the movement (motility) of food through the body. Food doesn't move down the esophagus and through the stomach and intestines on its own—it's pushed through by the contractions of the walls of these structures. But sometimes these food-moving muscles don't work as well as they should. By stimulating the action of these muscles, metoclopramide speeds the transit time of the food through the stomach and intestines. This is useful in treating the gastric stasis, or shutdown, sometimes seen following surgery or with diabetes and other ailments.

Possible Side Effects

The drug's more common side effects include weakness, drowsiness, and restlessness.

Which Nutrients Are Robbed

Taking this medicine may deplete your supply of, increase your need for, or interfere with the activity of:

- Riboflavin

Additional Ways This Drug May Upset Your Nutritional Balance

Metoclopramide can cause nausea, which can upset your eating habits and possibly interfere with good nutrition. It can also cause diarrhea, which can hamper nutrient absorption.

Restoring Your Nutritional Balance

To compensate for the nutrient loss caused by this drug, speak to your physician about taking 25–100 mg riboflavin per day.

You can also eat foods that contain the depleted nutrient:

- Riboflavin: dried sunflower seeds, orange juice, bulgur, spinach noodles, pine nuts

Consult with your physician before making any changes to your diet or supplemental regimen.

METOLAZONE (me-TOLE-uh-zone)

Brand Names: Diulo, Mykrox, Zaroxolyn

About Metolazone

Diuretics are "water pills" used to treat elevated blood pressure (hypertension). They work by forcing the kidneys to release extra water and sodium, thus reducing the blood volume. Less blood volume means less pressure exerted on the blood vessels and a lighter workload for the heart. Diuretics work well and have been a mainstay of hypertension treatment for many years.

Metolazone is a thiazide-like diuretic, which means that it lowers blood pressure by increasing the excretion of water and sodium, while encouraging small arteries called arterioles to relax and open wide. Just as the pressure in your water pipes at home will drop when the plumber installs wider pipes, so will the pressure in your internal pipes drop when the blood vessels relax and become wider.

These properties make metolazone effective in treating mild to moderate hypertension, as well as the accumulation of fluid seen in heart failure.

Possible Side Effects

Side effects include chest pain, dizziness, headache, anxiety, and muscle cramps.

Which Nutrients Are Robbed

Taking this medicine may deplete your supply of, increase your need for, or interfere with the activity of:

- Magnesium
- Phosphorus
- Potassium
- Sodium
- Zinc
- Coenzyme Q_{10}

Additional Ways This Drug May Upset Your Nutritional Balance

Metolazone can cause nausea, vomiting, abdominal pain, cramping, and bloating, all of which can upset your eating habits and possibly interfere with good nutrition. It can also cause diarrhea, which can hamper nutrient absorption.

This drug can also trigger hypercalcemia, or too much calcium in the blood.

Restoring Your Nutritional Balance

To compensate for the nutrient loss caused by this drug, speak to your physician about taking 500–1,000 mg magnesium, 700 mg phosphorus, 50–200 mg zinc, and 30–100 mg coenzyme Q_{10} per day. And ask your physician to consider the potential effects of sodium depletion.

A Note on Potassium: "Regular" diuretics lower potassium levels, while potassium-sparing diuretics do not—they may increase levels instead. It is not uncommon for doctors to prescribe two different diuretics. That's why you should speak to your physician about your potassium levels, and whether it is appropriate for you to take supplements or eat potassium-rich foods.

You can also eat foods that contain the depleted nutrients:

- Magnesium: Florida avocado, toasted wheat germ, almonds, shredded wheat cereal, pumpkin seeds
- Phosphorus: plain nonfat yogurt, lentils, salmon, milk, halibut
- Zinc: oysters, beef shank, chicken, pork tenderloin, plain yogurt
- Coenzyme Q_{10}: beef, chicken, trout, salmon, oranges, broccoli

Consult with your physician before making any changes to your diet or supplemental regimen.

METOPROLOL (me-TOE-proe-lole)

Brand Names: Apo-Metoprolol (Type L), Betaloc, Betaloc Durules,
Lopressor, Novo-Metoprolol, Nu-Metop, Toprol XL

About Metoprolol

A lot of people have watchdogs to protect their homes. Some of these
dogs aren't very selective; they'll bark at anyone invading their territory,
whether friend or foe, and try to keep everybody at bay. Other dogs are quite
selective, barking only at foes.

A group of medicines called the beta-blockers can be compared to both
of these kinds of dogs. The beta-blockers are used to treat elevated blood
pressure (hypertension), irregular heartbeat, angina, and other ailments.
While some beta-blockers are selective, others are not.

All of the beta-blockers work by blocking special areas called beta-receptors in various parts of the body, including the heart and the airways. The results can be both good and bad. If the beta-receptors in the heart are blocked,
for example, the heart slows a bit and blood pressure falls, which is good news
for hypertensives. But if the beta-receptors in the airways are blocked, these
passageways can become constricted, making it difficult to breathe—bad
news, especially for those who already have breathing problems.

Luckily, some beta-blockers are selective; that is, they "prefer" to block
beta-receptors in the heart. Although they do still block beta-receptors elsewhere, their preference for working in the heart makes them less likely to trigger breathing difficulties.

One of these selective beta-blockers, metoprolol, is useful for treating elevated blood pressure, angina, and certain irregular heartbeats, as well as reducing the risk of hospitalization or death in those with congestive heart
failure. It is often used when nonselective beta-blockers might cause breathing or other difficulties.

Possible Side Effects

The drug's more common side effects include drowsiness, insomnia, and
a decrease in sexual ability.

Which Nutrients Are Robbed

Taking this medicine may deplete your supply of, increase your need for,
or interfere with the activity of:

- Coenzyme Q_{10}
- Melatonin

Additional Ways This Drug May Upset Your Nutritional Balance

Metoprolol can cause nausea, vomiting, and stomach discomfort, all of which can upset your eating habits and possibly interfere with good nutrition. It can also cause diarrhea, which can hamper nutrient absorption.

Restoring Your Nutritional Balance

To compensate for the nutrient loss caused by this drug, speak to your physician about taking 30–100 mg coenzyme Q_{10} and 1–3 mg melatonin per day.

You can also eat foods that contain the depleted nutrient:

* Coenzyme Q_{10}: beef, chicken, trout, salmon, oranges, broccoli

Consult with your physician before making any changes to your diet or supplemental regimen.

METRONIDAZOLE (me-troe-NI-dah-zole)

Brand Names: Apo-Metronidazole, Flagyl, Flagyl ER, MetroCream, MetroGel Topical, MetroGel-Vaginal, Metro I.V. Injection, MetroLotion, Noritate Cream, Novo-Nidazol, Protostat Oral

About Metronidazole

Metronidazole is an antiprotozoal drug, which means it's designed to treat diseases caused by single-celled organisms from the subkingdom Protozoa. Taken as a pill or suppository or administered intravenously, metronidazole is used to treat all of these diseases:

* Trichomoniasis: A sexually transmitted disease caused by a parasite, it can trigger a yellow-green, frothy discharge from the vagina.
* Amebiasis: Caused by a single-celled parasite called *Entamoeba histolytica*, it may trigger no symptoms, or it may leave you with diarrhea, bowel gas, abdominal pain and cramps, or a fever. If the infection becomes chronic, anemia and emaciation can result.
* Bacterial vaginosis: This can leave the vagina feeling irritated and itchy, with a discharge and odor that may worsen following sexual intercourse.
* Giardiasis: This is caused by a microorganism called *Giardia*, which you can get from another person or from drinking contaminated water. It can

cause a loss of appetite, nausea, and diarrhea. If the disease continues, you may suffer from weight loss, abdominal bloating, gas, and greasy stools.

Inside the body, metronidazole is converted into another substance that burrows into offending organisms and destroys them by disrupting their DNA.

Possible Side Effects

The drug's more common side effects include dizziness and headache.

Which Nutrients Are Robbed

Taking this medicine may deplete your supply of, increase your need for, or interfere with the activity of:

- Vitamin K
- *Lactobacillus acidophilus*
- *Bifidobacterium bifidum*

Additional Ways This Drug May Upset Your Nutritional Balance

Metronidazole can cause loss of appetite, nausea, and vomiting, and the vaginal form of the drug can cause changes in taste, all of which can upset your eating habits and possibly interfere with good nutrition. It can also cause diarrhea, which can hamper nutrient absorption.

Restoring Your Nutritional Balance

To compensate for the nutrient loss caused by this drug, speak to your physician about taking 60–80 mcg vitamin K, 15 billion live *Bifidobacterium bifidum* organisms, and 15 billion live *Lactobacillus acidophilus* organisms per day.

You can also eat foods that contain the depleted nutrients:

- Vitamin K: kale, broccoli, parsley, Swiss chard, spinach
- *Bifidobacterium bifidum*: Jerusalem artichokes, asparagus, garlic, and onions may stimulate the growth or activity of this probiotic
- *Lactobacillus acidophilus*: yogurt containing live lactobacillus cultures, kefir, acidophilus milk

Consult with your physician before making any changes to your diet or supplemental regimen.

MINERAL OIL (MIN-er-ul oyl)

Brand Names: Agoral Plain, Fleet Mineral Oil Enema, Kondremul, Liqui-Doss, Milkinol, Neo-Cultol, Zymenol

About Mineral Oil

There is no normal number of weekly bowel movements: three, six, even a dozen times a week can all be considered normal. But if you move your bowels less than three times a week, strain a lot, or have great difficulty in passing stool, you're probably suffering from constipation. Constipation is a condition in which the stool becomes dry and hard, making it difficult to pass.

Many things can cause constipation, including poor bowel habits, lack of sufficient fluid or fiber in the diet, diabetes mellitus, Parkinson's disease, multiple sclerosis, paraplegia, irritable bowel syndrome, eating disorders, or the use of drugs such as calcium channel blockers or diuretics.

Mineral oil, an old remedy for constipation that can be administered orally or rectally, softens the stool, making it easier to pass.

Possible Side Effects

The drug's side effects include skin irritation near the rectal area.

Which Nutrients Are Robbed

Taking this medicine may deplete your supply of, increase your need for, or interfere with the activity of:

- Beta-carotene
- Vitamin A
- Vitamin D
- Vitamin E
- Vitamin K
- Calcium
- Phosphorus
- Potassium

Restoring Your Nutritional Balance

To compensate for the nutrient loss caused by this drug, speak to your physician about taking 25,000 IU beta-carotene, 5,000 IU vitamin A, 400 IU vitamin D, 400 IU vitamin E, 60–80 mcg vitamin K, 1,200 mg calcium, 700 mg phosphorus, and 100–300 mg potassium per day.

You can also eat foods that contain the depleted nutrients:

- Beta-carotene: carrot, spinach, mango, cantaloupe, apricot nectar
- Vitamin A: beef liver, chicken liver, cheese pizza, whole milk, cheddar cheese

- Vitamin D: salmon, mackerel, sardines, eel, fortified milk
- Vitamin E: wheat germ oil, almonds, safflower oil, corn oil, soybean oil
- Vitamin K: kale, broccoli, parsley, Swiss chard, spinach
- Calcium: milk, dried figs, Swiss cheese, yogurt, tofu
- Phosphorus: plain nonfat yogurt, lentils, salmon, milk, halibut
- Potassium: dried figs, California avocado, papaya, banana, dates

Consult with your physician before making any changes to your diet or supplemental regimen.

MINOCYCLINE (mi-noe-SYE-kleen)

Brand Names: Apo-Minocycline, Dynacin Oral, Gen-Minocycline, Minocin
IV Injection, Minocin Oral, Syn-Minocycline, Novo-Minocycline

About Minocycline

Acne is often the scourge of teenagers, but it can linger into the mid-20s or longer in some people. The problem arises when dead skin cells and oil (sebum) mix with bacteria inside a hair follicle, causing a blockage. Bacteria can then overgrow and interact with the sebum, prompting inflammation and infection. If the infection is severe, an abscess may develop, and if it ruptures, it can spread the offending substances underneath the skin, triggering even more inflammation.

Mild acne is usually treated with topical antibiotics or drugs that dry the skin or unclog the pores. For severe acne, doctors may recommend antibiotics such as minocycline. Although it doesn't kill bacteria, minocycline prevents the bacteria already present from manufacturing proteins necessary for reproduction. You may have to take minocycline (or other antibiotics) for months or years to keep severe acne under control. Fortunately for teens, the problem usually clears up by itself after a few years.

In addition to acne, minocycline is used to treat numerous bacterial infections, including anthrax.

Possible Side Effects

The drug's side effects include nausea, diarrhea, vertigo, and kidney and liver damage.

Which Nutrients Are Robbed

Taking this medicine may deplete your supply of, increase your need for, or interfere with the activity of:

- Biotin
- Folic acid
- Inositol
- Thiamin
- Riboflavin
- Niacin
- Vitamin B$_6$
- Vitamin B$_{12}$

- Vitamin C
- Vitamin K
- Calcium
- Iron
- Magnesium
- Zinc
- *Bifidobacterium bifidum*
- *Lactobacillus acidophilus*

Additional Ways This Drug May Upset Your Nutritional Balance

Minocycline can cause nausea, which can upset your eating habits and possibly interfere with good nutrition. It can also cause diarrhea, which can hamper nutrient absorption.

Restoring Your Nutritional Balance

To compensate for the nutrient loss caused by this drug, speak to your physician about taking 500–1,000 mcg biotin, 400–800 mcg folic acid, 250–1,000 mg inositol, 25–100 mg thiamin, 25–100 mg riboflavin, 50–100 mg niacin, 50–100 mg vitamin B$_6$, 500–1,000 mcg vitamin B$_{12}$, 250–1,500 mg vitamin C, 60–80 mcg vitamin K, 1,200 mg calcium, 500–1,000 mg magnesium, 50–200 mg zinc, 15 billion live *Bifidobacterium bifidum* organisms, and 15 billion live *Lactobacillus acidophilus* organisms per day. And ask your physician to consider the potential effects of iron depletion.

You can also eat foods that contain the depleted nutrients:

- Biotin: beef liver, soybeans, rice bran, peanut butter, barley
- Folic acid: beef liver, fortified breakfast cereals, spinach, great northern beans, asparagus
- Inositol: cantaloupe, oranges, green beans, grapefruit juice, limes
- Thiamin: braised liver, turkey heart, roasted chicken, gefilte fish, sardines
- Riboflavin: dried sunflower seeds, orange juice, bulgur, spinach noodles, pine nuts
- Niacin: chicken breast, beef liver, mackerel, barley, bulgur
- Vitamin B$_6$: potato, banana, garbanzo beans, chicken breast, fortified oatmeal
- Vitamin B$_{12}$: beef liver, rainbow trout, sockeye salmon, beef, haddock

- Vitamin C: papaya, guava, red pepper, cantaloupe, black currants
- Vitamin K: kale, broccoli, parsley, Swiss chard, spinach
- Calcium: milk, dried figs, Swiss cheese, yogurt, tofu
- Magnesium: Florida avocado, toasted wheat germ, almonds, shredded wheat cereal, pumpkin seeds
- Zinc: oysters, beef shank, chicken, pork tenderloin, plain yogurt
- *Bifidobacterium bifidum*: Jerusalem artichokes, asparagus, garlic, and onions may stimulate the growth or activity of this probiotic
- *Lactobacillus acidophilus*: yogurt containing live lactobacillus cultures, kefir, acidophilus milk

Consult with your physician before making any changes to your diet or supplemental regimen.

MOEXIPRIL, MOEXIPRIL PLUS HYDROCHLOROTHIAZIDE
(moe-EKS-i-pril, hye-droe-klor-oh-THYE-uh-zide)

Brand Names: Moexipril: Univasc
Moexipril plus hydrochlorothiazide: Uniretic

About Moexipril, Moexipril plus Hydrochlorothiazide

Many, many things can cause blood pressure to rise, but they all boil down to two physiological reactions: Either they increase the heart's output of blood, or they increase the blood vessels' resistance to the flow of blood. It's a simple formula: output times resistance equals pressure.

One of the ways the body raises the blood pressure is by producing a substance called angiotensin II, a powerful vasoconstrictor that encourages the blood vessels to "tighten up." This tightening-up increases the resistance to blood flow and pushes the pressure up.

Moexipril helps combat elevated blood pressure by slowing the production of angiotensin II. With less of this "tighten up" substance available, the blood vessels relax, resistance decreases, and blood pressure drops. Moexipril is also used to protect heart function following a heart attack.

Since it's often useful to attack hypertension from two directions at once, moexipril may be combined with hydrochlorothiazide, a diuretic that reduces the amount of fluid in the body, thereby decreasing the heart's output of blood. (For more on hydrochlorothiazide, see the entry on page 304.)

Possible Side Effects

Moexipril's side effects include muscle pain, dizziness, rash, and flushing. Hydrochlorothiazide's side effects include low blood pressure and skin sensitivity to light.

Which Nutrients Are Robbed

Taking moexipril may deplete your supply of, increase your need for, or interfere with the activity of:

- Zinc

Taking the combination of moexipril plus hydrochlorothiazide may deplete your supply of, increase your need for, or interfere with the activity of:

- Magnesium
- Phosphorus
- Potassium
- Sodium
- Zinc
- Coenzyme Q_{10}

Additional Ways This Drug May Upset Your Nutritional Balance

Moexipril can cause heartburn and nausea, while hydrochlorothiazide can cause loss of appetite. These side effects can upset your eating habits and possibly interfere with good nutrition.

Moexipril can also trigger hyperkalemia, or too much potassium in the blood.

Restoring Your Nutritional Balance

To compensate for the nutrient loss caused by moexipril, speak to your physician about taking 50–200 mg zinc per day.

To compensate for the nutrient loss caused by moexipril plus hydrochlorothiazide, speak to your physician about taking 500–1,000 mg magnesium, 700 mg phosphorus, 50–200 mg zinc, and 30–100 mg coenzyme Q_{10} per day. And ask your physician to consider the potential effects of sodium depletion.

A Note on Potassium: "Regular" diuretics lower potassium levels, while potassium-sparing diuretics do not—they may increase levels instead. It is not uncommon for doctors to prescribe two different diuretics. That's why you should speak to your physician about your potassium levels, and whether it is appropriate for you to take supplements or eat potassium-rich foods.

You can also eat foods that contain the depleted nutrients:

- Magnesium: Florida avocado, toasted wheat germ, almonds, shredded wheat cereal, pumpkin seeds
- Phosphorus: plain nonfat yogurt, lentils, salmon, milk, halibut
- Zinc: oysters, beef shank, chicken, pork tenderloin, plain yogurt
- Coenzyme Q_{10}: beef, chicken, trout, salmon, oranges and broccoli

Consult with your physician before making any changes to your diet or supplemental regimen.

MOMETASONE FUROATE (moe-MET-uh-sohn FYOOR-oh-ate)

Brand Names: Elocom, Elocon, Nasonex

About Mometasone Furoate

We call it hay fever even though there may be no hay within 100 miles. But it's really an allergy, or what doctors call allergic rhinitis (rhin- refers to the nose, -itis to inflammation). If you've got allergies, and you come into contact with certain allergens such as pollen, grass, dust mites, animal dander, or other substances, you can suffer from symptoms that include:

- Itching of your nose, the roof of your mouth and your throat
- Runny and stuffed nose
- Sneezing
- Watery eyes
- Swelling of the eyelids
- Headache
- Wheezing
- Irritability
- Insomnia

You can either live with these symptoms and wait for them to subside, or you can try to suppress them with medicines. One such medicine is mometasone furoate, a corticosteroid that comes in the form of a nasal spray and relieves nasal symptoms by suppressing inflammation. Mometasone furoate is also used in topical form to treat certain skin conditions.

Possible Side Effects

The drug's more common side effects include headache, cough, and inflammation of the throat.

Which Nutrients Are Robbed

Taking this medicine may deplete your supply of, increase your need for, or interfere with the activity of:

- Vitamin A
- Vitamin B$_6$
- Folic acid
- Vitamin C
- Vitamin D
- Vitamin K

- Calcium
- Magnesium
- Potassium
- Selenium
- Zinc
- Melatonin

Additional Ways This Drug May Upset Your Nutritional Balance

The nasal spray form of mometasone furoate can cause heartburn, a feeling of fullness, nausea, and vomiting, all of which can upset your eating habits and possibly interfere with good nutrition. It can also cause diarrhea, which can hamper nutrient absorption.

Restoring Your Nutritional Balance

To compensate for the nutrient loss caused by this drug, speak to your physician about taking 5,000 IU vitamin A, 50–100 mg vitamin B$_6$, 400–800 mcg folic acid, 250–1,500 mg vitamin C, 400 IU vitamin D, 60–80 mcg vitamin K, 1,200 mg calcium, 500–1,000 mg magnesium, 100–300 mg potassium, 20–100 mcg selenium, 50–200 mg zinc, and 1–3 mg melatonin per day.

You can also eat foods that contain the depleted nutrients:

- Vitamin A: beef liver, chicken liver, cheese pizza, whole milk, cheddar cheese
- Vitamin B$_6$: potato, banana, garbanzo beans, chicken breast, fortified oatmeal
- Folic acid: beef liver, fortified breakfast cereals, spinach, great northern beans, asparagus
- Vitamin C: papaya, guava, red pepper, cantaloupe, black currants
- Vitamin D: salmon, mackerel, sardines, eel, fortified milk
- Vitamin K: kale, broccoli, parsley, Swiss chard, spinach
- Calcium: milk, dried figs, Swiss cheese, yogurt, tofu
- Magnesium: Florida avocado, toasted wheat germ, almonds, shredded wheat cereal, pumpkin seeds
- Potassium: dried figs, California avocado, papaya, banana, dates

- Selenium: Brazil nuts, tuna, beef liver, turkey breast, spaghetti with meat sauce
- Zinc: oysters, beef shank, chicken, pork tenderloin, plain yogurt

Consult with your physician before making any changes to your diet or supplemental regimen.

MOXIFLOXACIN (moks-i-FLOKS-uh-sin)

Brand Name: Avelox

About Moxifloxacin

We tend to think of pneumonia as one disease, but it can stem from many different bacteria, viruses, or fungi, and produce slightly different arrays of symptoms. However, all forms of pneumonia infect the alveoli (tiny air sacs in the lungs) and the areas around them, causing an acute inflammation of the lungs.

Pneumonia is often classified according to the place in which it was contracted. There's hospital-acquired pneumonia, institutional pneumonia (which strikes those living in or visiting a nursing home or similar setting), and community-based pneumonia (which strikes those living at home). While this may seem like splitting epidemiological hairs, the distinction can be useful because certain places are more likely to cause certain types of pneumonia. For example, in community-acquired pneumonia, the bacteria *Streptococcus pneumoniae* is very likely the culprit.

Streptococcus pneumoniae often sneaks into your lungs after a cold or flu has damaged the natural defense system in your airways. The bacteria can move past the damaged biochemical defenses and find a place to settle, causing a fever, chills, shaking, shortness of breath, chest pain when breathing, and a sputum-producing cough. Fortunately, if it hasn't progressed too far and you are otherwise in good health, this form of pneumonia can be treated successfully.

Moxifloxacin helps combat several different types of community-acquired pneumonia, as well as bacterial sinusitis, uncomplicated skin infections, and other ailments.

Possible Side Effects

The drug's side effects include dizziness, nausea, allergic reactions, and low blood pressure.

Which Nutrients Are Robbed

Taking this medicine may deplete your supply of, increase your need for, or interfere with the activity of:

- Biotin
- Inositol
- Thiamin
- Riboflavin
- Niacin
- Vitamin B_6

- Vitamin B_{12}
- Vitamin K
- Zinc
- *Bifidobacterium bifidum*
- *Lactobacillus acidophilus*

Additional Ways This Drug May Upset Your Nutritional Balance

Moxifloxacin can cause low blood sugar (hypoglycemia) and nausea, which can upset your eating habits and possibly interfere with good nutrition. It can also cause diarrhea, which can hamper nutrient absorption.

Restoring Your Nutritional Balance

To compensate for the nutrient loss caused by this drug, speak to your physician about taking 500–1,000 mcg biotin, 250–1,000 mg inositol, 25–100 mg thiamin, 25–100 mg riboflavin, 50–100 mg niacin, 50–100 mg vitamin B_6, 500–1,000 mcg vitamin B_{12}, 60–80 mcg vitamin K, 50–200 mg zinc, 15 billion live *Bifidobacterium bifidum* organisms, and 15 billion live *Lactobacillus acidophilus* organisms per day.

You can also eat foods that contain the depleted nutrients:

- Biotin: beef liver, soybeans, rice bran, peanut butter, barley
- Inositol: cantaloupe, oranges, green beans, grapefruit juice, limes
- Thiamin: braised liver, turkey heart, roasted chicken, gefilte fish, sardines
- Riboflavin: dried sunflower seeds, orange juice, bulgur, spinach noodles, pine nuts
- Niacin: chicken breast, beef liver, mackerel, barley, bulgur
- Vitamin B_6: potato, banana, garbanzo beans, chicken breast, fortified oatmeal
- Vitamin B_{12}: beef liver, rainbow trout, sockeye salmon, beef, haddock
- Vitamin K: kale, broccoli, parsley, Swiss chard, spinach

- Zinc: oysters, beef shank, chicken, pork tenderloin, plain yogurt
- *Bifidobacterium bifidum*: Jerusalem artichokes, asparagus, garlic, and onions may stimulate the growth or activity of this probiotic
- *Lactobacillus acidophilus*: yogurt containing live lactobacillus cultures, kefir, acidophilus milk

Consult with your physician before making any changes to your diet or supplemental regimen.

MYCOPHENOLATE (mye-koe-FEN-oh-late)

Brand Name: CellCept

About Mycophenolate

Mycophenolate is one of the newer drugs designed to prevent the body from rejecting transplanted tissue. It works by suppressing the process necessary for T-cells and B-cells to amass in numbers large enough to destroy the transplant.

Your immune system has many different kinds of cells that you can think of as immune system soldiers. One way they can be grouped is according to those-who-know-exactly-what-to-do and those-who-have-to-learn. Macrophages belong to the those-who-know group. When these giant immune system soldiers discover foreign tissue, bacteria, or anything else that's not supposed to be in the body, they go into action, surrounding and swallowing the invaders. B-cells and certain T-cells, however, have to be taught exactly what the enemy "looks like" before they can swing into action. Other immune system cells teach these B- and T-cells what the enemy looks like by presenting them with a piece of the enemy. Once they have their orders, the B- and T-cells can rush into battle as powerful, highly focused soldiers bent on destroying this specific invader.

Suppressing the powerful B- and T-cells is key to preventing the body from rejecting transplanted tissue it considers to be a foreign invader.

Possible Side Effects

The drug's more common side effects include elevated or low blood pressure, rapid heartbeat, pain, stomach upset, anxiety, and fever.

Which Nutrients Are Robbed

Taking this medicine may deplete your supply of, increase your need for, or interfere with the activity of:

- Calcium
- Magnesium
- Phosphorus
- Potassium
- Sodium

Additional Ways This Drug May Upset Your Nutritional Balance

Mycophenolate can cause low blood sugar (hypoglycemia), abdominal pain, nausea, and vomiting, all of which can upset your eating habits and possibly interfere with good nutrition. It can also cause diarrhea, which can hamper nutrient absorption.

This drug can also trigger hyperkalemia, or too much potassium in the blood.

Restoring Your Nutritional Balance

To compensate for the nutrient loss caused by this drug, speak to your physician about taking 1,200 mg calcium, 500–1,000 mg magnesium, and 700 mg phosphorus per day. And ask your physician to consider the potential effects of sodium depletion and to monitor your potassium status.

You can also eat foods that contain the depleted nutrients:

- Calcium: milk, dried figs, Swiss cheese, yogurt, tofu
- Magnesium: Florida avocado, toasted wheat germ, almonds, shredded wheat cereal, pumpkin seeds
- Phosphorus: plain nonfat yogurt, lentils, salmon, milk, halibut

Consult with your physician before making any changes to your diet or supplemental regimen.

NABUMETONE (na-BYOO-me-tohn)

Brand Name: Relafen

About Nabumetone

Contrary to popular belief, osteoarthritis (OA) is not a necessary part of aging. And it *is* treatable.

The most common form of arthritis, OA strikes almost everyone to one degree or another by the age of seventy. It's a disease of the cartilage, the perfectly smooth and incredibly slick surface that cushions the ends of the bones within a joint. Cartilage allows the bone ends to slide smoothly across each other, and it absorbs the shock associated with weight-bearing movement. In OA, the cartilage becomes weak, pitted, rough, or cracked. It no longer cushions the bone ends properly or absorbs shock when you use the joint. The bone ends can rub against each other, weaken, and develop little bumps of bony overgrowth. The result is pain and difficulty moving the joint.

Sometimes the cause is clear; an injury to the joint may set the stage. But many times it's not so clear. For unknown reasons, the cells that manufacture the cartilage components—such as collagen and proteoglycans—begin to malfunction. Without sufficient collagen, which gives the cartilage structure, and without enough proteoglycans, which hold and release fluid, the cartilage dries out, weakens, and can't do its job properly.

Nabumetone can help by relieving pain and swelling in the joints. It doesn't cure the underlying disease process of OA, but if the problem hasn't progressed to the point where the joint has been seriously damaged, simply relieving the symptoms may be enough.

Possible Side Effects

Nabumetone's more common side effects include diarrhea, stomach upset, abdominal pain, dizziness, and rash.

Which Nutrients Are Robbed

Taking this medicine may deplete your supply of, increase your need for, or interfere with the activity of:

• Folic acid

Additional Ways This Drug May Upset Your Nutritional Balance

Nabumetone can cause heartburn, indigestion, nausea, and vomiting, all of which can upset your eating habits and possibly interfere with good nutrition. It can also cause diarrhea, which can hamper nutrient absorption.

Restoring Your Nutritional Balance

To compensate for the nutrient loss caused by this drug, speak to your physician about taking 400–800 mcg folic acid per day.

You can also eat foods that contain the depleted nutrient:

- Folic acid: beef liver, fortified breakfast cereals, spinach, great northern beans, asparagus

Consult with your physician before making any changes to your diet or supplemental regimen.

NAFCILLIN (naf-SIL-in)

Brand Names: Nafcil Injection, Nallpen Injection, Unipen Injection, Unipen Oral

About Nafcillin

Osteomyelitis is an infection of the bone that can be caused by either bacteria or fungi. When infection sets in, the marrow inside the bone can swell and press out in all directions, putting pressure on blood vessels inside the bone. This can slow or stop the flow of blood, and the parts of the bone supplied by the strangled blood vessels may die. In some cases, the infection can spread to nearby tissues.

If the osteomyelitis has been caused by bacteria, nafcillin may be prescribed. Nafcillin belongs to a group of antibiotics called beta-lactam antibiotics, which are so named because they're all built around what chemists call a lactam ring. Bacteria also "know" about this lactam ring and have created enzymes called beta-lactamases that are designed to deactivate these medicines. In fact, bacteria have developed more than 100 different beta-lactamases, rendering many antibiotics impotent.

Fortunately for us, nafcillin is relatively resistant to the beta-lactamases, which makes this drug useful for treating osteomyelitis and other infections caused by beta-lactamase–producing bacteria.

Possible Side Effects

The drug's side effects include pain, fever, rash, and swelling.

Which Nutrients Are Robbed

Taking this medicine may deplete your supply of, increase your need for, or interfere with the activity of:

- Biotin
- Inositol
- Vitamin B_{12}
- Vitamin K

- Thiamin
- Riboflavin
- Niacin
- Vitamin B$_6$

- Potassium
- *Bifidobacterium bifidum*
- *Lactobacillus acidophilus*

Additional Ways This Drug May Upset Your Nutritional Balance

Nafcillin can cause nausea, which can upset your eating habits and possibly interfere with good nutrition. It can also cause diarrhea, which can hamper nutrient absorption.

Restoring Your Nutritional Balance

To compensate for the nutrient loss caused by this drug, speak to your physician about taking 500–1,000 mcg biotin, 250–1,000 mg inositol, 25–100 mg thiamin, 25–100 mg riboflavin, 50–100 mg niacin, 50–100 mg vitamin B$_6$, 500–1,000 mcg vitamin B$_{12}$, 60–80 mcg vitamin K, 100–300 mg potassium, 15 billion live *Bifidobacterium bifidum* organisms, and 15 billion live *Lactobacillus acidophilus* organisms per day.

You can also eat foods that contain the depleted nutrients:

- Biotin: beef liver, soybeans, rice bran, peanut butter, barley
- Inositol: cantaloupe, oranges, green beans, grapefruit juice, limes
- Thiamin: braised liver, turkey heart, roasted chicken, gefilte fish, sardines
- Riboflavin: dried sunflower seeds, orange juice, bulgur, spinach noodles, pine nuts
- Niacin: chicken breast, beef liver, mackerel, barley, bulgur
- Vitamin B$_6$: potato, banana, garbanzo beans, chicken breast, fortified oatmeal
- Vitamin B$_{12}$: beef liver, rainbow trout, sockeye salmon, beef, haddock
- Vitamin K: kale, broccoli, parsley, Swiss chard, spinach
- Potassium: dried figs, California avocado, papaya, banana, dates
- *Bifidobacterium bifidum*: Jerusalem artichokes, asparagus, garlic, and onions may stimulate the growth or activity of this probiotic
- *Lactobacillus acidophilus*: yogurt containing live lactobacillus cultures, kefir, acidophilus milk

Consult with your physician before making any changes to your diet or supplemental regimen.

NALIDIXIC ACID (nal-i-DIKS-ik ASS-id)

Brand Name: NegGram

About Nalidixic Acid

Introduced in 1963, nalidixic acid was the first of a group of medicines called the quinolone antibiotics, which attack bacteria by preventing them from synthesizing DNA. Researchers soon found that nalidixic acid was excreted from the body too rapidly to make it useful in treating most infections, but it was effective in treating infections of the urinary tract. It may occasionally be used for this purpose today, although more modern drugs are usually prescribed instead.

Possible Side Effects

The drug's side effects include visual disturbances, drowsiness, and fever.

Which Nutrients Are Robbed

Taking this medicine may deplete your supply of, increase your need for, or interfere with the activity of:

- Biotin
- Inositol
- Thiamin
- Riboflavin
- Niacin
- Vitamin B$_6$
- Vitamin B$_{12}$
- Vitamin K
- *Bifidobacterium bifidum*
- *Lactobacillus acidophilus*

Additional Ways This Drug May Upset Your Nutritional Balance

Nalidixic acid can cause nausea and vomiting, which can upset your eating habits and possibly interfere with good nutrition.

Restoring Your Nutritional Balance

To compensate for the nutrient loss caused by this drug, speak to your physician about taking 500–1,000 mcg biotin, 250–1,000 mg inositol, 25–100 mg thiamin, 25–100 mg riboflavin, 50–100 mg niacin, 50–100 mg vitamin B$_6$, 500–1,000 mcg vitamin B$_{12}$, 60–80 mcg vitamin K, 15 billion live *Bifidobacterium bifidum* organisms, and 15 billion live *Lactobacillus acidophilus* organisms per day.

You can also eat foods that contain the depleted nutrients:

- Biotin: beef liver, soybeans, rice bran, peanut butter, barley
- Inositol: cantaloupe, oranges, green beans, grapefruit juice, limes

- Thiamin: braised liver, turkey heart, roasted chicken, gefilte fish, sardines
- Riboflavin: dried sunflower seeds, orange juice, bulgur, spinach noodles, pine nuts
- Niacin: chicken breast, beef liver, mackerel, barley, bulgur
- Vitamin B_6: potato, banana, garbanzo beans, chicken breast, fortified oatmeal
- Vitamin B_{12}: beef liver, rainbow trout, sockeye salmon, beef, haddock
- Vitamin K: kale, broccoli, parsley, Swiss chard, spinach
- *Bifidobacterium bifidum*: Jerusalem artichokes, asparagus, garlic, and onions may stimulate the growth or activity of this probiotic
- *Lactobacillus acidophilus*: yogurt containing live lactobacillus cultures, kefir, acidophilus milk

Consult with your physician before making any changes to your diet or supplemental regimen.

NAPROXEN (na-PROKS-en)

Brand Names: Aleve, Anaprox, Apo-Naproxen, EC-Naprosyn, Naprelan, Naprosyn, Naxen, Novo-Naprox, Nu-Naprox

About Naproxen

Naproxen is an a nonsteroidal anti-inflammatory drug (NSAID) that is available over-the-counter under brand names like Aleve and Anaprox. Or your doctor can prescribe it for you in stronger doses.

Like the other NSAIDs, naproxen relieves inflammation and pain (both the original pain and the pain caused by the inflammation). Naproxen does this by slowing the production of substances called prostaglandins, the heralds of inflammation. The prostaglandins help trigger the inflammation response when body tissue is damaged or invaded by germs. Very quickly, white blood cells swarm to the area, ready to fight the enemy and/or mop up damaged tissues. Unfortunately, the inflammatory process may go on too long or be too strong, leaving the affected area hot, red, and sore.

As an anti-inflammatory, naproxen is useful for treating some forms of arthritis, painful menstrual periods, and migraine headaches, as well for relieving fever.

Possible Side Effects

The drug's more common side effects include headache, fluid retention, stomach upset, rash, and ringing in the ears.

Which Nutrients Are Robbed

Taking this medicine may deplete your supply of, increase your need for, or interfere with the activity of:

- Folic acid

Additional Ways This Drug May Upset Your Nutritional Balance

Naproxen can cause abdominal discomfort, nausea, indigestion, and heartburn, all of which can upset your eating habits and possibly interfere with good nutrition. It can also cause diarrhea, which can hamper nutrient absorption.

Restoring Your Nutritional Balance

To compensate for the nutrient loss caused by this drug, speak to your physician about taking 400–800 mcg folic acid per day.

You can also eat foods that contain the depleted nutrient:

- Folic acid: beef liver, fortified breakfast cereals, spinach, great northern beans, asparagus

Consult with your physician before making any changes to your diet or supplemental regimen.

NEOMYCIN (nee-oh-MYE-sin)

Brand Names: Mycifradin Sulfate Oral, Mycifradin Sulfate Topical, Neo-Fradin Oral, Neo-Tabs Oral

About Neomycin

Neomycin is used both inside and outside the body: to cleanse the gut before surgery and to clear infections from the skin.

For a day or two before bowel surgery, you may be asked to take 1 gram of neomycin three or four times a day. The goal is to destroy certain aerobic germs that live in the bowels in order to keep them from spreading both during and after surgery.

Neomycin is also used on the skin to fight bacterial infections, or may be injected into infected joints, abscesses, or other infected areas.

Neomycin is a member of the aminoglycoside group of antibacterials. It destroys bacteria by penetrating their cellular walls and preventing them from forming certain protein structures. It does this, in part, by getting the bacteria to string together the wrong amino acids—fooling them into building useless proteins.

Possible Side Effects

The drug's more common side effects include nausea, diarrhea, vomiting, and soreness of the mouth or rectal area.

Which Nutrients Are Robbed

Taking this medicine may deplete your supply of, increase your need for, or interfere with the activity of:

- Beta-carotene
- Vitamin A
- Vitamin B$_6$
- Vitamin B$_{12}$
- Vitamin D
- Vitamin E
- Vitamin K
- Calcium
- Iron
- Magnesium
- Potassium
- Sodium
- *Bifidobacterium bifidum*
- *Lactobacillus acidophilus*

Additional Ways This Drug May Upset Your Nutritional Balance

Neomycin can cause nausea and vomiting, which can upset your eating habits and possibly interfere with good nutrition. It can also cause diarrhea, which can hamper nutrient absorption.

Restoring Your Nutritional Balance

To compensate for the nutrient loss caused by this drug, speak to your physician about taking 25,000 IU beta-carotene, 5,000 IU vitamin A, 50–100 mg vitamin B$_6$, 500–1,000 mcg vitamin B$_{12}$, 400 IU vitamin D, 400 IU vitamin E, 60–80 mcg vitamin K, 1,200 mg calcium, 500–1,000 mg magnesium, 100–300 mg potassium, 15 billion live *Bifidobacterium bifidum* organisms, and 15 billion live *Lactobacillus acidophilus* organisms per day. And ask your physician to consider the potential effects of iron and sodium depletion.

You can also eat foods that contain the depleted nutrients:

- Beta-carotene: carrot, spinach, mango, cantaloupe, apricot nectar
- Vitamin A: beef liver, chicken liver, cheese pizza, whole milk, cheddar cheese
- Vitamin B_6: potato, banana, garbanzo beans, chicken breast, fortified oatmeal
- Vitamin B_{12}: beef liver, rainbow trout, sockeye salmon, beef, haddock
- Vitamin D: salmon, mackerel, sardines, eel, fortified milk
- Vitamin E: wheat germ oil, almonds, safflower oil, corn oil, soybean oil
- Vitamin K: kale, broccoli, parsley, Swiss chard, spinach
- Calcium: milk, dried figs, Swiss cheese, yogurt, tofu
- Magnesium: Florida avocado, toasted wheat germ, almonds, shredded wheat cereal, pumpkin seeds
- Potassium: dried figs, California avocado, papaya, banana, dates
- *Bifidobacterium bifidum*: Jerusalem artichokes, asparagus, garlic, and onions may stimulate the growth or activity of this probiotic
- *Lactobacillus acidophilus*: yogurt containing live lactobacillus cultures, kefir, acidophilus milk

Consult with your physician before making any changes to your diet or supplemental regimen.

NEVIRAPINE (ne-VYE-ruh-peen)

Brand Name: Viramune

About Nevirapine

As if having acquired immunodeficiency syndrome (AIDS) were not enough, it's possible for a pregnant woman to transmit this disease to her unborn child. We don't yet have a cure for AIDS, but nevirapine, which is able to cross the placenta, has shown promise in preventing the spread of AIDS from mother to fetus. A dose of the drug is given when labor begins, and the newborn is given more of the drug later on.

Nevirapine is also used in combination with other antiviral drugs to combat AIDS in adults. It works by making it difficult for the human immunodeficiency virus (which causes AIDS) to replicate itself and spread.

Possible Side Effects

The drug's more common side effects include rash, diarrhea, headache, and fever.

Which Nutrients Are Robbed

Taking this medicine may deplete your supply of, increase your need for, or interfere with the activity of:

- Vitamin B_{12}
- Zinc
- Copper
- Carnitine

Additional Ways This Drug May Upset Your Nutritional Balance

Nevirapine can cause abdominal pain and nausea, which can upset your eating habits and possibly interfere with good nutrition. It can also cause diarrhea, which can hamper nutrient absorption.

Restoring Your Nutritional Balance

To compensate for the nutrient loss caused by this drug, speak to your physician about taking 500–1,000 mcg vitamin B_{12}, 2 mcg copper, 50–200 mg zinc, and 250–1,000 mg carnitine per day.

You can also eat foods that contain the depleted nutrients:

- Vitamin B_{12}: beef liver, rainbow trout, sockeye salmon, beef, haddock
- Copper: beef liver, almonds, raw mushrooms, hazelnuts, lentils
- Zinc: oysters, beef shank, chicken, pork tenderloin, plain yogurt
- Carnitine: ground beef, pork, Canadian bacon, whole milk, cod

Consult with your physician before making any changes to your diet or supplemental regimen.

NITROFURANTOIN (nye-troe-fyoor-AN-toyn)

Brand Names: Apo-Nitrofurantoin, Furadantin, Macrobid, Macrodantin, Nephronex, Novo-Furan

About Nitrofurantoin

Nitrofurantoin is an antibiotic that the body processes and excretes so quickly via the urine that it doesn't have time to build up to medicinal levels in the bloodstream or tissues.

Because nitrofurantoin reaches medicinal concentrations only in the urine, it's a good urinary antiseptic, useful for treating infections in the lower urinary tract (bladder and urethra). Another plus for this drug is that bacteria are relatively slow to develop a resistance to it, and there is little cross-resistance between nitrofurantoin and other antibiotics. Cross-resistance occurs when you take an antibiotic and the bacteria in your body not only become resistant to that drug but also to similar drugs at the same time. This means that after taking one drug, two or three others may become ineffective for you.

Nitrofurantoin is helpful in treating urinary tract infections caused by certain types of bacteria.

Possible Side Effects

The drug's side effects include chest pain, chills, dizziness, and fatigue.

Which Nutrients Are Robbed

Taking this medicine may deplete your supply of, increase your need for, or interfere with the activity of:

- *Bifidobacterium bifidum* - *Lactobacillus acidophilus*

Additional Ways This Drug May Upset Your Nutritional Balance

Nitrofurantoin can cause loss of appetite, stomach upset, nausea, and vomiting, all of which can upset your eating habits and possibly interfere with good nutrition. It can also cause diarrhea, which can hamper nutrient absorption.

Restoring Your Nutritional Balance

To compensate for the nutrient loss caused by this drug, speak to your physician about taking 15 billion live *Bifidobacterium bifidum* organisms and 15 billion live *Lactobacillus acidophilus* organisms per day.

You can also eat foods that contain the depleted nutrients:

- *Bifidobacterium bifidum*: Jerusalem artichokes, asparagus, garlic, and onions may stimulate the growth or activity of this probiotic
- *Lactobacillus acidophilus*: yogurt containing live lactobacillus cultures, kefir, acidophilus milk

Consult with your physician before making any changes to your diet or supplemental regimen.

NITROUS OXIDE (NYE-truss OKS-ide)

About Nitrous Oxide

We don't take nitrous oxide as a pill or a liquid. Instead, it comes in the form of an anesthetic gas used in dentistry and some forms of human and veterinary surgery. Nitrous oxide also makes whipped cream foamy and has other uses.

Patients who are exposed to nitrous oxide during surgery can suffer from nutrient depletions—as can the physicians, dentists, and veterinarians who inadvertently inhale this gas over and over again.

Possible Side Effects

The drug's side effects include a megaloblastic anemia and immune system impairment.

Which Nutrients Are Robbed

Being exposed to this medicine may deplete your supply of, increase your need for, or interfere with the activity of:

- Folic acid
- Vitamin B_{12}

Restoring Your Nutritional Balance

To compensate for the nutrient loss caused by this drug, speak to your physician about taking 400–800 mcg folic acid and 500–1,000 mcg vitamin B_{12} per day.

You can also eat foods that contain the depleted nutrients:

- Folic acid: beef liver, fortified breakfast cereals, spinach, great northern beans, asparagus
- Vitamin B_{12}: beef liver, rainbow trout, sockeye salmon, beef, haddock

Consult with your physician before making any changes to your diet or supplemental regimen.

NIZATIDINE (ni-ZA-ti-deen)

Brand Names: Apo-Nizatidine, Axid, Axid AR

About Nizatidine

Nizatidine is a member of a group of drugs known as H_2-receptor antagonists, which reduce stomach acid by competing with histamine for its place in the stomach.

Three substances are responsible for triggering production of much of the stomach acid that helps digest our food. One of these is histamine, which binds to specific sites on the lining of the stomach called H_2-receptors. In a sense, histamine is the key that fits into the H_2-receptor lock. With the key in place, the lock opens and stomach acid pours out.

Nizatidine acts a lot like the histamine key, but it doesn't turn to release the acid. Instead, it just sits there, preventing histamine from inserting itself. In everyday terms, nizatidine is referred to as a histamine blocker.

Thanks to its ability to reduce the production of stomach acid, nizatidine is used to treat certain ulcers, gastroesophageal reflux disease, acid indigestion, and sour stomach.

Possible Side Effects

The drug's more common side effects include headache, dizziness, rash, and stomach upset.

Which Nutrients Are Robbed

Taking this medicine may deplete your supply of, increase your need for, or interfere with the activity of:

- Thiamin
- Folic acid
- Vitamin B_{12}
- Vitamin D
- Calcium
- Iron
- Zinc

Additional Ways This Drug May Upset Your Nutritional Balance

Nizatidine can cause abdominal pain, nausea, vomiting, heartburn, dry mouth, and loss of appetite, all of which can upset your eating habits and possibly interfere with good nutrition. It can also cause diarrhea, which can hamper nutrient absorption.

Restoring Your Nutritional Balance

To compensate for the nutrient loss caused by this drug, speak to your physician about taking 25–100 mg thiamin, 400–800 mcg folic acid, 500–1,000 mcg vitamin B$_{12}$, 400 IU vitamin D, 1,200 mg calcium, and 50–200 mg zinc per day. And ask your physician to consider the potential effects of iron depletion.

You can also eat foods that contain the depleted nutrients:

- Thiamin: braised liver, turkey heart, roasted chicken, gefilte fish, sardines
- Folic acid: beef liver, fortified breakfast cereals, spinach, great northern beans, asparagus
- Vitamin B$_{12}$: beef liver, rainbow trout, sockeye salmon, beef, haddock
- Vitamin D: salmon, mackerel, sardines, eel, fortified milk
- Calcium: milk, dried figs, Swiss cheese, yogurt, tofu
- Zinc: oysters, beef shank, chicken, pork tenderloin, plain yogurt

Consult with your physician before making any changes to your diet or supplemental regimen.

NORETHINDRONE (nor-eth-IN-drohn)

Brand Names: Micronor, Nor-QD

About Norethindrone

Norethindrone is a synthetic version of the hormone progesterone. In the female body, this important hormone is made during the second half of the menstrual cycle by the discarded sac of a newly released egg. It's also manufactured by the adrenal glands and, during pregnancy, by the placenta. Men also make some progesterone, in their adrenal glands and their testes.

Norethindrone may be prescribed as a part of postmenopausal hormone replacement therapy (although this practice has recently fallen out of favor) or to prevent pregnancy. Although it's unclear exactly how norethindrone blocks conception, it may work by changing the lining of the uterus so that it's difficult for a fertilized egg to be implanted. It may also alter the cervical mucus, making it difficult for sperm to reach the eggs.

Possible Side Effects

The drug's side effects include headache, dizziness, irritability, and depression.

Which Nutrients Are Robbed

Taking this medicine may deplete your supply of, increase your need for, or interfere with the activity of:

- Folic acid
- Riboflavin
- Vitamin B_6
- Vitamin B_{12}
- Vitamin C
- Magnesium
- Zinc

Additional Ways This Drug May Upset Your Nutritional Balance

Norethindrone can cause nausea and vomiting, which can upset your eating habits and possibly interfere with good nutrition.

Restoring Your Nutritional Balance

To compensate for the nutrient loss caused by this drug, speak to your physician about taking 400–800 mcg folic acid, 25–100 mg riboflavin, 50–100 mg vitamin B_6, 500–1,000 mcg vitamin B_{12}, 250–1,500 mg vitamin C, 500–1,000 mg magnesium, and 50–200 mg zinc per day.

You can also eat foods that contain the depleted nutrients:

- Folic acid: beef liver, fortified breakfast cereals, spinach, great northern beans, asparagus
- Riboflavin: dried sunflower seeds, orange juice, bulgur, spinach noodles, pine nuts
- Vitamin B_6: potato, banana, garbanzo beans, chicken breast, fortified oatmeal
- Vitamin B_{12}: beef liver, rainbow trout, sockeye salmon, beef, haddock
- Vitamin C: papaya, guava, red pepper, cantaloupe, black currants
- Magnesium: Florida avocado, toasted wheat germ, almonds, shredded wheat cereal, pumpkin seeds
- Zinc: oysters, beef shank, chicken, pork tenderloin, plain yogurt

Consult with your physician before making any changes to your diet or supplemental regimen.

NORFLOXACIN (nor-FLOKS-uh-sin)

Brand Names: Chibroxin Ophthalmic, Noroxin Oral

About Norfloxacin

There are thousands of different kinds of bacteria, those tiny, single-celled organisms that live in and on our bodies, float though the air, and cover just about every surface.

One way that doctors classify bacteria is by their shape. Bacteria that have a spiral shape are called spirochetes; those with that are spherical are called cocci; and the rodlike ones are called bacilli. Another way to classify them is by the color they become after being exposed to Gram stain. If they turn blue, they're called gram-positive; if they turn pink, they're gram-negative.

Turning one color or the other may not sound like a big deal, but it tells doctors a lot about the characteristics of the bacteria. For example, gram-negative bacteria (which turn pink) have a tough outer coating that can ward off many drugs. This means that they are resistant to more medicines than their blue-colored, gram-positive counterparts. (And substances in that tough outer coating can cause the blood pressure to fall and the body temperature to soar, should those "pinkies" get into the bloodstream.)

On the other hand, the blue-turning, gram-positive bacteria are relatively slow to develop resistance to antibiotics, which means it's easier to destroy them.

Drugs are often categorized by their ability to slay gram-positive or gram-negative bacteria. Norfloxacin can do both, and as such is used to treat urinary tract infections caused by both "blue" and "pink" bacteria. It's also used for cystitis, an inflammation of the bladder and ureters (tubes that carry urine from the kidneys to the bladder).

Possible Side Effects

The drug's more common side effects include nausea, headache, and dizziness.

Which Nutrients Are Robbed

Taking this medicine may deplete your supply of, increase your need for, or interfere with the activity of:

- Biotin
- Inositol
- Vitamin B_{12}
- Vitamin K

- Thiamin
- Riboflavin
- Niacin
- Vitamin B$_6$

- Zinc
- *Bifidobacterium bifidum*
- *Lactobacillus acidophilus*

Additional Ways This Drug May Upset Your Nutritional Balance

Norfloxacin can cause nausea, which can upset your eating habits and possibly interfere with good nutrition.

Restoring Your Nutritional Balance

To compensate for the nutrient loss caused by this drug, speak to your physician about taking 500–1,000 mcg biotin, 250–1,000 mg inositol, 25–100 mg thiamin, 25–100 mg riboflavin, 50–100 mg niacin, 50–100 mg vitamin B$_6$, 500–1,000 mcg vitamin B$_{12}$, 60–80 mcg vitamin K, 50–200 mg zinc, 15 billion live *Bifidobacterium bifidum* organisms, and 15 billion live *Lactobacillus acidophilus* organisms per day.

You can also eat foods that contain the depleted nutrients:

- Biotin: beef liver, soybeans, rice bran, peanut butter, barley
- Inositol: cantaloupe, oranges, green beans, grapefruit juice, limes
- Thiamin: braised liver, turkey heart, roasted chicken, gefilte fish, sardines
- Riboflavin: dried sunflower seeds, orange juice, bulgur, spinach noodles, pine nuts
- Niacin: chicken breast, beef liver, mackerel, barley, bulgur
- Vitamin B$_6$: potato, banana, garbanzo beans, chicken breast, fortified oatmeal
- Vitamin B$_{12}$: beef liver, rainbow trout, sockeye salmon, beef, haddock
- Vitamin K: kale, broccoli, parsley, Swiss chard, spinach
- Zinc: oysters, beef shank, chicken, pork tenderloin, plain yogurt
- *Bifidobacterium bifidum*: Jerusalem artichokes, asparagus, garlic, and onions may stimulate the growth or activity of this probiotic
- *Lactobacillus acidophilus*: yogurt containing live lactobacillus cultures, kefir, acidophilus milk

Consult with your physician before making any changes to your diet or supplemental regimen.

NORTRIPTYLINE (nor-TRIP-ti-leen)

Brand Names: Apo-Nortriptyline, Aventyl Hydrochloride, Pamelor

About Nortriptyline

It's normal to be anxious when a threat arises, we're stressed, or we think about possible dangers. Anxiety is a survival mechanism that helps us respond to danger by triggering the fight-or-flight response. Sometimes, however, anxiety arises when there is no danger or threat, or it comes on too strong or lasts too long. If that happens to you, you may have an anxiety disorder.

Intense anxiety can take the form of panic attacks or panic disorder. Panic attacks are sudden, fairly brief, fearful reactions. They may come in response to a specific situation or thing. For example, if you're terribly afraid of snakes and you come across one, you may find yourself suffering from chest pain, a feeling of choking, dizziness, chills, nausea, tingling sensations, a rapid heart rate, or shortness of breath. You'll most likely have an incredible urge to get away from the offending situation or thing. Within about 10 minutes, these symptoms will peak and soon thereafter begin to fade away. But panic attacks can also strike for no obvious reason.

You may have one panic attack and then never be troubled again. Or you may develop panic disorder, with multiple panic attacks and new problems to worry about: When will the next attack hit? What will happen when it does?

One of the treatments for panic disorder is the drug nortriptyline. Also used for depression, bedwetting, and ADHD (attention deficit hyperactivity disorder), this drug shields serotonin from being broken down in the central nervous system. It's believed that keeping more serotonin in play in the nervous system can help ease anxiety.

Possible Side Effects

The drug's side effects include insomnia, nightmares, rash, and irregular heartbeat.

Which Nutrients Are Robbed

Taking this medicine may deplete your supply of, increase your need for, or interfere with the activity of:

- Riboflavin
- Coenzyme Q_{10}
- Sodium

Additional Ways This Drug May Upset Your Nutritional Balance

Nortriptyline can cause nausea, vomiting, loss of appetite, abdominal cramps, and changes in taste, all of which can upset your eating habits and possibly interfere with good nutrition. It can also cause diarrhea, which can hamper nutrient absorption.

Restoring Your Nutritional Balance

To compensate for the nutrient loss caused by this drug, speak to your physician about taking 25–100 mg riboflavin and 30–100 mg coenzyme Q_{10} per day. And ask your physician to consider the potential effects of sodium depletion.

You can also eat foods that contain the depleted nutrients:

- Riboflavin: dried sunflower seeds, orange juice, bulgur, spinach noodles, pine nuts
- Coenzyme Q_{10}: beef, chicken, trout, salmon, oranges, broccoli

Consult with your physician before making any changes to your diet or supplemental regimen.

OCTREOTIDE (ok-TREE-oh-tide)

Brand Names: Sandostatin, Sandostatin LAR Depot

About Octreotide

Everybody experiences diarrhea once in a while, but did you know it's not defined by how often you run to the bathroom? The presence of diarrhea is defined by the percentage of water the stool contains, not the frequency of bowel movements. If your stool is 60 to 90 percent water, it's normal. If it's more than 90 percent water, it's probably diarrhea.

Diarrhea that comes on suddenly and lasts a couple days is probably caused by food that wasn't prepared or stored properly, drinking or swimming in impure water, or a viral or bacterial infection (think traveler's diarrhea). In many cases, the diarrhea clears up once the underlying problem is resolved, perhaps with the aid of an over-the-counter remedy.

Then there are more serious kinds of diarrhea, caused by inflammatory bowel disease, an inability to digest food properly, cancerous tumors, infectious organisms, chronic parasitic infections, laxative abuse, and other problems. These kinds of diarrhea may require therapy with prescription medicines.

Octreotide is used when diarrhea is caused by certain tumors. It works by stimulating the intestines to absorb more fluid, thus drying the stool.

Possible Side Effects

The drug's more common side effects include slow heartbeat, elevated blood sugar, diarrhea, constipation, abdominal pain, and flatulence.

Which Nutrients Are Robbed

Taking this medicine may deplete your supply of, increase your need for, or interfere with the activity of:

- Beta-carotene

Additional Ways This Drug May Upset Your Nutritional Balance

Octreotide can cause abdominal pain, nausea, and vomiting, all of which can upset your eating habits and possibly interfere with good nutrition. It can also cause diarrhea, which can hamper nutrient absorption.

Restoring Your Nutritional Balance

To compensate for the nutrient loss caused by this drug, speak to your physician about taking 25,000 IU beta-carotene per day.

You can also eat foods that contain the depleted nutrient:

- Beta-carotene: carrot, spinach, mango, cantaloupe, apricot nectar

Consult with your physician before making any changes to your diet or supplemental regimen.

OFLOXACIN (oh-FLOKS-uh-sin)

Brand Names: Floxin, Floxin IV, Ocuflox Ophthalmic

About Ofloxacin

Pelvic inflammatory disease (PID) is the most common preventable cause of infertility in American women. About 20 percent of those who have the disease will lose the ability to bear children.

PID tends to strike young, sexually active women who do not use a diaphragm or other form of barrier contraception, and who have many sexual partners. It's usually caused by bacteria, which enter the vagina during sexual intercourse, while douching, during childbirth or abortions, or through certain medical procedures.

The bacteria that cause PID are often the same as those that cause gonorrhea and chlamydia. They move up the vagina to the cervix, uterus, and fallopian tubes, and sometimes into the ovaries. The symptoms of PID may include fever, abdominal pain, vaginal bleeding, foul-smelling vaginal discharge, nausea, and vomiting. If the infection breaks out of the reproductive system and spreads into the abdominal cavity, it can cause a severe infection called peritonitis.

Doctors typically attack pelvic inflammatory disease with two antibiotics at once. The idea is to make sure that at least one (but preferably both) will kill the offending bacteria and knock the infection out ASAP. Ofloxacin destroys bacteria by interfering with their ability to repair and replicate their DNA.

Ofloxacin is also used to treat infections of the skin, eyes, and ears, as well as the respiratory and urinary tracts.

Possible Side Effects

The drug's more common side effects include fainting, burning or irritation of the eye, and crusts or crystals forming in the eye.

Which Nutrients Are Robbed

Taking this medicine may deplete your supply of, increase your need for, or interfere with the activity of:

- Biotin
- Inositol
- Thiamin
- Riboflavin
- Niacin
- Vitamin B_6
- Vitamin B_{12}
- Vitamin K
- Zinc
- *Bifidobacterium bifidum*
- *Lactobacillus acidophilus*

Additional Ways This Drug May Upset Your Nutritional Balance

Ofloxacin can cause nausea, vomiting, gastrointestinal distress, changes in taste, and a decreased appetite, all of which can upset your eating habits and possibly interfere with good nutrition. It can also cause diarrhea, which can hamper nutrient absorption.

Restoring Your Nutritional Balance

To compensate for the nutrient loss caused by this drug, speak to your physician about taking 500–1,000 mcg biotin, 250–1,000 mg inositol, 25–100 mg thiamin, 25–100 mg riboflavin, 50–100 mg niacin, 50–100 mg vitamin B_6, 500–1,000 mcg vitamin B_{12}, 60–80 mcg vitamin K, 50–200 mg zinc, 15 billion live *Bifidobacterium bifidum* organisms, and 15 billion live *Lactobacillus acidophilus* organisms per day.

You can also eat foods that contain the depleted nutrients:

- Biotin: beef liver, soybeans, rice bran, peanut butter, barley
- Inositol: cantaloupe, oranges, green beans, grapefruit juice, limes
- Thiamin: braised liver, turkey heart, roasted chicken, gefilte fish, sardines
- Riboflavin: dried sunflower seeds, orange juice, bulgur, spinach noodles, pine nuts
- Niacin: chicken breast, beef liver, mackerel, barley, bulgur
- Vitamin B_6: potato, banana, garbanzo beans, chicken breast, fortified oatmeal
- Vitamin B_{12}: beef liver, rainbow trout, sockeye salmon, beef, haddock
- Vitamin K: kale, broccoli, parsley, Swiss chard, spinach
- Zinc: oysters, beef shank, chicken, pork tenderloin, plain yogurt
- *Bifidobacterium bifidum:* Jerusalem artichokes, asparagus, garlic, and onions may stimulate the growth or activity of this probiotic
- *Lactobacillus acidophilus:* yogurt containing live lactobacillus cultures, kefir, acidophilus milk

Consult with your physician before making any changes to your diet or supplemental regimen.

OLSALAZINE (ole-SAL-uh-zeen)

Brand Name: Dipentum

About Olsalazine

Ulcerative colitis is an inflammatory disease of the large intestines, that final section of the digestive tract that reabsorbs water and forms digestive waste products into stool. The disease often begins at the end of the large intestines—in the rectum or sigmoid colon—and works its way backward, possibly affecting the entire large intestine over time.

When ulcerative colitis strikes, your large intestine becomes ulcerated and inflamed, causing cramps, fever, and diarrhea, which may be bloody. Because vitamin K is created by bacteria in the large intestines, ulcerative colitis can lead to a deficiency of this vitamin, which may interfere with your blood's ability to coagulate. Ulcerative colitis also increases your risk of developing different types of arthritis, as well as cancer, if you developed the disease in childhood and have had it for a long time.

Treatment for ulcerative colitis includes diet, drugs, and possibly surgery. One of the drugs that may be prescribed is olsalazine, which helps reduce inflammation.

Olsalazine is really more of a vehicle for a drug than an active drug. One of the better medicines for intestinal inflammation is 5-aminosalicylic acid. But it's hard to take enough of this medication to ease inflammation without causing too many side effects. Olsalazine solves this problem by combining two 5-aminosalicylic acid molecules. (When combined, molecules of 5-aminosalicylic acid don't cause the problems they do when they're free and single.) Inside the large intestines, bacteria split the two molecules, so they can get to work.

This action makes olsalazine useful in preventing flare-ups of ulcerative colitis.

Possible Side Effects

The drug's more common side effects include abdominal pain and diarrhea.

Which Nutrients Are Robbed

Taking this medicine may deplete your supply of, increase your need for, or interfere with the activity of:

• Folic acid

Additional Ways This Drug May Upset Your Nutritional Balance

Olsalazine can cause heartburn, bloating, loss of appetite, abdominal pain, and nausea, all of which can upset your eating habits and possibly interfere with good nutrition. It can also cause diarrhea, which can hamper nutrient absorption.

Restoring Your Nutritional Balance

To compensate for the nutrient loss caused by this drug, speak to your physician about taking 400–800 mcg folic acid per day.

You can also eat foods that contain the depleted nutrient:

- Folic acid: beef liver, fortified breakfast cereals, spinach, great northern beans, asparagus

Consult with your physician before making any changes to your diet or supplemental regimen.

OMEPRAZOLE (oh-MEP-rah-zole)

Brand Names: Losec, Prilosec

About Omeprazole

Heartburn is a fairly common problem. According to some studies, as many as 17 percent of Americans have heartburn (partial regurgitation of the stomach contents) at least once a week. Heartburn is more than just a pain; it disrupts sleep, depresses the mood, decreases the sense of well-being, and can interfere with work and social activities. According to a 2000 Gallup Poll, over one third of those afflicted with heartburn find that it affects what and when they eat, as well as when and how well they sleep.[4]

Heartburn is perhaps the most noticeable symptom of GERD, or gastroesophageal reflux disease. GERD arises because of the weakening of the sphincter, or the "gate" that normally keeps the food and digestive juices in the stomach. This allows the powerful stomach acids to splash back into the esophagus, causing pain, esophageal inflammation, and other symptoms. In more severe cases, GERD can cause pre-cancerous changes in the lining of the esophagus.

For some people, heartburn is a brief problem that resolves itself in a few days or weeks and doesn't return for a long time. For others, the problem can recur for 10 years or longer. It's no wonder that over 70 percent of those with heartburn take medicines, prescription or over-the-counter, to control it.

Omeprazole, which comes in both prescription and nonprescription forms, is a proton pump inhibitor. It interferes with the action of the proton pumps in the stomach lining that secrete digestive acid, thereby reducing the acid production. Omeprazole and the other proton pump inhibitors are considered first-line therapy for heartburn and other symptoms of GERD and associated problems.

Possible Side Effects

The drug's more common side effects include stomach or abdominal pain, headache, and diarrhea.

Which Nutrients Are Robbed

Taking this medicine may deplete your supply of, increase your need for, or interfere with the activity of:

- Beta-carotene
- Folic acid
- Thiamin
- Vitamin B_{12}
- Iron
- Sodium
- Zinc

Additional Ways This Drug May Upset Your Nutritional Balance

Omeprazole can cause abdominal pain, nausea, and vomiting, all of which can upset your eating habits and possibly interfere with good nutrition. It can also cause diarrhea, which can hamper nutrient absorption.

Restoring Your Nutritional Balance

To compensate for the nutrient loss caused by this drug, speak to your physician about taking 25,000 IU beta-carotene, 400–800 mcg folic acid, 25–100 mg thiamin, 500–1,000 mcg vitamin B_{12}, and 50–200 mg zinc per day. And ask your physician to consider the potential effects of iron and sodium depletion.

You can also eat foods that contain the depleted nutrients:

- Beta-carotene: carrot, spinach, mango, cantaloupe, apricot nectar
- Folic acid: beef liver, fortified breakfast cereals, spinach, great northern beans, asparagus
- Thiamin: braised liver, turkey heart, roasted chicken, gefilte fish, sardines
- Vitamin B_{12}: beef liver, rainbow trout, sockeye salmon, beef, haddock
- Zinc: oysters, beef shank, chicken, pork tenderloin, plain yogurt

Consult with your physician before making any changes to your diet or supplemental regimen.

ONDANSETRON (on-DAN-se-tron)

Brand Names: Zofran, Zofran ODT

About Ondansetron

Vomiting can be triggered by a variety of things, including infections, peptic ulcer disease, certain cancers, Crohn's disease, scleroderma, appendicitis, hepatitis, acute pancreatitis, various drugs, heart attacks, motion sickness, migraine headaches, tumors in the central nervous system, pregnancy, and hypothyroidism. Chemotherapy and the drugs used during surgery can also trigger an irresistible urge to empty the stomach.

These things do not act directly on the stomach to make you vomit. Instead, they stimulate the vomiting center in the brain, which then sends out the order to vomit. For example, certain nerve fibers in the gastrointestinal tract may detect that the stomach is terribly distended and pass that message up to the vomit center, which solves the problem by sending back the order to vomit.

One way to prevent vomiting is to stop the messages from getting to the vomit center. Ondansetron can do that by inserting itself into certain receptor sites in the brain, thus preventing the proper neurotransmitters from getting into the receptors and passing on the message. Ondansetron is useful in quelling the vomiting associated with surgery and certain types of chemotherapy and radiation treatments.

Possible Side Effects

The drug's more common side effects include diarrhea, fatigue, and headache.

Which Nutrients Are Robbed

Taking this medicine may deplete your supply of, increase your need for, or interfere with the activity of:

• Potassium

Additional Ways This Drug May Upset Your Nutritional Balance

Ondansetron can diarrhea, which can hamper nutrient absorption.

Restoring Your Nutritional Balance

To compensate for the nutrient loss caused by this drug, speak to your physician about taking 100–300 mg potassium per day.

You can also eat foods that contain the depleted nutrient:

- Potassium: dried figs, California avocado, papaya, banana, dates

Consult with your physician before making any changes to your diet or supplemental regimen.

ORLISTAT (OR-li-stat)

Brand Name: Xenical

About Orlistat

The fat from the food you eat isn't absorbed as is. Instead, it's attacked by various substances that break it down into smaller pieces called fatty acids, which are absorbed by the body and reassembled into various forms that the body can either use or store.

Fat is a big issue in the United States today, with nearly two-thirds of the adult population either overweight or obese. Obesity contributes in a major way to the development of many diseases, as well as some 400,000 deaths annually.

One of the strategies for reducing weight is to prevent the body from absorbing much of the fat in the diet. Orlistat accomplishes this by interfering with the action of enzymes that break down dietary fat and make it available for absorption in the digestive tract. As a result, less fat can be absorbed, and much of it is carried out along with the stool. Orlistat is typically used in conjunction with a weight-control diet to treat obese patients who also have diabetes, elevated blood pressure, or other serious conditions.

Possible Side Effects

The drug's more common side effects include headache, abdominal pain, fecal urgency, and fatty, oily stool.

Which Nutrients Are Robbed

Taking this medicine may deplete your supply of, increase your need for, or interfere with the activity of:

- Beta-carotene
- Vitamin A
- Vitamin D
- Vitamin E
- Vitamin K

Additional Ways This Drug May Upset Your Nutritional Balance

Orlistat can cause abdominal discomfort and pain, nausea, and vomiting, all of which can upset your eating habits and possibly interfere with good nutrition. It can also cause diarrhea, which can hamper nutrient absorption.

Restoring Your Nutritional Balance

To compensate for the nutrient loss caused by this drug, speak to your physician about taking 25,000 IU beta-carotene, 5,000 IU vitamin A, 400 IU vitamin D, 400 IU vitamin E, and 60–80 mcg vitamin K per day.

You can also eat foods that contain the depleted nutrients:

- Beta-carotene: carrot, spinach, mango, cantaloupe, apricot nectar
- Vitamin A: beef liver, chicken liver, cheese pizza, whole milk, cheddar cheese
- Vitamin D: salmon, mackerel, sardines, eel, fortified milk
- Vitamin E: wheat germ oil, almonds, safflower oil, corn oil, soybean oil
- Vitamin K: kale, broccoli, parsley, Swiss chard, spinach

Consult with your physician before making any changes to your diet or supplemental regimen.

OXALIPLATIN (oks-al-i-PLAT-in)

Brand Name: Eloxatin

About Oxaliplatin

Cancer of the large intestine (colon) and rectum is the second leading cause of cancer deaths, with women more likely to develop the former and men the latter. The colon, a big, upside-down U-shape tube inside your belly, carries the food you eat through its final digestive and processing procedures. The food is in a liquid state when it enters the colon, but as it travels up, across, and down this large tube, bacteria convert it into stool.

Colorectal cancer may not cause any symptoms for quite a while, and those that it does trigger will depend on the cancer's type, location, and stage, and how far it has spread. Possible symptoms include internal bleeding that causes weakness and fatigue, and bloody and painful bowel movements.

If the cancer is caught while still in the inner linings of the colon, surgeons may be able to remove the cancerous tissue and attack any remaining cancer cells with chemotherapy. In more advanced cases, surgery, chemotherapy, and other treatments may make the symptoms more manageable or modestly extend survival time.

Oxaliplatin is one of the drugs that may be used to track down and destroy remaining cancer cells following surgery. Used in combination with other medications, it works by binding to the DNA and RNA in cancer cells, gumming up their works, and killing them.

Possible Side Effects

The drug's more common side effects include fatigue, diarrhea, vomiting, and nerve damage.

Which Nutrients Are Robbed

Taking this medicine may deplete your supply of, increase your need for, or interfere with the activity of:

- Potassium

Additional Ways This Drug May Upset Your Nutritional Balance

Oxaliplatin can cause abdominal pain, changes in taste, nausea, and vomiting, all of which can upset your eating habits and possibly interfere with good nutrition. It can also cause diarrhea, which can hamper nutrient absorption.

Restoring Your Nutritional Balance

To compensate for the nutrient loss caused by this drug, speak to your physician about taking 100–300 mg potassium per day.

You can also eat foods that contain the depleted nutrient:

- Potassium: dried figs, California avocado, papaya, banana, dates

Consult with your physician before making any changes to your diet or supplemental regimen.

OXAPROZIN (oks-uh-PROE-zin)

Brand Name: Daypro

About Oxaprozin

A medicine's longevity is measured by its half-life, or the amount of time it takes for half of it to be metabolized by the body and deactivated.

Aspirin has a half-life of less than half an hour, so you may have to take it several times a day. Other nonsteroidal anti-inflammatory drugs (NSAIDs) last longer. For example:

- Ibuprofen (Advil) has a half-life of 2 hours.
- Indomethacin (Indocin) has a half-life of 4 to 5 hours.
- Ketorolac (Orudis) has a half-life of 4 to 10 hours.
- Naproxen (Aleve) has a half-life of 14 hours.
- Nabumetone (Relafen) has a half-life of 26 hours.

But the winner is oxaprozin, an NSAID with a half-life of 58 hours. This makes it a convenient medication for people suffering from the chronic pain of osteoarthritis, rheumatoid arthritis, and juvenile rheumatoid arthritis.

Possible Side Effects

The drug's more common side effects include water retention, confusion, sleep disturbances, ulcers, and anemia.

Which Nutrients Are Robbed

Taking this medicine may deplete your supply of, increase your need for, or interfere with the activity of:

- Folic acid

Additional Ways This Drug May Upset Your Nutritional Balance

Oxaprozin can cause abdominal distress, loss of appetite, heartburn, nausea, and vomiting, all of which can upset your eating habits and possibly interfere with good nutrition. It can also cause diarrhea, which can hamper nutrient absorption.

Restoring Your Nutritional Balance

To compensate for the nutrient loss caused by this drug, speak to your physician about taking 400–800 mcg folic acid per day.

You can also eat foods that contain the depleted nutrient:

- Folic acid: beef liver, fortified breakfast cereals, spinach, great northern beans, asparagus

Consult with your physician before making any changes to your diet or supplemental regimen.

OXCARBAZEPINE (oks-kar-BAZ-e-peen)

Brand Name: Trileptal

About Oxcarbazepine

For many years, medical researchers searched for a drug that would effectively control seizure disorder, or epilepsy, as it was sometimes called in the past. Potassium bromide helped some people after being introduced in 1857, and phenobarbital, which became available in 1912, helped even more. Then, in the late 1930s, phenytoin gave even more people hope.

But the one drug that could control or prevent all seizures has never emerged, because seizures are not a single problem with a single cause. They have symptoms in common, most notably jerking, uncoordinated muscle movements, and they share an obvious trigger, which is uncontrolled and inappropriate firing of certain brain cells. But many different things seem to bring about this firing, which can occur in different parts of the brain, last for varying amounts of time, strike in different forms at different ages, and so on. Because of these differences, the search for the magic bullet against seizure disorder has been abandoned in favor of developing various medicines that can treat different manifestations of the problem.

Oxcarbazepine is used alone or together with another drug to treat partial seizures in adults and children. Partial seizures are "limited" seizures that strike on only one side of the brain.

Possible Side Effects

The drug's more common side effects include dizziness, sleepiness, vomiting, and vision problems.

Which Nutrients Are Robbed

Taking this medicine may deplete your supply of, increase your need for, or interfere with the activity of:

- Biotin
- Folic acid
- Vitamin D
- Calcium
- Sodium

Additional Ways This Drug May Upset Your Nutritional Balance

Oxcarbazepine can cause abdominal pain, nausea, and vomiting, all of which can upset your eating habits and possibly interfere with good nutrition. It can also cause diarrhea, which can hamper nutrient absorption.

Restoring Your Nutritional Balance

To compensate for the nutrient loss caused by this drug, speak to your physician about taking 500–1,000 mcg biotin, 400 IU vitamin D, and 1,200 mg calcium per day. And ask your physician to consider the potential effects of sodium depletion. Taking folic acid can increase the risk of seizures in some people, so discuss the use of this nutrient with your physician.

You can also eat foods that contain the depleted nutrients:

- Biotin: beef liver, soybeans, rice bran, peanut butter, barley
- Vitamin D: salmon, mackerel, sardines, eel, fortified milk
- Calcium: milk, dried figs, Swiss cheese, yogurt, tofu

Consult with your physician before making any changes to your diet or supplemental regimen.

OXYCODONE PLUS ACETAMINOPHEN (oks-i-KOE-dohn, uh-seet-uh-MIN-oh-fen)

Brand Names: Endocet, Oxycocet, Percocet-Demi, Percocet 2.5/325, Percocet 5/325, Percocet 7.5/500, Percocet 10/650, Roxicet 5/500, Roxilox, Tylox

About Oxycodone plus Acetaminophen

Opioid analgesics are the most powerful painkillers we have, the workhorses that handle both severe acute and severe chronic pain. Acute pain is an immediate response to being cut, burned, or scraped, to breaking a bone, and so on. It's a message telling us to get away from or fix the source of trouble, right now! Chronic pain, however, is a long-lasting pain that seems to serve no real purpose. Many times we don't even know what's causing these pain messages; they're simply there, making us miserable.

Oxycodone is an opioid painkiller that works in the central nervous system to quell pain. The drug doesn't actually make the pain disappear, but it does change the way we perceive and respond to the pain signals. It can be used for moderate to severe pain, whether acute or chronic.

Oxycodone is often paired with another painkiller such as acetaminophen, which slows the production of the prostaglandins that encourage pain. (For more on acetaminophen, see the entry on page 90.)

Possible Side Effects

Oxycodone's more common side effects include low blood pressure, fatigue, weakness, nausea, and vomiting. Acetaminophen's side effects include liver and kidney damage.

Which Nutrients Are Robbed

Taking this medicine may deplete your supply of, increase your need for, or interfere with the activity of:

- Glutathione

Additional Ways This Drug May Upset Your Nutritional Balance

Oxycodone can cause nausea and vomiting, which can upset your eating habits and possibly interfere with good nutrition.

Restoring Your Nutritional Balance

To compensate for the nutrient loss caused by this drug, speak to your physician about taking 800–2,000 mg n-acetyl cysteine (a precursor to glutathione) per day.

Consult with your physician before making any changes to your diet or supplemental regimen.

OXYCODONE PLUS ASPIRIN (oks-i-KOE-dohn, ASS-pir-in)

Brand Names: Codoxy, Endodan, Oxycodan, Percodan, Percodan-Demi, Roxiprin

About Oxycodone plus Aspirin

Managing pain can be difficult. You want the painkiller to be strong enough and last long enough to do the job, but you don't want to experience uncomfortable or dangerous side effects or become addicted to it.

Narcotics like oxycodone are our strongest painkillers, changing our perception of pain by stimulating certain receptors in the central nervous system. So although they don't cure the underlying problem, ease inflammation, or make the pain go away, they do make it feel different—less painful and less of an urgent problem.

Oxycodone is typically combined with another painkiller, such as aspirin, the popular and universal medicine that inhibits pain and eases inflammation, which can cause or worsen the pain.

Possible Side Effects

Oxycodone's more common side effects include low blood pressure, fatigue, weakness, nausea, and vomiting. Side effects seen with aspirin include anemia, insomnia, rapid heartbeat, and liver damage.

Which Nutrients Are Robbed

Taking this medicine may deplete your supply of, increase your need for, or interfere with the activity of:

- Folic acid
- Vitamin C
- Iron
- Potassium
- Sodium

Additional Ways This Drug May Upset Your Nutritional Balance

Oxycodone can cause nausea and vomiting, while aspirin can cause heartburn, nausea, and vomiting. These side effects can upset your eating habits and possibly interfere with good nutrition.

Aspirin can also trigger hyperkalemia, or too much potassium in the blood.

Restoring Your Nutritional Balance

To compensate for the nutrient loss caused by this drug, speak to your physician about taking 400–800 mcg folic acid and 250–1,500 mg vitamin C per day. And ask your physician to consider the potential effects of iron and sodium depletion and to monitor your potassium status.

You can also eat foods that contain the depleted nutrients:

- Folic acid: beef liver, fortified breakfast cereals, spinach, great northern beans, asparagus
- Vitamin C: papaya, guava, red pepper, cantaloupe, black currants

Consult with your physician before making any changes to your diet or supplemental regimen.

PAMIDRONATE (pa-mi-DROE-nate)

Brand Name: Aredia

About Pamidronate

The mineral calcium is vitally important; it is needed to build strong bones, keep the heart beating regularly, make the blood clot, and ensure that the muscles contract and release properly. A lack of calcium can cause muscle aches, muscle cramps, osteoporosis, and other problems.

But too much calcium, a condition called hypercalcemia, can be just as dangerous as too little. With this disease, excess calcium gets into the bloodstream and upsets the delicate balance between minerals and other substances. Depending on the degree of hypercalcemia, there may be no symptoms at all, or there may be abdominal pain, nausea and vomiting, loss of appetite, constipation, and excessive urination. In more severe cases, there can be confusion, hallucinations, delirium, muscle weakness, irregular heartbeat, coma, and even death.

A number of things can cause excessively high calcium levels in the blood, including destruction of bone tissue and taking too many antacids that contain calcium.

Pamidronate is one of the medicines that can be used to counteract hypercalcemia. It works by slowing the rate at which calcium is released from the bones.

Possible Side Effects

The drug's more common side effects include fever, nausea, and fatigue.

Which Nutrients Are Robbed

Taking this medicine may deplete your supply of, increase your need for, or interfere with the activity of:

- Calcium
- Magnesium
- Phosphorus
- Potassium

Additional Ways This Drug May Upset Your Nutritional Balance

Pamidronate can cause loss of appetite and nausea, which can upset your eating habits and possibly interfere with good nutrition.

Restoring Your Nutritional Balance

To compensate for the nutrient loss caused by this drug, speak to your physician about taking 500–1,000 mg magnesium, 700 mg phosphorus, and 100–300 mg potassium per day. And ask your physician to monitor your calcium status.

You can also eat foods that contain the depleted nutrients:

- Magnesium: Florida avocado, toasted wheat germ, almonds, shredded wheat cereal, pumpkin seeds
- Phosphorus: plain nonfat yogurt, lentils, salmon, milk, halibut
- Potassium: dried figs, California avocado, papaya, banana, dates

Consult with your physician before making any changes to your diet or supplemental regimen.

PANTOPRAZOLE (pan-TOE-prah-zole)

Brand Names: Pantoloc, Protonix

About Pantoprazole

That burning pain centered behind your breastbone, perhaps spreading to your chest, neck, throat, and face, may be caused by gastroesophageal reflux disease, or GERD. If you have GERD, the contents of your stomach, including some powerful acids and digestive juices, can splash back up into your esophagus.

Besides pain, GERD can cause some serious problems with your esophagus, including bleeding, painful ulcers, precancerous changes in its lining, narrowing of this "food tube," and difficulty swallowing.

You may feel the stomach acid eating away at your esophagus or, surprisingly, you may not, for GERD can be "silent." Or you may have the symptoms of GERD but your esophageal lining remains normal, a condition called nonerosive reflux disease, or NERD.

The treatment for GERD usually starts with a medicine such as pantoprazole, which reduces the amount of acid produced in your stomach after you eat by blocking the biochemical acid "switches" in the lining of the stomach.

Pantoprazole is used to treat the esophageal inflammation seen in GERD and to reduce heartburn and associated problems.

Possible Side Effects

The drug's side effects include chest pain, migraine headaches, dizziness, and urinary tract infections.

Which Nutrients Are Robbed

Taking this medicine may deplete your supply of, increase your need for, or interfere with the activity of:

- Beta-carotene
- Thiamin
- Vitamin B_{12}
- Iron

Additional Ways This Drug May Upset Your Nutritional Balance

Pantoprazole can cause loss of appetite, nausea, vomiting, and abdominal discomfort and pain, all of which can upset your eating habits and possibly interfere with good nutrition. It can also cause diarrhea, which can hamper nutrient absorption.

Restoring Your Nutritional Balance

To compensate for the nutrient loss caused by this drug, speak to your physician about taking 25,000 IU beta-carotene, 25–100 mg thiamin, and 500–1,000 mcg vitamin B_{12} per day. And ask your physician to consider the potential effects of iron depletion.

You can also eat foods that contain the depleted nutrients:

- Beta-carotene: carrot, spinach, mango, cantaloupe, apricot nectar
- Thiamin: braised liver, turkey heart, roasted chicken, gefilte fish, sardines
- Vitamin B_{12}: beef liver, rainbow trout, sockeye salmon, beef, haddock

Consult with your physician before making any changes to your diet or supplemental regimen.

PENBUTOLOL (pen-BYOO-toe-lole)

Brand Name: Levatol

About Penbutolol

Penbutolol is an imposter. It acts like a chemical messenger from the brain, but it's really a medicine that fools the body into thinking that it has received a certain message from the brain and has responded accordingly. And that can be a good thing. For example, your blood pressure rises in response to messages sent to the heart telling it to work harder. But if your blood pressure is already too high, you don't want your heart to receive and respond to the "work harder" messages. Instead, you want the heart to relax a bit, slow down, and let the pressure ease back toward normal.

Penbutolol helps resolve this problem by pretending to be one of those "work hard" messages sent from the brain to the heart. It fits into the proper receptor sites on the heart and tells it to work, but the message it delivers is more like "work slightly hard" instead of "work really hard." As a result, the heart works less energetically and the blood pressure drops, thanks to this "phony messenger."

Penbutolol is used to treat elevated blood pressure, irregular heartbeat, and angina, which triggers pain in the chest and possibly the left arm, neck, jaw, and shoulder.

Possible Side Effects

The drug's more common side effects include weakness, fatigue, and impotence.

Which Nutrients Are Robbed

Taking this medicine may deplete your supply of, increase your need for, or interfere with the activity of:

- Coenzyme Q_{10}

Restoring Your Nutritional Balance

To compensate for the nutrient loss caused by this drug, speak to your physician about taking 30–100 mg coenzyme Q_{10} per day.

You can also eat foods that contain the depleted nutrient:

- Coenzyme Q_{10}: beef, chicken, trout, salmon, oranges, broccoli

Consult with your physician before making any changes to your diet or supplemental regimen.

PENICILLAMINE (pen-i-SIL-uh-meen)

Brand Names: Cuprimine, Depen

About Penicillamine

An uncommon hereditary ailment called Wilson's disease causes the body to absorb too much copper from food and excrete too little of this mineral via the liver into the bile. As a result, excess copper builds up in various parts of the body, especially in the brain and liver, causing major problems.

In almost half of the victims of Wilson's disease, the brain suffers first. As the brain becomes overloaded with copper, there may be difficulty in swallowing and speaking, jerky movements, changes in personality, and schizophrenia or other psychoses. In an equally large but different group of people, the liver becomes overloaded, causing hepatitis and the degenerative disease called cirrhosis. Unless treated, Wilson's disease is fatal.

Penicillamine is the preferred treatment for Wilson's disease. It works by attaching itself to copper in the body, making it easier for the mineral to be carried away via the urine.

Penicillamine may also be used to treat toxicity caused by excessive amounts of other minerals in the body.

Possible Side Effects

The drug's more common side effects include rash, itching, joint pain, and decreased sense of taste.

Which Nutrients Are Robbed

Taking this medicine may deplete your supply of, increase your need for, or interfere with the activity of:

- Vitamin B_6
- Copper
- Iron
- Magnesium
- Zinc

Additional Ways This Drug May Upset Your Nutritional Balance

Penicillamine can cause changes in taste, which can upset your eating habits and possibly interfere with good nutrition.

Restoring Your Nutritional Balance

To compensate for the nutrient loss caused by this drug, speak to your physician about taking 50–100 mg vitamin B_6, 500–1,000 mg magnesium, and 50–200 mg zinc per day. And ask your physician to consider the potential effects of iron depletion and to monitor your copper status. (People with Wilson's disease should avoid supplements containing copper.)

You can also eat foods that contain the depleted nutrients:

- Vitamin B_6: potato, banana, garbanzo beans, chicken breast, fortified oatmeal
- Magnesium: Florida avocado, toasted wheat germ, almonds, shredded wheat cereal, pumpkin seeds
- Zinc: oysters, beef shank, chicken, pork tenderloin, plain yogurt

Consult with your physician before making any changes to your diet or supplemental regimen.

PENICILLIN
PENICILLIN G BENZATHINE, PENICILLIN G BENZATHINE PLUS PROCAINE, PENICILLIN G PROCAINE, PENICILLIN V POTASSIUM (pen-i-SIL-in jee BENZ-uh-theen, PROE-kane, vee poe-TASS-ee-um)

Brand Names: Penicillin G benzathine: Bicillin L-A, Permapen
Penicillin G benzathine plus penicillin G procaine: Bicillin C-R
Penicillin G procaine: Pfizerpen-AS, Wycillin
Penicillin V potassium: Novo-Pen-VK, Suspen, Truxcillin

About Penicillin

The era of antibiotics began back in 1928, when Sir Alexander Fleming noticed that staphylococci colonies flourished in a culture except in the areas where there was some *Penicillium notatum* fungi. The medicine penicillin, which was derived from that fungi, was developed in 1940 and was soon put to use on the battlefield, where it was credited with saving many Allied soldiers during World War II.

Penicillin combats bacteria by interfering with their ability to build their cellular walls. Without this protective coating, the cell dies. Penicillin proved so effective in fighting bacterial infections that by the 1950s, it was being produced in great quantities in the United States and given freely to patients—often when they didn't need it. Many patients demanded a shot of some sort of medicine when they weren't feeling well, and doctors felt that giving penicillin was, at the very least, a good preventive measure. Unfortunately, this overuse led to the rise of penicillin-resistant bacteria, as the germs "learned" how to produce mutated strains that were increasingly difficult to destroy. Because of this rise of penicillin-resistant bacteria, medical researchers have been forced to develop newer, stronger medicines.

Despite the rise of resistant bacteria, penicillin is still used to treat a wide variety of ailments, including syphilis and certain pneumococcal, streptococcal, and other infections. Several different forms of penicillin are designed for different purposes. For example, penicillin V can withstand stomach acid, so it can be taken in pill form rather than via injection. Other formulations have added procaine to reduce the pain of injection.

Possible Side Effects

Side effects for the various forms of penicillin include convulsions, fever, rash, and confusion.

Which Nutrients Are Robbed

Taking these forms of penicillin may deplete your supply of, increase your need for, or interfere with the activity of:

- Biotin
- Inositol
- Thiamin
- Riboflavin
- Niacin
- Vitamin B_6

- Vitamin B_{12}
- Vitamin K
- Potassium
- *Bifidobacterium bifidum*
- *Lactobacillus acidophilus*

Additional Ways This Drug May Upset Your Nutritional Balance

Penicillin V potassium can cause nausea and vomiting, which can upset your eating habits and possibly interfere with good nutrition. It can also cause diarrhea, which can hamper nutrient absorption.

Restoring Your Nutritional Balance

To compensate for the nutrient loss caused by these drugs, speak to your physician about taking 500–1,000 mcg biotin, 250–1,000 mg inositol, 25–100 mg thiamin, 25–100 mg riboflavin, 50–100 mg niacin, 50–100 mg vitamin B_6,

500–1,000 mcg vitamin B_{12}, 60–80 mcg vitamin K, 100–300 mg potassium, 15 billion live *Bifidobacterium bifidum* organisms, and 15 billion live *Lactobacillus acidophilus* organisms per day.

You can also eat foods that contain the depleted nutrients:

- Biotin: beef liver, soybeans, rice bran, peanut butter, barley
- Inositol: cantaloupe, oranges, green beans, grapefruit juice, limes
- Thiamin: braised liver, turkey heart, roasted chicken, gefilte fish, sardines
- Riboflavin: dried sunflower seeds, orange juice, bulgur, spinach noodles, pine nuts
- Niacin: chicken breast, beef liver, mackerel, barley, bulgur
- Vitamin B_6: potato, banana, garbanzo beans, chicken breast, fortified oatmeal
- Vitamin B_{12}: beef liver, rainbow trout, sockeye salmon, beef, haddock
- Vitamin K: kale, broccoli, parsley, Swiss chard, spinach
- Potassium: dried figs, California avocado, papaya, banana, dates
- *Bifidobacterium bifidum*: Jerusalem artichokes, asparagus, garlic, and onions may stimulate the growth or activity of this probiotic
- *Lactobacillus acidophilus*: yogurt containing live lactobacillus cultures, kefir, acidophilus milk

Consult with your physician before making any changes to your diet or supplemental regimen.

PENTAMIDINE (pen-TAM-i-deen)

Brand Names: NebuPent Inhalation, Pentacarinat Injection, Pentam-300 Injection, Pneumopent

About Pentamidine

We humans coexist with a host of deadly bacteria, including *Pneumocystis carinii* (*P. carinii*), part of the normal collection of bacteria, fungi, and other things that live within our bodies. *P. carinii* isn't usually a problem because the immune system easily keeps it in check.

Unfortunately, an HIV-ravaged immune system cannot suppress *P. carinii*, which multiplies in the lungs, taking up residence in the tiny air sacs (alveoli) where oxygen and carbon dioxide are exchanged. *P. carinii* bacteria make the alveoli thicken and wither, triggering shortness of breath, cough, fatigue, loss of appetite, fever, and other problems. The overwhelming majority of people infected with HIV eventually develop *P. carinii* pneumonia, and the disease can be fatal.

Pentamidine is one of the drugs used to treat *P. carinii* pneumonia, by hindering the germs' manufacture of protein, DNA and RNA. Pentamidine can be taken intravenously or as an aerosol.

Pentamidine is also used to treat African sleeping sickness (trypanosomiasis).

Possible Side Effects

The drug's more common side effects include chest pain, rash, wheezing, and coughing.

Which Nutrients Are Robbed

Taking this medicine may deplete your supply of, increase your need for, or interfere with the activity of:

- Folic acid
- Calcium
- Magnesium

Additional Ways This Drug May Upset Your Nutritional Balance

Pentamidine can cause low blood sugar (hypoglycemia), loss of appetite, changes in taste, nausea, and vomiting, all of which can upset your eating habits and possibly interfere with good nutrition. It can also cause diarrhea, which can hamper nutrient absorption.

Restoring Your Nutritional Balance

To compensate for the nutrient loss caused by this drug, speak to your physician about taking 400–800 mcg folic acid, 500–1,000 mg magnesium, and 1,200 mg calcium per day.

You can also eat foods that contain the depleted nutrients:

- Folic acid: beef liver, fortified breakfast cereals, spinach, great northern beans, asparagus
- Magnesium: Florida avocado, toasted wheat germ, almonds, shredded wheat cereal, pumpkin seeds
- Calcium: milk, dried figs, Swiss cheese, yogurt, tofu

Consult with your physician before making any changes to your diet or supplemental regimen.

PERINDOPRIL ERBUMINE (per-IN-doe-pril er-BYOO-meen)

Brand Name: Aceon

About Perindopril Erbumine

Imagine a group of dominoes, all standing on end in a line. When one falls, it knocks over the next, which knocks over the next, and so on. A similar cascading action takes place in the body when the blood pressure falls too low. A substance called angiotensinogen is converted into angiotensin I, which is converted into angiotensin II, which causes the blood vessels to constrict. This increases the resistance to the flow of blood, which raises the blood pressure. The angiotensin II also prompts the release of a substance called aldosterone, which makes the kidneys retain sodium, causing the body to retain water. The blood volume increases and blood pressure rises.

Unfortunately, too many Americans have blood pressure that's already too high, and that can be dangerous, or even deadly. Doctors use perindopril erbumine and similar drugs to lower high blood pressure by blocking the conversion of angiotensin I to angiotensin II. This has the same effect as stopping one domino from falling; the cascade halts at that point. So instead of rising, the blood pressure stays at more normal levels.

Thanks to this effect and others, perindopril is used to treat elevated blood pressure, congestive heart failure, and other ailments.

Possible Side Effects

The drug's more common side effects include headache, dizziness, weakness, and pain in the lower extremities.

Which Nutrients Are Robbed

Taking this medicine may deplete your supply of, increase your need for, or interfere with the activity of:

- Zinc

Additional Ways This Drug May Upset Your Nutritional Balance

Perindopril erbumine can cause nausea, vomiting, heartburn, a feeling of fullness, and abdominal pain, all of which can upset your eating habits and possibly interfere with good nutrition. It can also cause diarrhea, which can hamper nutrient absorption.

This drug can also trigger hyperkalemia, or too much potassium in the blood.

Restoring Your Nutritional Balance

To compensate for the nutrient loss caused by this drug, speak to your physician about taking 50–200 mg zinc per day.

You can also eat foods that contain the depleted nutrient:

- Zinc: oysters, beef shank, chicken, pork tenderloin, plain yogurt

Consult with your physician before making any changes to your diet or supplemental regimen.

PERPHENAZINE (per-FEN-uh-zeen)

Brand Names: Apo-Perphenazine, PMS-Perphenazine, Trilafon

About Perphenazine

Some time after your bout with chicken pox has faded into memory, you may be hit with a reminder called shingles. Technically known as herpes zoster, shingles is a reemergence of the virus that caused your chicken pox, and has been hiding quietly in certain nerves ever since. Now it surfaces again, streaking along the nerves and out to the skin, where it triggers painful sores, blisters, and rash, and possibly bladder and bowel problems, and other symptoms. Antiviral drugs may be given to strengthen the immune system's ability to fight back during the attack, and medicines for pain and other problems are generally prescribed to handle the symptoms. A small percentage of people hit by shingles will suffer through more attacks, but most people only go through it once.

Unfortunately, perhaps 10 percent of those hit by shingles are struck again, this time by postherpetic neuralgia ("nerve pain"), or lingering chronic pain in the area where the shingles had been. The pain, which can be bad and even incapacitating, may last for months or years. We don't fully understand what causes this "second time around" probem.

Perphenazine is one of the drugs used to treat postherpetic neuralgia. Also used to treat schizophrenia, nausea, and vomiting, the drug works by changing the way the neurotransmitter dopamine is handled in the brain, and by slowing the release of certain hormones.

Possible Side Effects

The drug's side effects include seizures, headache, drowsiness, and liver damage.

Which Nutrients Are Robbed

Taking this medicine may deplete your supply of, increase your need for, or interfere with the activity of:

- Riboflavin
- Coenzyme Q_{10}

Additional Ways This Drug May Upset Your Nutritional Balance

Perphenazine can cause low blood sugar (hypoglycemia), loss of appetite, stomach pain, nausea, and vomiting, all of which can upset your eating habits and possibly interfere with good nutrition. It can also cause diarrhea, which can hamper nutrient absorption.

Restoring Your Nutritional Balance

To compensate for the nutrient loss caused by this drug, speak to your physician about taking 25–100 mg riboflavin and 30–100 mg coenzyme Q_{10} per day.

You can also eat foods that contain the depleted nutrients:

- Riboflavin: dried sunflower seeds, orange juice, bulgur, spinach noodles, pine nuts
- Coenzyme Q_{10}: beef, chicken, trout, salmon, oranges, broccoli

Consult with your physician before making any changes to your diet or supplemental regimen.

PHENELZINE (FEN-el-zeen)

Brand Name: Nardil

About Phenelzine

Phenelzine is a monoamine oxidase inhibitor (MAOI), one of a group of drugs used to treat depression. Back in the 1950s, researchers noted that interfering with the actions of amine neurotransmitters (brain messengers) such as serotonin or norepinephrine caused people to become depressed. This led to the idea that depression is triggered by problems with amine transmitters. Perhaps fewer are manufactured in the nervous systems of the depressed, or they're being used improperly, or they are broken down too quickly.

Monoamine oxidase is a substance that "chews up" these amines. This destruction is normal, for the body continually manufactures and disassembles many substances. But too much of a good thing can be harmful. Phenelzine and other MAOIs interfere with the chewing up process, allowing more serotonin and other amines to accumulate in the nervous system and lift the mood.

Possible Side Effects

The drug's side effects include dizziness, sleep disturbances, mania, and twitching.

Which Nutrients Are Robbed

Taking this medicine may deplete your supply of, increase your need for, or interfere with the activity of:

- Vitamin B_6

Restoring Your Nutritional Balance

To compensate for the nutrient loss caused by this drug, speak to your physician about taking 50–100 mg vitamin B_6 per day.

You can also eat foods that contain the depleted nutrient:

- Vitamin B_6: potato, banana, garbanzo beans, chicken breast, fortified oatmeal

Consult with your physician before making any changes to your diet or supplemental regimen.

PHENOBARBITAL (fee-noe-BAR-bi-tall)

Brand Names: Ancalixir, Barbita, Barbilixir, Luminal, Solfoton

About Phenobarbital

Introduced in 1912, phenobarbital was the first modern drug used for epilepsy, and it's still in use today for different types of seizures. (Today, the word "epilepsy" is reserved for a pattern of chronic seizures, rather than for an isolated seizure.)

We don't know exactly how phenobarbital works to prevent or control seizures. It appears to inhibit the action of abnormal nerve cells that trigger random, uncontrolled firing of the electrical circuits in the brain and to encourage the brain's natural dampening mechanisms.

Phenobarbital is used to treat partial seizures, which affect only one side, or half, of the brain. The symptoms of a partial seizure can vary. For example:

- In a *simple partial seizure*, only a small area of the brain is involved, and only the part of the body that it controls is affected. For example, your right leg may jerk and shake.
- In a *Jacksonian seizure,* the problem begins in one part of the brain, then spreads. Thus, the jerking and shaking may begin in your right foot, then move up your right leg.
- In a *complex partial seizure*, the symptoms aren't limited to shaking and jerking. You may stare without comprehension, move your limbs in a meaningless way, and be unable to understand what others are saying. That may be the extent of the seizure, and you may be fine within several minutes. Or, the problem may spread to other parts of the brain, triggering a generalized seizure complete with jerking limbs and loss of consciousness.

These and other partial seizures are different from generalized seizures, which strike on both sides—right and left halves—of the brain at once.

In addition to partial seizures, phenobarbital is approved for the treatment of grand mal seizures and for use as a sedative.

Possible Side Effects

The drug's side effects include fainting, lethargy, and a slow heartbeat.

Which Nutrients Are Robbed

Taking this medicine may deplete your supply of, increase your need for, or interfere with the activity of:

- Biotin
- Folic acid
- Vitamin B_6
- Vitamin B_{12}
- Vitamin D
- Vitamin K
- Calcium
- Carnitine

Additional Ways This Drug May Upset Your Nutritional Balance

Phenobarbital can cause nausea and vomiting, which can upset your eating habits and possibly interfere with good nutrition.

Restoring Your Nutritional Balance

To compensate for the nutrient loss caused by this drug, speak to your physician about taking 500–1,000 mcg biotin, 50–100 mg vitamin B_6, 500–1,000 mcg vitamin B_{12}, 400 IU vitamin D, 60–80 mcg vitamin K, 1,200 mg calcium, and 250–1,000 mg carnitine per day. Taking folic acid can increase the risk of seizures in some people, so speak to your physician about the use of this nutrient.

You can also eat foods that contain the depleted nutrients:

- Biotin: beef liver, soybeans, rice bran, peanut butter, barley
- Vitamin B_6: potato, banana, garbanzo beans, chicken breast, fortified oatmeal
- Vitamin B_{12}: beef liver, rainbow trout, sockeye salmon, beef, haddock
- Vitamin D: salmon, mackerel, sardines, eel, fortified milk
- Vitamin K: kale, broccoli, parsley, Swiss chard, spinach
- Calcium: milk, dried figs, Swiss cheese, yogurt, tofu
- Carnitine: ground beef, pork, Canadian bacon, whole milk, cod

Consult with your physician before making any changes to your diet or supplemental regimen.

PHENYTOIN (FEN-i-toyn)

Brand Names: Dilantin, Diphenylan Sodium, Phenytek, Tremytoine

About Phenytoin

Grand mal seizures may begin when a little part of the brain is blanketed by random, excessive electrical discharges. You may have difficulty communicating with and understanding others, and your limbs may move without reason. This "electrical storm" soon spreads to larger areas of your brain. Depending on how far it spreads and which parts of the brain are affected, you may experience loss of consciousness, powerful muscle spasms, clenched teeth, and loss of bladder control. Your head may jerk to one side and remain fixed there. In a couple of minutes, it all passes, leaving you confused and tired, with a headache and no memory of what has just happened.

Phenytoin is one of the drugs used to treat grand mal seizures. As with many other drugs, we can't pinpoint the exact mechanism(s) it employs to quell seizures. We do know that it changes the way electrolytes are handled in the nervous system, as well as the relative amounts of several amino acids. It also has some effects on the fats that reside in cell walls, which may help to "calm" the cells, and it changes the way serotonin, dopamine, and norepinephrine are released and accepted within the brain.

Introduced in 1928, phenytoin is the oldest antiseizure drug in existence that does *not* have a sedative effect. It's an effective medicine for treating grand mal seizures and is also used to treat partial seizures and to prevent seizures in people who have had brain surgery or a head injury.

Possible Side Effects

The drug's side effects include low blood pressure, irregular heart rhythms, slurred speech, and blurred vision.

Which Nutrients Are Robbed

Taking this medicine may deplete your supply of, increase your need for, or interfere with the activity of:

- Biotin
- Folic acid
- Thiamin
- Vitamin B_{12}
- Vitamin D
- Vitamin K
- Calcium
- Phosphorus
- Carnitine

Additional Ways This Drug May Upset Your Nutritional Balance

Phenytoin can cause nausea and vomiting, which can upset your eating habits and possibly interfere with good nutrition.

Restoring Your Nutritional Balance

To compensate for the nutrient loss caused by this drug, speak to your physician about taking 500–1,000 mcg biotin, 25–100 mg thiamin, 500–1,000 mcg vitamin B_{12}, 400 IU vitamin D, 60–80 mcg vitamin K, 1,200 mg calcium, 700 mg phosphorus, and 250–1,000 mg carnitine per day. Taking folic acid can increase the risk of seizures in some people, so discuss the use of this nutrient with your physician.

You can also eat foods that contain the depleted nutrients:

- Biotin: beef liver, soybeans, rice bran, peanut butter, barley
- Thiamin: braised liver, turkey heart, roasted chicken, gefilte fish, sardines
- Vitamin B_{12}: beef liver, rainbow trout, sockeye salmon, beef, haddock
- Vitamin D: salmon, mackerel, sardines, eel, fortified milk
- Vitamin K: kale, broccoli, parsley, Swiss chard, spinach
- Calcium: milk, dried figs, Swiss cheese, yogurt, tofu
- Phosphorus: plain nonfat yogurt, lentils, salmon, milk, halibut
- Carnitine: ground beef, pork, Canadian bacon, whole milk, cod

Consult with your physician before making any changes to your diet or supplemental regimen.

PINDOLOL (PIN-doe-lole)

Brand Names: Syn-Pindolol, Visken

About Pindolol

Just about everyone who drives a car has used the horn to hurry another driver along. But you can honk the horn in more than one way. You can hit it hard and hold it down for a long time, or you can tap it gently.

The brain has its own way of sending a hurry-up signal to the heart to tell it to beat faster and stronger. It sends messengers called neurotransmitters to specialized areas in the heart called beta-receptors, where they insert themselves and "honk the horn" to make the heart speed up. And they'll do this as long and as hard as it takes to make the heart shift into high gear.

Normally, it's safe to let the brain decide how fast and hard the heart should beat. But if you have elevated blood pressure, you don't want your heart to beat any faster or pump any harder than necessary. In other words, you don't want those neurotransmitters "leaning on the horn." In fact, you may not want them anywhere near the horn.

Drugs called beta-blockers are specially designed to keep the neurotransmitters from leaning on those horns. Some of these drugs, such as pindolol, move right into the beta-receptors and "blow the horn"—but they do it very gently. As a result, the heart doesn't shift into high gear, just beats slightly harder, which keeps blood pressure from rising to unhealthy levels.

Pindolol is used to treat hypertension. It's also sometimes used to treat irregular heartbeats and anxiety, as well as aggression in people suffering from dementia.

Possible Side Effects

The drug's more common side effects include insomnia, nervousness, and joint and muscle pain.

Which Nutrients Are Robbed

Taking this medicine may deplete your supply of, increase your need for, or interfere with the activity of:

- Coenzyme Q_{10}
- Melatonin

Additional Ways This Drug May Upset Your Nutritional Balance

Pindolol can cause nausea and abdominal discomfort, which can upset your eating habits and possibly interfere with good nutrition.

Restoring Your Nutritional Balance

To compensate for the nutrient loss caused by this drug, speak to your physician about taking 30–100 mg coenzyme Q_{10} and 1–3 mg melatonin per day.

You can also eat foods that contain the depleted nutrient:

- Coenzyme Q_{10}: beef, chicken, trout, salmon, oranges, broccoli

Consult with your physician before making any changes to your diet or supplemental regimen.

PIPERACILLIN, PIPERACILLIN PLUS TAZOBACTAM SODIUM (pi-PER-uh-sil-in, ta-zoe-BAK-tam SOE-dee-um)

Brand Names: Piperacillin: Pipracil
Piperacillin plus tazobactam sodium: Tazocin, Zosyn

About Piperacillin, Piperacillin plus Tazobactam Sodium

Bacteria are not supposed to be in the bloodstream. Of course, small numbers of them do manage to sneak in, perhaps through a cut in your skin. But as soon as your body notices the presence of bacteria, it mounts a vigorous counterattack, sending white blood cells scurrying to the area to wage war.

Yet sometimes—fortunately, not very often—large numbers of bacteria from an infection in the lungs, the skin, or elsewhere find their way into the bloodstream and prove to be too much for the immune system to handle. These bloodborne germs can then spread throughout the bloodstream, a condition called septicemia.

Still, the immune system doesn't give up, but sends out more white blood cells to destroy the bacteria. As the battle between the immune system and the invaders grows, toxins released by either side to destroy the other can cause the blood vessels to dilate, which can trigger a severe drop in blood pressure. Deprived of adequate blood, the brain, kidneys, and other organs may begin to malfunction.

The heart then tries to crank up the blood pressure by pumping fast and furiously, to no avail. Eventually, the combination of overwork and toxins makes the heart weaken. Meanwhile, the toxins cause leaks in the blood vessel walls, so nearby tissues swell with fluid. If this happens in the lungs, breathing can be impaired. This combination of symptoms, called septic shock, can be fatal.

Doctors treat septicemia aggressively with antibiotics such as piperacillin, a chemical cousin to penicillin. The drug destroys bacteria by preventing them from constructing their cellular walls. Piperacillin may be combined with tazobactam sodium, which inhibits enzymes that bacteria make to destroy penicillins.

Piperacillin is also used to treat respiratory, skin, and urinary tract infections.

Possible Side Effects

Side effects seen with piperacillin plus tazobactam sodium include rash, diarrhea, seizures, and drug-induced hepatitis.

Which Nutrients Are Robbed

Taking this combination medicine may deplete your supply of, increase your need for, or interfere with the activity of:

- Biotin
- Inositol
- Thiamin
- Riboflavin
- Vitamin B_{12}
- Vitamin K
- Potassium
- *Bifidobacterium bifidum*

- Niacin
- Vitamin B$_6$

- *Lactobacillus acidophilus*

Additional Ways These Drugs May Upset Your Nutritional Balance

The combination of piperacillin plus tazobactam sodium can cause nausea, vomiting, heartburn, and bloating, all of which can upset your eating habits and possibly interfere with good nutrition. It can also cause diarrhea, which can hamper nutrient absorption.

Your need for potassium may decrease when you're taking piperacillin plus tazobactam.

Restoring Your Nutritional Balance

To compensate for the nutrient loss caused by these drugs, speak to your physician about taking 500–1,000 mcg biotin, 250–1,000 mg inositol, 25–100 mg thiamin, 25–100 mg riboflavin, 50–100 mg niacin, 50–100 mg vitamin B$_6$, 500–1,000 mcg vitamin B$_{12}$, 60–80 mcg vitamin K, 15 billion live *Bifidobacterium bifidum* organisms, and 15 billion live *Lactobacillus acidophilus* organisms per day. And ask your physician to monitor your potassium status.

You can also eat foods that contain the depleted nutrients:

- Biotin: beef liver, soybeans, rice bran, peanut butter, barley
- Inositol: cantaloupe, oranges, green beans, grapefruit juice, limes
- Thiamin: braised liver, turkey heart, roasted chicken, gefilte fish, sardines
- Riboflavin: dried sunflower seeds, orange juice, bulgur, spinach noodles, pine nuts
- Niacin: chicken breast, beef liver, mackerel, barley, bulgur
- Vitamin B$_6$: potato, banana, garbanzo beans, chicken breast, fortified oatmeal
- Vitamin B$_{12}$: beef liver, rainbow trout, sockeye salmon, beef, haddock
- Vitamin K: kale, broccoli, parsley, Swiss chard, spinach
- *Bifidobacterium bifidum*: Jerusalem artichokes, asparagus, garlic, and onions may stimulate the growth or activity of this probiotic
- *Lactobacillus acidophilus*: yogurt containing live lactobacillus cultures, kefir, acidophilus milk

Consult with your physician before making any changes to your diet or supplemental regimen.

PIROXICAM (peer-OKS-i-kam)

Brand Names: Apo-Piroxicam, Feldene, Novo-Piroxicam, Nu-Pirox, Pro-Piroxicam

About Piroxicam

What do a ballerina's ankles, a football player's knees, and a data processor's wrists have in common? They're all prone to repetitive motion injury, the kind of damage that occurs when joints are used—or abused—in the same way over and over again, day after day, year after year.

Repetitive motion injury is one of the risk factors for osteoarthritis, the most common form of arthritis today. Osteoarthritis is a disease in which the cartilage breaks down. It no longer serves as an incredibly slick shock absorber that caps and protects the ends of the bones, allowing them to glide smoothly across each other. Without this protective and buffering surface, the bones rub against each other and may develop bone spurs or even crack. Osteoarthritis causes pain and sometimes inflammation and disability.

Your doctor may prescribe piroxicam as part of the treatment for your osteoarthritis. Piroxicam, an NSAID (nonsteroidal anti-inflammatory drug) that quells pain and inflammation, won't cure the disease, but it can help you regain the use of the afflicted joint and improve your quality of life.

By the way, it's not just ballerinas, football players, and data processors who are at risk of developing osteoarthritis. Anyone who has injured a joint, suffered damage to the end of a bone, contracted certain bone diseases, or is overweight is a candidate for osteoarthritis.

Piroxican may also be used to treat rheumatold arthritis and other inflammatory ailments.

Possible Side Effects

The drug's more common side effects include water retention, headache, dizziness, and stomach upset.

Which Nutrients Are Robbed

Taking this medicine may deplete your supply of, increase your need for, or interfere with the activity of:

- Folic acid

Additional Ways This Drug May Upset Your Nutritional Balance

Piroxicam can cause low blood sugar (hypoglycemia), loss of appetite, indigestion, nausea, and abdominal discomfort, all of which can upset your eating habits and possibly interfere with good nutrition. It can also cause diarrhea, which can hamper nutrient absorption.

Restoring Your Nutritional Balance

To compensate for the nutrient loss caused by this drug, speak to your physician about taking 400–800 mcg folic acid per day.

You can also eat foods that contain the depleted nutrient:

- Folic acid: beef liver, fortified breakfast cereals, spinach, great northern beans, asparagus

Consult with your physician before making any changes to your diet or supplemental regimen.

PLICAMYCIN (plye-kuh-MYE-sin)

Brand Name: Mithracin

About Plicamycin

A cell's DNA contains all the information the cell needs to live, work, and replicate. But DNA is not set up like a book; it's more like an amazingly long, very thin sheet of paper that's tightly twisted and coiled. To read some of the instructions—say, those detailing how to make a protein—the DNA has to untwist the portion that contains those directions and let the cell use them as a kind of template to make RNA. The RNA, in turn, serves as a template for making the necessary protein.

Plicamycin helps fight cancer by binding to the DNA in a cancer cell, making it difficult for the cell to make RNA and various proteins. The drug is used to treat advanced tumors of the testicles.

Plicamycin has another interesting property. It lowers the amount of calcium in the blood, possibly by acting on the body's bone-building and bone-destroying cells. This makes it useful for treating high levels of calcium in the blood (hypercalcemia), a condition that may be seen in conjunction with different kinds of cancer.

Possible Side Effects

The drug's more common side effects include nausea, vomiting, diarrhea, and loss of appetite.

Which Nutrients Are Robbed

Taking this medicine may deplete your supply of, increase your need for, or interfere with the activity of:

- Calcium
- Potassium
- Phosphorus

Additional Ways This Drug May Upset Your Nutritional Balance

Plicamycin can cause loss of appetite, nausea, and vomiting, all of which can upset your eating habits and possibly interfere with good nutrition. It can also cause diarrhea, which can hamper nutrient absorption.

Restoring Your Nutritional Balance

To compensate for the nutrient loss caused by this drug, speak to your physician about taking 700 mg phosphorus and 100–300 mg potassium per day. And ask your physician to monitor your calcium status.

You can also eat foods that contain the depleted nutrients:

- Phosphorus: plain nonfat yogurt, lentils, salmon, milk, halibut
- Potassium: dried figs, California avocado, papaya, banana, dates

Consult with your physician before making any changes to your diet or supplemental regimen.

POTASSIUM AND SODIUM PHOSPHATES (poe-TASS-ee-um, SOE-dee-um FOSS-fates)

Brand Names: K-Phos Neutral, Neutra-Phos, Uro-KP-Neutral

About Potassium and Sodium Phosphates

We need the mineral potassium to keep our muscles, nerves, and cells in good working order. Potassium plays an important part in muscle contraction and relaxation and in maintaining the fluid and electrolyte balance in the body's cells. It also helps the nerves conduct messages, and assists in the release of energy from the protein, fat, and carbohydrates that we eat. Most of the potassium in the human body resides in the cells; only a relatively small amount circulates in the blood.

When levels of potassium in the blood fall below a certain level—a condition called hypokalemia—you may suffer from generalized weakness, twitching of the muscles, or muscle paralysis. Your heart, that all-important muscle, can begin to beat irregularly.

A loss of potassium may be caused by diarrhea, vomiting, polyps in the colon, Cushing's syndrome, or the chronic use of laxatives, diuretics, or other medicines. Even eating large amounts of licorice root (the real thing, not the synthetic kind found in most candies) can deplete you of potassium.

Eating potassium-rich foods may solve the problem if you have a mild potassium deficiency. For more severe cases, medicines like potassium phosphate plus sodium phosphate may be prescribed.

Possible Side Effects

The drug's more common side effects include diarrhea, nausea, vomiting, flatulence, and stomach pain.

Which Nutrients Are Robbed

Taking this combination medicine may deplete your supply of, increase your need for, or interfere with the activity of:

- Calcium   • Magnesium

Additional Ways This Drug May Upset Your Nutritional Balance

Potassium and sodium phosphates can cause abdominal pain, nausea, and vomiting, all of which can upset your eating habits and possibly interfere with good nutrition. It can also cause diarrhea, which can hamper nutrient absorption.

This drug can also trigger hyperkalemia, or too much potassium in the blood, and hyperphosphatemia, or too much phosphate in the blood.

Restoring Your Nutritional Balance

To compensate for the nutrient loss caused by this drug, speak to your physician about taking 1,200 mg calcium and 500–1,000 mg magnesium per day.

You can also eat foods that contain the depleted nutrients:

- Calcium: milk, dried figs, Swiss cheese, yogurt, tofu
- Magnesium: Florida avocado, toasted wheat germ, almonds, shredded wheat cereal, pumpkin seeds

Consult with your physician before making any changes to your diet or supplemental regimen.

POTASSIUM CHLORIDE (poe-TASS-ee-um KLOR-ide)

Brand Names: Apo-K, Cena-K, Gen-K, K-Dur, K-Long, Kaochlor, Kaon-Cl, Kato, Micro-K

About Potassium Chloride

Potassium is an important mineral that helps maintain proper fluid levels in the body as well as the acid-base balance. It's the third most common mineral body in the body (after calcium and phosphorus).

Excessive diarrhea or vomiting, prolonged use of laxatives, the use of various drugs, and diseases such as Cushing's syndrome can deplete your body of potassium, resulting in low blood levels of this vital mineral, a condition called hypokalemia.

The symptoms of hypokalemia include muscle twitching, irregular heartbeat, nausea, vomiting, paralysis, and heart attack.

Physicians may prescribe potassium chloride to replace the missing mineral or to prevent the problem from occurring in those at risk.

Possible Side Effects

The drug's more common side effects include nausea, vomiting, stomach pain, flatulence, and diarrhea.

Which Nutrients Are Robbed

Taking this medicine may deplete your supply of, increase your need for, or interfere with the activity of:

- Vitamin B_{12}
- Magnesium

Additional Ways This Drug May Upset Your Nutritional Balance

Potassium chloride can cause nausea, vomiting, and stomach pain, all of which can upset your eating habits and possibly interfere with good nutrition. It can also cause diarrhea, which can hamper nutrient absorption.

This drug can also trigger hyperkalemia, or too much potassium in the blood.

Restoring Your Nutritional Balance

To compensate for the nutrient loss caused by this drug, speak to your physician about taking 500–1,000 mcg vitamin B_{12} and 500–1,000 mg magnesium per day.

You can also eat foods that contain the depleted nutrients:

- Vitamin B_{12}: beef liver, rainbow trout, sockeye salmon, beef, haddock
- Magnesium: Florida avocado, toasted wheat germ, almonds, shredded wheat cereal, pumpkin seeds

Consult with your physician before making any changes to your diet or supplemental regimen.

PRAVASTATIN (PRAH-vuh-stat-in)

Brand Name: Pravachol

About Pravastatin

Many of us are familiar with the statin drugs used to lower cholesterol. One of these is pravastatin, popularly known by the brand name Pravachol.

To physicians, the statins are known as HMG-CoA reductase inhibitors, so-named because they interfere with the creation of cholesterol at a point that requires the enzyme HMG-CoA reductase. The statin drugs inhibit the action of this enzyme, derailing the process and reducing the amount of cholesterol in the body.

Unfortunately, this same enzyme is also needed for the production of coenzyme Q_{10} (or CoQ_{10}, for short). CoQ_{10} is a naturally occurring enzyme required for the production of cellular energy. Heart cells are particularly dependent on CoQ_{10} since they are rich in mitochondria—tiny cellular energy factories—which need good amounts of the coenzyme to function properly. In Japan, CoQ_{10} is used to treat congestive heart failure.

Ironically, pravastatin and the other statin drugs used to prevent or treat heart disease may actually contribute to heart problems by reducing the levels of CoQ_{10} in the body—particularly in the heart. During the course of many months of treatment with statins, CoQ_{10} levels fall, and you may begin to experience fatigue, muscle weakness, and other problems—including, possibly, heart failure. Some physicians call this problem statin cardiomyopathy, or heart failure caused by statin-induced loss of CoQ_{10}. One strategy for avoiding this is to take CoQ_{10} supplements along with your statin drug.

Pravastatin is used to treat elevated cholesterol and blood fats, as well as to prevent heart attacks in certain patients.

Possible Side Effects

The drug's more common side effects include nausea, vomiting, diarrhea, chest pain, and fatigue.

Which Nutrients Are Robbed

Taking this medicine may deplete your supply of, increase your need for, or interfere with the activity of:

- Coenzyme Q_{10}

Additional Ways This Drug May Upset Your Nutritional Balance

Pravastatin can cause heartburn, nausea, and vomiting, all of which can upset your eating habits and possibly interfere with good nutrition. It can also cause diarrhea, which can hamper nutrient absorption.

This drug may cause blood levels of vitamin A to rise.

Restoring Your Nutritional Balance

To compensate for the nutrient loss caused by this drug, speak to your physician about taking 30–100 mg coenzyme Q_{10} per day.

You can also eat foods that contain the depleted nutrient:

- Coenzyme Q_{10}: beef, chicken, trout, salmon, oranges, broccoli

Consult with your physician before making any changes to your diet or supplemental regimen.

PRAZOSIN PLUS POLYTHIAZIDE (PRAH-zoe-sin, pol-ee-THYE-uh-zide)

Brand Name: Minizide

About Prazosin plus Polythiazide

Imagine a grown man trying to wedge himself through a doggy door. It's a tight squeeze, so there's a lot of pressure where his belly meets the edges of the opening. But if you could magically make the door opening a little wider, the pressure would drop and he could move on through more easily.

Something similar happens with your blood pressure. It goes up when the blood vessels narrow, making it harder for the blood to flow through. But if you could widen them, the blood would slip through more easily and blood pressure would fall.

Prazosin lowers elevated blood pressure by blocking what are called alpha-1 receptors in the smaller arteries and veins, forcing these blood vessels to open wider. This reduces their resistance to the flow of blood, and pressure drops.

Prazosin can be used either alone or in conjunction with other drugs, such as the diuretic polythiazide, which increases the output of urine, thereby reducing the amount of fluid in the blood. Less fluid means a lower volume of blood, which reduces the heart's workload and allows it to relax a bit.

The combination of prazosin plus polythiazide is used to treat mildly to moderately elevated blood pressure.

Possible Side Effects

The more common side effects of prazosin include dizziness, headache, drowsiness, and weakness. Side effects seen with polythiazide include elevated total cholesterol and LDL "bad" cholesterol, weakness, and fatigue.

Which Nutrients Are Robbed

Taking this medicine may deplete your supply of, increase your need for, or interfere with the activity of:

- Magnesium
- Phosphorus
- Potassium
- Sodium
- Zinc
- Coenzyme Q_{10}

Additional Ways This Drug May Upset Your Nutritional Balance

Prazosin can cause nausea and vomiting, which can upset your eating habits and possibly interfere with good nutrition. It can also cause diarrhea, which can hamper nutrient absorption.

Restoring Your Nutritional Balance

To compensate for the nutrient loss caused by this drug, speak to your physician about taking 500–1,000 mg magnesium, 700 mg phosphorus, 50–200 mg zinc, and 30–100 mg coenzyme Q_{10} per day. And ask your physician to consider the effects of sodium depletion.

A Note on Potassium: "Regular" diuretics lower potassium levels, while potassium-sparing diuretics do not—they may increase levels instead. It is not uncommon for doctors to prescribe two different diuretics. That's why you should speak to your physician about your potassium levels, and whether it is appropriate for you to take supplements or eat potassium-rich foods.

You can also eat foods that contain the depleted nutrients:

- Magnesium: Florida avocado, toasted wheat germ, almonds, shredded wheat cereal, pumpkin seeds
- Phosphorus: plain nonfat yogurt, lentils, salmon, milk, halibut
- Zinc: oysters, beef shank, chicken, pork tenderloin, plain yogurt
- Coenzyme Q_{10}: beef, chicken, trout, salmon, oranges, broccoli

Consult with your physician before making any changes to your diet or supplemental regimen.

PREDNISOLONE (pred-NISS-oh-lohn)

Brand Names: Delta-Cortef, Key-Pred, Predalone-50, Predate S, Pediapred, Prelone

About Prednisolone

Many people think that the eyelid is just a single layer of tissue designed to cover and protect the eye. It does protect, but it's made of more than one layer. On the inside of the eyelid is a lining called the conjunctiva, which helps to protect the eye from microorganisms and small objects like a piece of sand. But the conjunctiva can easily become inflamed due to allergies, bacteria, or even too much sunlight, causing a common condition called conjunctivitis. Many cases of conjunctivitis are self-limiting; that is, they clear up on their own. But sometimes the body needs help, perhaps because chronic irritation or dryness of the eye keeps the problem alive.

Prednisolone, which has anti-inflammatory properties, is used to treat certain cases of conjunctivitis, as well as injuries to the cornea. It's also used for a variety of inflammatory diseases involving the skin, collagen, joints, and glands.

Possible Side Effects

The drug's more common side effects include insomnia, nervousness, indigestion, and increased appetite.

Which Nutrients Are Robbed

Taking this medicine may deplete your supply of, increase your need for, or interfere with the activity of:

- Vitamin A
- Vitamin B_6
- Folic acid
- Vitamin C
- Vitamin D
- Vitamin K
- Calcium
- Magnesium
- Phosphorus
- Potassium
- Selenium
- Zinc

Additional Ways This Drug May Upset Your Nutritional Balance

Prednisolone can cause indigestion, which can upset your eating habits and possibly interfere with good nutrition.

Restoring Your Nutritional Balance

To compensate for the nutrient loss caused by this drug, speak to your physician about taking 5,000 IU vitamin A, 50–100 mg vitamin B_6, 400–800 mcg folic acid, 250–1,500 mg vitamin C, 400 IU vitamin D, 60–80 mcg vitamin K, 1,200 mg calcium, 500–1,000 mg magnesium, 700 mg phosphorus, 100–300 mg potassium, 20–100 mcg selenium, and 50–200 mg zinc per day.

You can also eat foods that contain the depleted nutrients:

- Vitamin A: beef liver, chicken liver, cheese pizza, whole milk, cheddar cheese
- Vitamin B_6: potato, banana, garbanzo beans, chicken breast, fortified oatmeal

- Folic acid: beef liver, fortified breakfast cereals, spinach, great northern beans, asparagus
- Vitamin C: papaya, guava, red pepper, cantaloupe, black currants
- Vitamin D: salmon, mackerel, sardines, eel, fortified milk
- Vitamin K: kale, broccoli, parsley, Swiss chard, spinach
- Calcium: milk, dried figs, Swiss cheese, yogurt, tofu
- Magnesium: Florida avocado, toasted wheat germ, almonds, shredded wheat cereal, pumpkin seeds
- Phosphorus: plain nonfat yogurt, lentils, salmon, milk, halibut
- Potassium: dried figs, California avocado, papaya, banana, dates
- Selenium: Brazil nuts, tuna, beef liver, turkey breast, spaghetti with meat sauce
- Zinc: oysters, beef shank, chicken, pork tenderloin, plain yogurt

Consult with your physician before making any changes to your diet or supplemental regimen.

PREDNISONE (PRED-ni-sohn)

Brand Names: Apo-Prednisone, Cordrol, Deltasone, Liquid Pred, Meticorten, Orasone, Prednicen-M, Prednisone, Winpred

About Prednisone

Inflammation, a complex process involving cytokines, macrophages, monocytes, T-cells, B-cells, and other immune system "soldiers," is one of the body's chief weapons for fighting off bacteria and other invaders. But sometimes inflammation can be harmful, particularly if it is triggered unnecessarily, goes on too long, or seriously damages body tissues. Such is the case in autoimmune diseases like rheumatoid arthritis, when the body mistakenly sets off the inflammation process and attacks itself.

Prednisone is one of the glucocorticoids, a group of drugs used to treat diseases in which inflammation is a problem. It puts a damper on inflammation in several ways, including:

- "Muzzling" the cytokines, chemokines, and other substances that call the immune system cells into battle
- Decreasing the amounts of T-cells, B-cells, and other immune system soldiers in the blood

- Calming the macrophages, the giant cells that literally engulf invaders

All in all, prednisone is a powerful anti-inflammatory. The medicine is an effective treatment for a variety of diseases, including allergic contact dermatitis, which arises when the skin comes in contact with chemicals or other substances (such as perfume, soap, or detergent) that trigger an allergic reaction. The skin becomes red, inflamed, and swollen and may ooze and become crusty. If the skin breaks open, germs can enter the body and trigger a secondary infection. Prednisone is used in severe cases of allergic contact dermatitis to turn off the inflammation so that the area can heal.

Prednisone is prescribed for inflammatory ailments of the skin, eye, respiratory tract, gastrointestinal tract, and other areas of the body. The drug may also be used in organ transplants to prevent the body from rejecting the new part, or when the adrenal glands aren't producing enough hormones.

Possible Side Effects

The drug's more common side effects include insomnia, nervousness, indigestion, and increased appetite.

Which Nutrients Are Robbed

Taking this medicine may deplete your supply of, increase your need for, or interfere with the activity of:

- Vitamin A
- Vitamin B_6
- Folic acid
- Vitamin C
- Vitamin D
- Vitamin K
- Calcium
- Magnesium
- Potassium
- Selenium
- Zinc

Additional Ways This Drug May Upset Your Nutritional Balance

Prednisone can cause indigestion, which can upset your eating habits and possibly interfere with good nutrition.

Restoring Your Nutritional Balance

To compensate for the nutrient loss caused by this drug, speak to your physician about taking 5,000 IU vitamin A, 50–100 mg vitamin B_6, 400–800 mcg folic acid, 250–1,500 mg vitamin C, 400 IU vitamin D, 60–80 mcg vitamin K, 1,200 mg calcium, 500–1,000 mg magnesium, 100–300 mg potassium, 20–100 mcg selenium, and 50–200 mg zinc per day.

You can also eat foods that contain the depleted nutrients:

- Vitamin A: beef liver, chicken liver, cheese pizza, whole milk, cheddar cheese
- Vitamin B_6: potato, banana, garbanzo beans, chicken breast, fortified oatmeal
- Folic acid: beef liver, fortified breakfast cereals, spinach, great northern beans, asparagus
- Vitamin C: papaya, guava, red pepper, cantaloupe, black currants
- Vitamin D: salmon, mackerel, sardines, eel, fortified milk
- Vitamin K: kale, broccoli, parsley, Swiss chard, spinach
- Calcium: milk, dried figs, Swiss cheese, yogurt, tofu
- Magnesium: Florida avocado, toasted wheat germ, almonds, shredded wheat cereal, pumpkin seeds
- Potassium: dried figs, California avocado, papaya, banana, dates
- Selenium: Brazil nuts, tuna, beef liver, turkey breast, spaghetti with meat sauce
- Zinc: oysters, beef shank, chicken, pork tenderloin, plain yogurt

Consult with your physician before making any changes to your diet or supplemental regimen.

PRIMIDONE (PRI-mi-dohn)

Brand Names: Apo-Primidone, Myidone, Mysoline, Sertan

About Primidone

The brain is a very complex, remarkably orderly organ with a bewildering number and variety of duties. In order for its machinery to work, brain cells (neurons) have to fire at just the right time, sending messages from one neuron to the next. But sometimes the system breaks down, and the cells fire at the wrong time. If this happens in the part of your brain that controls awareness, you may not know what's happening to you or around you. If it happens in the part of your brain responsible for the muscle movement in your right leg, that leg may jerk uncontrollably. The more parts of your brain affected by the uncontrolled firing of the neurons, the more symptoms you'll experience.

Doctors call the uncontrolled firing of brain cells and the resulting symptoms a seizure. Many things can cause a seizure, including infections, rabies, syphilis, elevated levels of sodium or sugar in the blood, kidney failure, head injuries, an overdose of cocaine, a brain tumor, a stroke, and various prescription drugs.

Primidone is one of the drugs used to treat seizures. We don't know exactly how it works, but it's been used for about 50 years to treat people suffering from the generalized seizures that attack both halves of the brain. It is also used to treat partial seizures (those that involve just one side of the brain).

Possible Side Effects

The drug's side effects include drowsiness, lethargy, fatigue, and impotence.

Which Nutrients Are Robbed

Taking this medicine may deplete your supply of, increase your need for, or interfere with the activity of:

- Biotin
- Folic acid
- Vitamin B_6
- Vitamin B_{12}
- Vitamin D
- Vitamin K
- Calcium
- Carnitine

Additional Ways This Drug May Upset Your Nutritional Balance

Primidone can cause loss of appetite, nausea, and vomiting, all of which can upset your eating habits and possibly interfere with good nutrition.

Restoring Your Nutritional Balance

To compensate for the nutrient loss caused by this drug, speak to your physician about taking 500–1,000 mcg biotin, 50–100 mg vitamin B_6, 500–1,000 mcg vitamin B_{12}, 400 IU vitamin D, 60–80 mcg vitamin K, 1,200 mg calcium, and 250–1,000 mg carnitine per day. Taking folic acid can increase the risk of seizures in some people, so speak to your physician about the use of this nutrient.

You can also eat foods that contain the depleted nutrients:

- Biotin: beef liver, soybeans, rice bran, peanut butter, barley
- Vitamin B_6: potato, banana, garbanzo beans, chicken breast, fortified oatmeal
- Vitamin B_{12}: beef liver, rainbow trout, sockeye salmon, beef, haddock
- Vitamin D: salmon, mackerel, sardines, eel, fortified milk
- Vitamin K: kale, broccoli, parsley, Swiss chard, spinach

- Calcium: milk, dried figs, Swiss cheese, yogurt, tofu
- Carnitine: ground beef, pork, Canadian bacon, whole milk, cod

Consult with your physician before making any changes to your diet or supplemental regimen.

PROCHLORPERAZINE (proe-klor-PAIR-uh-zeen)

Brand Names: Compazine, Nu-Prochlor, PMS-Prochlorperazine, Prorazin, Stemetil

About Prochlorperazine

Nausea and vomiting can strike anyone, particularly those who are taking certain drugs; are pregnant; are suffering from ulcers or gastrointestinal obstructions; have migraines or hepatitis; or are undergoing chemotherapy. In fact, some people on chemotherapy start feeling nauseous even before they get their medicine, because they know what's coming. Emesis is the medical term for vomiting, but when you're in the middle of it, you don't care.

Although the physiologic processes that stir the nausea-vomiting process are still something of a mystery, it appears that the neurotransmitters serotonin and dopamine play important roles. Prochlorperazine helps to quell the urge to vomit by interfering with dopamine receptors in the brain. The drug is also used to treat anxiety.

Possible Side Effects

The drug's side effects include dizziness, heart attack, insomnia, and tremor.

Which Nutrients Are Robbed

Taking this medicine may deplete your supply of, increase your need for, or interfere with the activity of:

- Riboflavin
- Coenzyme Q_{10}

Additional Ways This Drug May Upset Your Nutritional Balance

Prochlorperazine can cause low blood sugar (hypoglycemia), loss of appetite, stomach pain, nausea, and vomiting, all of which can upset your eating habits and possibly interfere with good nutrition. It can also cause diarrhea, which can hamper nutrient absorption.

Restoring Your Nutritional Balance

To compensate for the nutrient loss caused by this drug, speak to your physician about taking 25–100 mg riboflavin and 30–100 mg coenzyme Q_{10} per day.

You can also eat foods that contain the depleted nutrients:

- Riboflavin: dried sunflower seeds, orange juice, bulgur, spinach noodles, pine nuts
- Coenzyme Q_{10}: beef, chicken, trout, salmon, oranges, broccoli

Consult with your physician before making any changes to your diet or supplemental regimen.

PROMETHAZINE (proe-METH-uh-zeen)

Brand Names: Anergan, Histantil, Phenazine, Phenergan, Prorex

About Promethazine

Promethazine is a multitalented medicine that can help:

- Relieve the symptoms of various allergies
- Ease motion sickness
- Treat nausea and vomiting
- Serve as an adjunct to anesthesia
- Relieve postsurgical pain

It can perform these diverse duties because it has several actions within the body, including interfering with the action of histamine, which plays a key role in allergies.

Possible Side Effects

The drug's side effects include drowsiness, seizures, lactation, and impotence.

Which Nutrients Are Robbed

Taking this medicine may deplete your supply of, increase your need for, or interfere with the activity of:

- Riboflavin
- Coenzyme Q_{10}

Additional Ways This Drug May Upset Your Nutritional Balance

Promethazine can cause low blood sugar (hypoglycemia) and nausea, which can upset your eating habits and possibly interfere with good nutrition.

Restoring Your Nutritional Balance

To compensate for the nutrient loss caused by this drug, speak to your physician about taking 25–100 mg riboflavin and 30–100 mg coenzyme Q_{10} per day.

You can also eat foods that contain the depleted nutrients:

- Riboflavin: dried sunflower seeds, orange juice, bulgur, spinach noodles, pine nuts
- Coenzyme Q_{10}: beef, chicken, trout, salmon, oranges, broccoli

Consult with your physician before making any changes to your diet or supplemental regimen.

PROPAFENONE (proe-pah-FEEN-ohn)

Brand Name: Rythmol

About Propafenone

Your heart runs on electricity: It won't pump unless an electrical current originating in your heart's pacemaker jolts it into action. This current races through your heart in a prescribed manner that makes the two atria (smaller upper chambers) and ventricles (larger lower chambers) contract in a coordinated rhythm.

But all too often, something goes wrong with the flow of electricity. It may be that the pacemaker fires too often, creating an overly rapid heart rate, or it may not fire often enough. Perhaps one part of the heart contracts rapidly, while another works at a more leisurely pace. Or it may be that one part of the heart contracts before the electrical current reaches it, because it's generating its own electrical current.

Propafenone is used to regulate the heart rate by slowing the conduction of electricity and increasing the resting period between beats, among other things. This makes propafenone useful for treating atrial fibrillation. When atrial fibrillation strikes, the two atria contract so rapidly that their walls quiver, and the chambers do not empty completely. The ventricles may begin to beat irregularly and out of synch with the atria. The net result is that blood is poorly pumped throughout the body, blood pressure falls, and the heart may fail. Another problem with atrial fibrillation is that blood may sit too long in the atrium and begin to clot. If a clot escapes the heart and moves into the brain, you may suffer a stroke.

Possible Side Effects

The drug's more common side effects include dizziness, fatigue, the worsening of irregular heartbeats, and the creation of new ones.

Which Nutrients Are Robbed

Taking this medicine may deplete your supply of, increase your need for, or interfere with the activity of:

- Coenzyme Q_{10}

Additional Ways This Drug May Upset Your Nutritional Balance

Propafenone can cause nausea, vomiting, changes in taste, abdominal pain, and loss of appetite, all of which can upset your eating habits and possibly interfere with good nutrition. It can also cause diarrhea, which can hamper nutrient absorption.

Restoring Your Nutritional Balance

To compensate for the nutrient loss caused by this drug, speak to your physician about taking 30–100 mg coenzyme Q_{10} per day.

You can also eat foods that contain the depleted nutrient:

- Coenzyme Q_{10}: beef, chicken, trout, salmon, oranges, broccoli

Consult with your physician before making any changes to your diet or supplemental regimen.

PROPOXYPHENE PLUS ACETAMINOPHEN (pro-POKS-i-feen, uh-seet-uh-MIN-oh-fen)

Brand Names: Darvocet-N, Darvocet-N 100, E-Lor, Propacet, Wygesic

About Propoxyphene plus Acetaminophen

Pain can be aching, agonizing, burning, crushing, grinding, nauseating, numbing, piercing, pounding, pulsing, racking, ripping, sharp, shooting, stabbing, and throbbing. And those are just a few of the words we use to describe it.

Pain is a big problem. The American Pain Foundation reports that "over 50 million Americans suffer from chronic pain" and an additional 25 million develop acute pain following surgery or injuries. The American Pain Society agrees that 50 million Americans suffer from chronic pain, and counts 25 million more who suffer from "moderate-to-severe pain," plus another 8 million who suffer with cancer pain.[5]

With all this pain, it's no wonder that our national medicine chest contains a variety of painkillers, from aspirin to morphine.

Propoxyphene is one of those painkillers. A chemical cousin of methadone, it's a narcotic painkiller that acts on the central nervous system to alter the perception of pain. Used for mild to moderate pain, propoxyphene is often combined with other painkillers, such as acetaminophen, which slows production of the prostaglandins that encourage pain. (For more on acetaminophen, see the entry on page 90.) The combination of propoxyphene and acetaminophen is used to treat mild to moderate pain.

Possible Side Effects

Propoxyphene's side effects include low blood pressure, dizziness, sedation, and rash. Acetaminophen's side effects include liver and kidney damage.

Which Nutrients Are Robbed

Taking this combination of medicines may deplete your supply of, increase your need for, or interfere with the activity of:

- Glutathione

Additional Ways This Drug May Upset Your Nutritional Balance

Propoxyphene can cause loss of appetite, nausea, vomiting, and stomach cramps, all of which can upset your eating habits and possibly interfere with good nutrition.

Restoring Your Nutritional Balance

To compensate for the nutrient loss caused by this drug, speak to your physician about taking 800–2,000 mg n-acetyl cysteine (a precursor to glutathione) per day.

Consult with your physician before making any changes to your diet or supplemental regimen.

PROPRANOLOL (proe-PRAN-oh-lole)

Brand Names: Apo-Propranolol, Betachron E-R Capsule, Detensol, Inderal, Inderal LA, Nu-Propranolol

About Propranolol

A staple in the physician's little black bag for many years, propranolol is used to treat a variety of heart and blood pressure problems, including the very common problem of mildly to moderately elevated blood pressure. In case of severe hypertension, it is used to slow the overly rapid heartbeat that may be caused by other hypertension medicines. Propranolol is also used to combat migraine headaches, angina, and certain tremors and may be useful in treating anxiety and panic.

Propranolol is a beta-blocker, which means that it blocks off beta-receptors in the heart and elsewhere. You can think of these receptors as tiny mailboxes. Normally, your brain sends messages to your heart that tell it to beat faster and harder. But sometimes it sends too many. If you have elevated blood pressure, you'd like to stop receiving some of these messages so your heart could beat more slowly and your blood pressure could fall. Propranolol jams itself into the mailboxes in your heart, so that letters telling it to work harder don't get delivered. Thus, the heart relaxes a bit, and elevated blood pressure falls.

Possible Side Effects

The drug's side effects include irregular heartbeat, chest pain, low blood pressure, weakness, vertigo, and fainting.

Which Nutrients Are Robbed

Taking this medicine may deplete your supply of, increase your need for, or interfere with the activity of:

- Coenzyme Q_{10}
- Melatonin

Additional Ways This Drug May Upset Your Nutritional Balance

Propranolol can cause low blood sugar (hypoglycemia), loss of appetite, stomach discomfort, nausea, and vomiting, all of which can upset your eating habits and possibly interfere with good nutrition.

This drug can also trigger hyperkalemia, or too much potassium in the blood.

Restoring Your Nutritional Balance

To compensate for the nutrient loss caused by this drug, speak to your physician about taking 30–100 mg coenzyme Q_{10} and 1–3 mg melatonin per day.

You can also eat foods that contain the depleted nutrient:

- Coenzyme Q_{10}: beef, chicken, trout, salmon, oranges, broccoli

Consult with your physician before making any changes to your diet or supplemental regimen.

PROPRANOLOL PLUS HYDROCHLOROTHIAZIDE

(proe-PRAN-oh-lole, hye-droe-klor-oh-THYE-uh-zide)

Brand Name: Inderide

About Propranolol plus Hydrochlorothiazide

Propranolol plus hydrochlorothiazide is a "one-two" punch that doctors use to knock out hypertension.

Propranolol is a beta-blocker that prevents the brain's "beat harder" messages from getting through to the heart. This allows the heart to relax a bit.

Hydrochlorothiazide is a diuretic that instructs the kidneys to skim more water out of the bloodstream and get rid of it via the urine. This reduces the amount of fluid in the bloodstream, which means there's less for the heart to pump.

Allowing the heart to relax a little and lightening its workload lowers blood pressure. (For more information, see the drugs' individual entries on pages 461 and 304.)

Possible Side Effects

The side effects seen with propranolol plus hydrochlorothiazide include irregular heartbeat, chest pain, low blood pressure, weakness, vertigo, and fainting. The side effects of hydrochlorothiazide include low blood pressure, photosensitivity, and allergic reactions.

Which Nutrients Are Robbed

Taking this medicine may deplete your supply of, increase your need for, or interfere with the activity of:

- Magnesium
- Phosphorus
- Potassium
- Sodium
- Zinc
- Coenzyme Q_{10}

Additional Ways This Drug May Upset Your Nutritional Balance

Propranolol can cause low blood sugar (hypoglycemia), loss of appetite, stomach discomfort, nausea, and vomiting, while hydrochlorothiazide can cause loss of appetite. These side effects can upset your eating habits and possibly interfere with good nutrition.

Propranolol can also trigger hyperkalemia, or too much potassium in the blood.

Restoring Your Nutritional Balance

To compensate for the nutrient loss caused by this drug, speak to your physician about taking 500-1,000 mg magnesium, 700 mg phosphorus, 50–200 mg zinc, and 30–100 mg coenzyme Q_{10} per day. And ask your physician to consider the potential effects of sodium depletion.

A Note on Potassium: "Regular" diuretics lower potassium levels, while potassium-sparing diuretics do not—they may increase levels instead. It is not uncommon for doctors to prescribe two different diuretics. That's why you should speak to your physician about your potassium levels, and whether it is appropriate for you to take supplements or eat potassium-rich foods.

You can also eat foods that contain the depleted nutrients:

- Magnesium: Florida avocado, toasted wheat germ, almonds, shredded wheat cereal, pumpkin seeds
- Phosphorus: plain nonfat yogurt, lentils, salmon, milk, halibut
- Zinc: oysters, beef shank, chicken, pork tenderloin, plain yogurt
- Coenzyme Q_{10}: beef, chicken, trout, salmon, oranges, broccoli

Consult with your physician before making any changes to your diet or supplemental regimen.

PROTRIPTYLINE (proe-TRIP-ti-leen)

Brand Names: Triptil, Vivactil

About Protriptyline

If you were to freeze time right now and go around the country observing everybody's mood, you'd find that 5 to 6 percent of Americans are depressed. That's somewhere between 14 and 16.8 million of us who feel intensely sad, often for no obvious reason.

We have all suffered (or will suffer) from the reactive or situational depression that strikes when a loved one dies, a job is lost, a marriage fails, and so on. This depression is a very normal response to the difficulties of life, and with time the depression fades away.

The more difficult problem is the melancholia, or endogenous depression, that isn't a typical response to life's problems. It may be caused by or related to hormonal changes, certain drugs, brain tumors, a stroke, or a lack of vitamin B_6 or B_{12}. A disease such as AIDS can cause depression directly by damaging the brain or indirectly by making the person fear for his or her health and future.

Many times, a depressive episode will clear up on its own in six months or so, although in some cases the problem may persist for a couple of years. Protriptyline is one of the drugs used to treat depression. It's classified as a tricyclic antidepressant, an older group of drugs that became less popular when newer drugs like Prozac were introduced. Protriptyline works at the synapses in the nervous system, those gaps between cells where neurotransmitters shuttle back and forth to keep messages flowing to and from the brain. Specifically, it slows the reabsorption of serotonin and perhaps other neurotransmitters, ensuring that there are more of them available to keep their "everything-is-OK" message flowing.

Possible Side Effects

Protriptyline's side effects include irregular heartbeat, heart attack, stroke, and breast enlargement.

Which Nutrients Are Robbed

Taking this medicine may deplete your supply of, increase your need for, or interfere with the activity of:

- Riboflavin
- Coenzyme Q_{10}
- Sodium

Additional Ways This Drug May Upset Your Nutritional Balance

Protriptyline can cause changes in taste, nausea, vomiting, heartburn, loss of appetite and gum problems, all of which can upset your eating habits and possibly interfere with good nutrition. It can also cause diarrhea, which can hamper nutrient absorption.

Restoring Your Nutritional Balance

To compensate for the nutrient loss caused by this drug, speak to your physician about taking 25–100 mg riboflavin and 30–100 mg coenzyme Q_{10} per day. And ask your physician to consider the potential effects of sodium depletion.

You can also eat foods that contain the depleted nutrients:

- Riboflavin: dried sunflower seeds, orange juice, bulgur, spinach noodles, pine nuts
- Coenzyme Q_{10}: beef, chicken, trout, salmon, oranges, broccoli

Consult with your physician before making any changes to your diet or supplemental regimen.

PSEUDOEPHEDRINE PLUS IBUPROFEN (soo-doe-e-FED-rin, eye-byoo-PRO-fen)

Brand Names: Advil Cold & Sinus Caplets, Dimetapp Sinus Caplets, Dristan Sinus Caplets, Motrin IB Sinus, Sine-Aid IB

About Pseudoephedrine plus Ibuprofen

Being cold does not give you a cold, and having a cold does not make you cold: The common cold has little to do with cold temperatures.

Colds are caused by viruses, and the rhinovirus is the usual suspect. This virus leaves an infected body via the nasal secretions, typically by hitching a ride on the individual's hands, which pass it the next victim's hands. When the second victim touches his or her own nose, mouth, or eyes, the rhinovirus moves right in.

We're all very familiar with the symptoms of a cold, which can include a sore throat, runny nose, sneezing, and general feeling of being under the weather. Without treatment, it normally takes anywhere from several days to three weeks for a cold to disappear.

Pseudoephedrine plus ibuprofen may be given to relieve some of the symptoms of a cold. Pseudoephedrine is a decongestant that helps improve breathing by constricting the blood vessels in the mucosa of the respiratory tract and relaxing the bronchial (breathing) tubes. These two actions allow air to flow in and out more freely. Ibuprofen helps reduce inflammation and relieve pain.

Possible Side Effects

Pseudoephedrine's side effects include rapid heartbeat, irregular heartbeat, weakness, and tremor. Ibuprofen's side effects include headache, fluid retention, rash, and kidney failure.

Which Nutrients Are Robbed

Taking this combination of medicines may deplete your supply of, increase your need for, or interfere with the activity of:

• Folic acid

Additional Ways This Drug May Upset Your Nutritional Balance

Pseudoephedrine can cause nausea and vomiting, while ibuprofen can cause nausea, vomiting, peptic ulcer, heartburn, and indigestion. These side effects can upset your eating habits and possibly interfere with good nutrition.

Restoring Your Nutritional Balance

To compensate for the nutrient loss caused by this drug, speak to your physician about taking 400–800 mcg folic acid per day.

You can also eat foods that contain the depleted nutrient:

• Folic acid: beef liver, fortified breakfast cereals, spinach, great northern beans, asparagus

Consult with your physician before making any changes to your diet or supplemental regimen.

QUINAPRIL (KWIN-uh-pril)

Brand Name: Accupril

About Quinapril

Heart failure, the potentially fatal inability of the heart to pump enough blood to meet the body's demands, afflicts some 5 million Americans. Although it's not surprising that heart failure makes you tired, you might not know that when your heart fails, you can become waterlogged. That's because when the heart isn't pumping blood as powerfully and efficiently as it should, the body attempts to compensate in various ways. One of these ways is to have the kidneys hold on to sodium, which makes the body retain water. This extra water gives more volume to the blood, which helps the heart perform better. But over time, this extra fluid begins to seep out of the blood vessels and pool in various places in the body.

Just where the extra fluid goes is determined by which half of the heart is failing. If the right side of the heart is weak, the fluid will accumulate and cause swelling in the feet, ankles, legs or abdomen. If the left side is weak, the fluid will gather in the lungs (pulmonary edema), causing shortness of breath.

To combat the fluid buildup and other symptoms of heart failure, doctors may prescribe quinapril, which helps in two ways. First, it reduces the tired heart's workload by causing the blood vessels to relax and open wider, making it easier for the heart to pump blood through them. Second, the drug encourages the body to rid itself of excess fluid.

Quinapril is used to treat heart failure, as well as elevated blood pressure.

Possible Side Effects

The drug's more common side effects include cough, dizziness, muscle pain, low blood pressure, and headache.

Which Nutrients Are Robbed

Taking this medicine may deplete your supply of, increase your need for, or interfere with the activity of:

- Zinc

Additional Ways This Drug May Upset Your Nutritional Balance

Quinapril can cause nausea and vomiting, which can upset your eating habits and possibly interfere with good nutrition. It can also cause diarrhea, which can hamper nutrient absorption.

This drug can also trigger hyperkalemia, or too much potassium in the blood.

Restoring Your Nutritional Balance

To compensate for the nutrient loss caused by this drug, speak to your physician about taking 50–200 mg zinc per day.

You can also eat foods that contain the depleted nutrient:

- Zinc: oysters, beef shank, chicken, pork tenderloin, plain yogurt

Consult with your physician before making any changes to your diet or supplemental regimen.

RABEPRAZOLE (rah-BEP-ruh-zole)

Brand Name: Aciphex

About Rabeprazole

Scattered throughout the lining of your stomach are numerous "biochemical pumps," called parietal cell proton pumps, which produce stomach acid. When you have a duodenal or gastric ulcer, heartburn, or gastroesophageal reflux disease, you may want to reduce the level of acid in your stomach and give things a chance to heal.

One approach is to slow down the action of the acid pumps by using medicines called proton pump inhibitors. Rabeprazole is a proton pump inhibitor that can bind to the pumps and drastically reduce the amount of acid they produce. It works well, reducing acid secretion by 90 percent or more over a 24-hour period. If taken every day for four weeks, it will lead to a 90 percent healing of the ulcers in an area of the small intestine called the duodenum, and if taken for eight weeks will lead to a 90 percent healing of stomach ulcers.

Possible Side Effects

The drug's side effects include headache, asthma, jaundice, and rapid heartbeat.

Which Nutrients Are Robbed

Taking this medicine may deplete your supply of, increase your need for, or interfere with the activity of:

- Beta-carotene
- Iron
- Folic acid
- Zinc
- Vitamin B$_{12}$

Restoring Your Nutritional Balance

To compensate for the nutrient loss caused by this drug, speak to your physician about taking 25,000 IU beta-carotene, 400–800 mcg folic acid, 500–1,000 mcg vitamin B$_{12}$, and 50–200 mg zinc per day. And ask your physician to consider the potential effects of iron depletion.

You can also eat foods that contain the depleted nutrients:

- Beta-carotene: carrot, spinach, mango, cantaloupe, apricot nectar
- Folic acid: beef liver, fortified breakfast cereals, spinach, great northern beans, asparagus
- Vitamin B$_{12}$: beef liver, rainbow trout, sockeye salmon, beef, haddock
- Zinc: oysters, beef shank, chicken, pork tenderloin, plain yogurt

Consult with your physician before making any changes to your diet or supplemental regimen.

RALOXIFENE (ral-OKS-i-feen)

Brand Name: Evista

About Raloxifene

Some 8 million American women (and 2 million men) have osteoporosis, the thinning of the bones that makes them much more susceptible to fracture. The dramatic decrease in bone density seen in postmenopausal women indicates that decreased estrogen is an important factor in bone loss. But race is also a factor, with white and Asian women at greater risk of developing osteoporosis than Hispanic or African American women. And thinner women are more at risk than their heavier counterparts for two reasons: Their bones tend to be thinner to begin with, and because they have less body fat, they tend to produce less estrogen.

Osteoporosis may produce no symptoms at all. The first sign that something is wrong could be the wrist that unexpectedly snaps or a collapsing vertebra that causes back pain.

Until recently, estrogen replacement therapy was used as a preventive measure against osteoporosis, but new studies have highlighted the dangers associated with taking hormones, especially over the long term. Raloxifene is an estrogen agonist, which means that it plugs into estrogen receptors and triggers a little bit of estrogen activity—not the full dose. And it only plugs into certain estrogen receptors, such as those affecting the bones and cholesterol levels, which limits its actions even more. The net result is that the drug helps to prevent bone loss and improve cholesterol levels without encouraging breast or uterine cancer.

Possible Side Effects

The drug's more common side effects include hot flashes, muscle pain, flu syndrome, and inflammation of the sinuses.

Which Nutrients Are Robbed

Taking this medicine may deplete your supply of, increase your need for, or interfere with the activity of:

- Vitamin B_6
- Magnesium

Additional Ways This Drug May Upset Your Nutritional Balance

Raloxifene can cause loss of appetite, heartburn, abdominal discomfort, nausea, and vomiting, all of which can upset your eating habits and possibly interfere with good nutrition.

Restoring Your Nutritional Balance

To compensate for the nutrient loss caused by this drug, speak to your physician about taking 50–100 mg vitamin B_6 and 500–1,000 mg magnesium per day.

You can also eat foods that contain the depleted nutrients:

- Vitamin B_6: potato, banana, garbanzo beans, chicken breast, fortified oatmeal
- Magnesium: Florida avocado, toasted wheat germ, almonds, shredded wheat cereal, pumpkin seeds

Consult with your physician before making any changes to your diet or supplemental regimen.

RAMIPRIL (ra-MI-pril)

Brand Name: Altace

About Ramipril

A study published in 2003 in the American Heart Association's journal, *Circulation*, reported that ramipril reduces high-risk patients' chances of developing heart failure.[6] Heart failure—the inability of the heart to pump enough blood throughout the body—is a major health problem that afflicts some 5 million Americans. When you think of heart failure, imagine a CD player with dying batteries struggling to keep the disc spinning.

Doctors used to focus on trying to get the failing heart to beat more energetically—they wanted to make the heart work harder. But today's treatments emphasize *reducing* the heart's workload. They do this in two ways: by reducing the amount of fluid in the blood, so there's less for the heart to pump, and by opening up the blood vessels, so the heart doesn't have to work as hard to pump blood through them.

Ramipril does both of these things, reducing the blood volume and making the blood vessels open wider. This makes it easier for the heart to do its job.

In addition to heart failure, ramipril is used to treat elevated blood pressure and to reduce the risk of heart attacks, stroke, and death in high-risk patients.

Possible Side Effects

The drug's more common side effects include low blood pressure, cough, dizziness, and headache.

Which Nutrients Are Robbed

Taking this medicine may deplete your supply of, increase your need for, or interfere with the activity of:

• Zinc

Additional Ways This Drug May Upset Your Nutritional Balance

Ramipril can cause nausea and vomiting, which can upset your eating habits and possibly interfere with good nutrition.

This drug can also trigger hyperkalemia, or too much potassium in the blood.

Restoring Your Nutritional Balance

To compensate for the nutrient loss caused by this drug, speak to your physician about taking 50–200 mg zinc per day.

You can also eat foods that contain the depleted nutrient:

• Zinc: oysters, beef shank, chicken, pork tenderloin, plain yogurt

Consult with your physician before making any changes to your diet or supplemental regimen.

RANITIDINE (rah-NI-ti-deen)

Brand Names: Apo-Rinitidine, Novo-Ranidine, Nu-Ranit, Zantac, Zantac 75

About Ranitidine

Do you remember walking around construction sites when you were a kid? Sometimes you could find little round pieces of metal about the size of a nickel that were called slugs. You probably picked up a slug and dropped it into a candy machine, just to see what happened, and it didn't work. Although it was enough like a nickel to fit into the slot, it wasn't similar enough to make the machine surrender any candy.

Ranitidine is a "biochemical slug," enough like the real thing to fit into the biochemical "slot," but not close enough to make anything happen. And in this case, that's a good thing.

Let's back up a minute to see why. Certain cells in the lining of the stomach produce very powerful acid that helps to digest food. Ordinarily this acid would eat away at the lining of the stomach, as well as the esophagus (if the stomach contents splashed back up into this "food tube") and the duodenum, the first part of the small intestines. Luckily, the stomach, duodenum, and esophagus are protected by layers of mucus. But sometimes, for various reasons, the protection breaks down. When that happens, a variety of ailments can crop up, ranging from occasional heartburn to life-threatening ulcers.

A substance called histamine stimulates the production of stomach acid by plugging itself into specific spots in the lining of the stomach called H_2-receptors. One way to slow down the production of stomach acid is to use the biochemical slug, ranitidine. This drug resembles histamine enough to fit into the H_2-receptors, but not enough to cause the production of stomach acid. Instead, ranitidine just sits there, preventing histamine from dropping into the slot and thus reducing the production of stomach acid.

Ranitidine is used to treat duodenal and gastric ulcers, gastroesophageal disease, esophagitis, and related ailments. The over-the-counter version of this medicine is used for heartburn, acid indigestion, and sour stomach.

Possible Side Effects

The drug's side effects include irregular heartbeat, hallucinations, headache, and liver failure.

Which Nutrients Are Robbed

Taking this medicine may deplete your supply of, increase your need for, or interfere with the activity of:

- Thiamin
- Folic acid
- Vitamin B_{12}
- Vitamin D
- Calcium
- Iron
- Zinc

Restoring Your Nutritional Balance

To compensate for the nutrient loss caused by this drug, speak to your physician about taking 25–100 mg thiamin, 400–800 mcg folic acid, 500–1,000 mcg vitamin B_{12}, 400 IU vitamin D, 1,200 mg calcium, and 50–200 mg zinc per day. And ask your physician to consider the potential effects of iron depletion.

You can also eat foods that contain the depleted nutrients:

- Thiamin: braised liver, turkey heart, roasted chicken, gefilte fish, sardines
- Folic acid: beef liver, fortified breakfast cereals, spinach, great northern beans, asparagus
- Vitamin B_{12}: beef liver, rainbow trout, sockeye salmon, beef, haddock
- Vitamin D: salmon, mackerel, sardines, eel, fortified milk
- Calcium: milk, dried figs, Swiss cheese, yogurt, tofu
- Zinc: oysters, beef shank, chicken, pork tenderloin, plain yogurt

Consult with your physician before making any changes to your diet or supplemental regimen.

REPAGLINIDE (re-PAG-li-nide)

Brand Name: Prandin

About Repaglinide

One of the main duties of the hormone insulin is to escort glucose from the blood into specific body cells where it's used for fuel or stored for later use. It works like a traffic cop, guiding cars off the road and into garages. Insulin usually does its job well, but its effect can be blunted or even lost in people who develop insulin resistance.

This problem can progress to type 2 diabetes, in which the insulin simply can't round up the glucose and put it where it belongs, so it remains in circulation and builds up, eventually spilling over into the urine. This excess glucose draws water along with it, causing frequent urination and intense thirst. Because the cells aren't getting their fuel, intense hunger can also be triggered. Other symptoms of type 2 diabetes include fatigue, drowsiness, blurred vision, and nausea. Over time, the excess sugar in the bloodstream damages the blood vessels, leading to atherosclerosis ("clogged arteries"), poor circulation, damage to the kidneys and retinas, and a host of other problems.

Repaglinide attacks the problem by encouraging the pancreas to produce more insulin, a solution that's comparable to sending out more traffic cops to get things under control. It's used alone or in combination with drugs such as metformin.

Possible Side Effects

The drug's more common side effects include low blood sugar (hypoglycemia), upper respiratory tract infections, and headache.

Which Nutrients Are Robbed

Taking this medicine may deplete your supply of, increase your need for, or interfere with the activity of:

- Coenzyme Q_{10}

Additional Ways This Drug May Upset Your Nutritional Balance

Repaglinide can cause low blood sugar (hypoglycemia), heartburn, nausea, and vomiting, all of which can upset your eating habits and possibly interfere with good nutrition. It can also cause diarrhea, which can hamper nutrient absorption.

Restoring Your Nutritional Balance

To compensate for the nutrient loss caused by this drug, speak to your physician about taking 30–100 mg coenzyme Q_{10} per day.

You can also eat foods that contain the depleted nutrient:

- Coenzyme Q_{10}: beef, chicken, trout, salmon, oranges, broccoli

Consult with your physician before making any changes to your diet or supplemental regimen.

RIFABUTIN (rif-uh-BYOO-tin)

Brand Name: Mycobutin

About Rifabutin

A group of germs called *Mycobacterium avium* complex (MAC) can cause an uncommon disease known as a MAC infection.

A MAC infection resembles tuberculosis (TB). Its early symptoms include coughing and spitting up mucus, and later there may be difficulty breathing and blood in the sputum. In fact, it may be difficult to tell the difference between a MAC infection and TB; laboratory examination of your sputum may be necessary to make the diagnosis.

If your immune system has been weakened by AIDS or another disease, the infection may spread to other parts of your body, causing stomach pain, diarrhea, anemia, and fever, among other problems.

Only a few drugs are effective treatments for MAC, including rifabutin, which is used to treat mycobacteria infections in those infected with HIV.

Possible Side Effects

The drug's more common side effects include rash, nausea and vomiting, and a reddish-orange discoloration of the urine, sweat, saliva, and tears.

Which Nutrients Are Robbed

Taking this medicine may deplete your supply of, increase your need for, or interfere with the activity of:

- Vitamin D

Additional Ways This Drug May Upset Your Nutritional Balance

Rifabutin can cause abdominal pain, loss of appetite, nausea, and vomiting, all of which can upset your eating habits and possibly interfere with good nutrition. It can also cause diarrhea, which can hamper nutrient absorption.

Restoring Your Nutritional Balance

To compensate for the nutrient loss caused by this drug, speak to your physician about taking 400 IU vitamin D per day.

You can also eat foods that contain the depleted nutrient:

- Vitamin D: salmon, mackerel, sardines, eel, fortified milk

Consult with your physician before making any changes to your diet or supplemental regimen.

RIFAMPIN, RIFAMPIN PLUS ISONIAZID (RIF-am-pin, eye-soe-NYE-uh-zid)

Brand Names: Rifampin: Rifadin (Injection, Oral), Rimactane, Rimactane Oral, Rofact
Rifampin plus isoniazid: Rifamate

About Rifampin, Rifampin plus Isoniazid

The immune system has different ways of defeating invading bacteria. One approach is to destroy the invaders; another is for white blood cells called macrophages to literally engulf them. The macrophages serve as cellular jailhouses, walling off the bacteria and preventing them from damaging the body.

This is what happens to many of the *Mycobacterium tuberculosis* bacteria that trigger tuberculosis (TB). At least 90 percent of the time, these imprisoned bacteria remain quietly trapped inside the macrophages. But if the immune system weakens because of advancing age, disease, the use of certain steroids, or other problems, the mycobacteria can "bust out of jail" and begin to reproduce, triggering the potentially fatal spread of TB. Depending on where the infection spreads, the symptoms can include a cough, night sweats, loss of appetite, painful urination, kidney damage, fever, headache, and, in severe cases, death.

Rifampin is one of the antibacterial drugs used to combat tuberculosis.

Unlike many other drugs, rifampin is able to get inside the macrophage to kill the trapped *Mycobacterium tuberculosis*. It can also hunt for and destroy these organisms when they're residing in lung cavities and abscesses, areas that are difficult for other drugs to reach. When it finds the TB-causing bacteria, it destroys them by interfering with their ability to make new RNA.

In addition to combating tuberculosis, rifampin may be used to treat *Haemophilus influenzae B* infection, certain staphylococcal infections, and *Legionella pneumonia*.

All tuberculosis drugs are used in combination. Doctors don't like to use one drug at a time, for that might encourage the spread of *Mycobacterium tuberculosis* strains that are resistant to any one drug. For this reason, rifampin and isoniazid are often used in combination: a one-two punch against TB. (For more on isoniazid, see the entry on page 323.)

Possible Side Effects

Rifampin's side effects include muscle and bone pain, hepatitis, dizziness, and flushing. Isoniazid's side effects include weakness, dizziness, and slurred speech.

Which Nutrients Are Robbed

Taking these medicines may deplete your supply of, increase your need for, or interfere with the activity of:

> Rifamin: vitamin D, calcium
> Rifampin plus isoniazid: niacin, vitamin B_6, vitamin D, calcium

Additional Ways These Drugs May Upset Your Nutritional Balance

Rifampin can cause loss of appetite, nausea, and vomiting, all of which can upset your eating habits and possibly interfere with good nutrition. It can also cause diarrhea, which can hamper nutrient absorption.

Isoniazid can cause loss of appetite, nausea, vomiting, and stomach pain, all of which can upset your eating habits and possibly interfere with good nutrition.

Restoring Your Nutritional Balance

To compensate for the nutrient loss caused by rifampin, speak to your physician about taking 400 IU vitamin D, and 1,200 mg calcium per day.

To compensate for the nutrient loss caused by rifampin plus isoniazid, speak to your physician about taking 50–100 mg niacin, 50–100 mg vitamin B_6, 400 IU vitamin D, and 1,200 mg calcium per day.

You can also eat foods that contain the depleted nutrients:

- Niacin: chicken breast, beef liver, mackerel, barley, bulgur
- Vitamin B$_6$: potato, banana, garbanzo beans, chicken breast, fortified oatmeal
- Vitamin D: salmon, mackerel, sardines, eel, fortified milk
- Calcium: milk, dried figs, Swiss cheese, yogurt, tofu

Consult with your physician before making any changes to your diet or supplemental regimen.

RIFAPENTINE (RIF-uh-pen-teen)

Brand Name: Priftin

About Rifapentine

You may have heard your doctor talk about first-line and second-line drugs. The first-line drugs are the ones that doctors expect—or at least hope—will handle the problem. But sometimes these drugs don't do the trick. It may be that the bacteria have developed a resistance to a "first-liner," or perhaps you're allergic to it or it has intolerable side effects. In such cases, doctors will turn to the second-line selections.

Rifapentine is a second-line drug for treating tuberculosis (TB)—second choice because many of the strains of the *Mycobacterium tuberculosis* bacteria that cause TB are resistant to it. It works by interfering with the bacteria as they attempt to manufacture RNA. It's used only in combination with other anti-TB drugs.

Possible Side Effects

The drug's side effects include elevated blood pressure, joint pain, gout, dizziness, and headache.

Which Nutrients Are Robbed

Taking this medicine may deplete your supply of, increase your need for, or interfere with the activity of:

- Vitamin D

Additional Ways This Drug May Upset Your Nutritional Balance

Rifapentine can cause loss of appetite, nausea, and vomiting, which can upset your eating habits and possibly interfere with good nutrition. It can also cause diarrhea, which can hamper nutrient absorption.

Rifapentine can also trigger hyperkalemia, or too much potassium in the blood.

Restoring Your Nutritional Balance

To compensate for the nutrient loss caused by this drug, speak to your physician about taking 400 IU vitamin D per day.

You can also eat foods that contain the depleted nutrient:

- Vitamin D: salmon, mackerel, sardines, eel, fortified milk

Consult with your physician before making any changes to your diet or supplemental regimen.

ROFECOXIB (roe-fe-KOKS-ib)

Brand Name: Vioxx

Special Note: In October 2004, rofecoxib was recalled because of fears that it increased the risk of heart attack and stroke if taken for eighteen months or longer. It *may* be used in the future as a short-term treatment for select ailments.

About Rofecoxib

One of the reasons that medicines cause side effects is that they're not very selective. Selectivity is key in the minuscule, delicately balanced world of biochemistry. But from a medicine's point of view, a lot of things look alike in the body. For example, many cancer drugs are designed to seek out and destroy rapidly growing cancer cells. Since they can't tell the difference between a rapidly growing healthy cell in the lining of the stomach, a rapidly growing hair follicle, or a rapidly growing cancer cell, these drugs kill them all.

For years, this lack of selectivity has bedeviled millions of Americans with arthritis and other painful or inflammatory conditions. That's because the medicines typically used to treat these problems, called nonsteroidal anti-inflammatory drugs (NSAIDs), work by interfering with COX (cyclooxygenase). But there are two forms of COX, one that promotes inflammation and one that protects the stomach lining. To the NSAIDs, the two COXes look pretty much alike, so both are targeted. As a result, we get the benefits (the relief of pain and inflammation), but also get the side effects (stomach ulcers, gastrointestinal bleeding, and other problems).

Fortunately, the relatively new kind of NSAID called rofecoxib is fairly good at telling the difference between the two COXes and generally goes after the one that causes pain and inflammation, rather than the one that protects the stomach lining. As a result, pain and inflammation are relieved, but there is less risk of developing ulcers and stomach bleeding.

Possible Side Effects

The drug's more common side effects include high blood pressure, diarrhea, upper respiratory tract infections, and flu-like syndrome.

Which Nutrients Are Robbed

Taking this medicine may deplete your supply of, increase your need for, or interfere with the activity of:

• Folic acid

Additional Ways This Drug May Upset Your Nutritional Balance

Rofecoxib can cause heartburn, abdominal pain, esophageal reflux, and nausea, all of which can upset your eating habits and possibly interfere with good nutrition. It can also cause diarrhea, which can hamper nutrient absorption.

Restoring Your Nutritional Balance

To compensate for the nutrient loss caused by this drug, speak to your physician about taking 400–800 mcg folic acid per day.

You can also eat foods that contain the depleted nutrient:

• Folic acid: beef liver, fortified breakfast cereals, spinach, great northern beans, asparagus

Consult with your physician before making any changes to your diet or supplemental regimen.

SALSALATE (SAL-suh-late)

Brand Names: Amigesic, Argesic-SA, Artha-G, Disalcid, Marthritic, Mono-
Gesic, Salflex, Salgesic, Salsitab

About Salsalate

Salsalate is a salicylate, which makes it a chemical cousin to aspirin. Like aspirin, salsalate interferes with the production of the prostaglandins that play an important role in producing inflammation. Because inflammation can be painful, dampening this process can relieve pain.

Salsalate also works via the hypothalamus to lower fever and helps reduce the odds that blood platelets will clump together unnecessarily and thicken the blood.

These properties make salsalate helpful for treating rheumatoid arthritis and other inflammatory ailments, as well as mild to moderate pain.

Possible Side Effects

The drug's more common side effects include nausea, heartburn, and stomach pain.

Which Nutrients Are Robbed

Taking this medicine may deplete your supply of, increase your need for, or interfere with the activity of:

- Folic acid   • Potassium

Additional Ways This Drug May Upset Your Nutritional Balance

Salsalate can cause heartburn, stomach pain, and nausea, all of which can upset your eating habits and possibly interfere with good nutrition.

Restoring Your Nutritional Balance

To compensate for the nutrient loss caused by this drug, speak to your physician about taking 400–800 mcg folic acid and 100–300 mg potassium per day.

You can also eat foods that contain the depleted nutrients:

- Folic acid: beef liver, fortified breakfast cereals, spinach, great northern beans, asparagus
- Potassium: dried figs, California avocado, papaya, banana, dates

Consult with your physician before making any changes to your diet or supplemental regimen.

THE SARTANS
CANDESARTAN, IRBESARTAN, LOSARTAN, TELMISARTAN, AND VALSARTAN (kan-de-SAR-tan, ir-be-SAR-tan, loe-SAR-tan, tel-mi-SAR-tan, val-SAR-tan)

Brand Names: Candesartan plus hydrochlorothiazide: Atacand HCT
Irbesartan plus hydrochlorothiazide: Avalide
Losartan plus hydrochlorothiazide: Hyzaar
Telmisartan plus hydrochlorothiazide: Micardis HCT
Valsartan plus hydrochlorothiazide: Diovan HCT

About the Sartans

Believe it or not, the kidneys play a major role in controlling blood pressure. When arterial blood pressure falls too low, or the blood levels of sodium are subpar, or the sympathetic nervous system issues certain orders, the kidneys trigger a cascade of complex biochemical reactions that include production of a substance called angiotensin II.

Angiotensin II causes the muscles surrounding the blood vessels to constrict, which makes them narrower and increases their resistance to the flow of blood. It also encourages the body to retain water and sodium. Both of these actions—narrowing the blood vessels and retaining fluid—push the blood pressure up.

Because angiotensin II increases blood pressure, it makes sense that interfering with its action could lower blood pressure. A group of medications called the sartans are designed to do just that. By taking up space in the angiotensin receptor sites, they can put angiotensin II out of business. The sartans include candesartan, irbesartan, losartan, telmisartan, and valsartan. Technically, they're called angiotensin receptor-blocking agents because they block the receptor sites where angiotensin would otherwise plug in to increase blood pressure.

Like many medicines used to treat elevated blood pressure, the sartans are often combined with other drugs. All of the sartans discussed on this page are combined with hydrochlorothiazide, a diuretic discussed on page 304.

Possible Side Effects

Some of the more common side effects seen with the sartans include fatigue, dizziness, upper respiratory tract infections, and chest pain. Hydrochlorothiazide's more common side effects include low blood pressure and skin sensitivity to light.

Which Nutrients Are Robbed

Taking these medicines may deplete your supply of, increase your need for, or interfere with the activity of:

- Magnesium
- Phosphorus
- Potassium
- Sodium
- Zinc
- Coenzyme Q_{10}

Additional Ways These Drugs May Upset Your Nutritional Balance

Candesartan can cause nausea, vomiting, heartburn, and loss of appetite; irbesartan can cause heartburn and nausea; losartan can cause low blood sugar (hypoglycemia); telmisartan can cause abdominal pain and nausea; and valsartan can cause abdominal pain. Hydrochlorothiazide can cause loss of appetite. All of these side effects can upset your eating habits and possibly interfere with good nutrition.

All of the sartans can also cause diarrhea, which can hamper nutrient absorption.

In addition, irbesartan, losartan, and valsartan can trigger hyperkalemia, or too much potassium in the blood.

Restoring Your Nutritional Balance

To compensate for the nutrient loss caused by these drugs, speak to your physician about taking 500–1,000 mg magnesium, 700 mg phosphorus, 50–200 mg zinc, and 30–100 mg coenzyme Q_{10} per day. And ask your physician to consider the effects of sodium depletion.

A Note on Potassium: "Regular" diuretics lower potassium levels, while potassium-sparing diuretics do not—they may increase levels instead. It is not uncommon for doctors to prescribe two different diuretics. That's why you should speak to your physician about your potassium levels, and whether it is appropriate for you to take supplements or eat potassium-rich foods.

You can also eat foods that contain the depleted nutrients:

- Magnesium: Florida avocado, toasted wheat germ, almonds, shredded wheat cereal, pumpkin seeds

- Phosphorus: plain nonfat yogurt, lentils, salmon, milk, halibut
- Zinc: oysters, beef shank, chicken, pork tenderloin, plain yogurt
- Coenzyme Q_{10}: beef, chicken, trout, salmon, oranges, broccoli

Consult with your physician before making any changes to your diet or supplemental regimen.

SEVELAMER (se-VEL-uh-mer)

Brand Name: Renagel

About Sevelamer

We need the mineral phosphorus to help the body's cells generate energy, to maintain strong bones and teeth, and otherwise stay healthy. But too much of a good thing—including phosphorus—can be dangerous. Excessive levels of phosphorus in the blood (a condition called hyperphosphatemia) are generally seen in people whose weakened kidneys can't filter the mineral out and excrete it with the urine. Over time, high levels of phosphorus can weaken the bones, leading to fractures and pain. Combined with calcium, phosphorus can harden the arteries, causing poor circulation, heart attack, and stroke, and can also crystallize in the skin and cause itching.

Sevelamer, which is used to treat hyperphosphatemia, binds to the phosphorus from food within your gastrointestinal tract and prevents this mineral from being absorbed.

Possible Side Effects

The drug's more common side effects include low blood pressure, muscle and bone pain, headache, and diarrhea.

Which Nutrients Are Robbed

Taking this medicine may deplete your supply of, increase your need for, or interfere with the activity of:

- Folic acid
- Vitamin D
- Vitamin E
- Vitamin K
- Phosphorus

Additional Ways This Drug May Upset Your Nutritional Balance

Sevelamer can cause heartburn, nausea, and vomiting, which can upset your eating habits and possibly interfere with good nutrition. It can also cause diarrhea, which can hamper nutrient absorption.

Restoring Your Nutritional Balance

To compensate for the nutrient loss caused by this drug, speak to your physician about taking 400–800 mcg folic acid, 400 IU vitamin D, 400 IU vitamin E, and 60–80 mcg vitamin K per day. And ask your physician to monitor your phosphorus status.

You can also eat foods that contain the depleted nutrients:

- Folic acid: beef liver, fortified breakfast cereals, spinach, great northern beans, asparagus
- Vitamin D: salmon, mackerel, sardines, eel, fortified milk
- Vitamin E: wheat germ oil, almonds, safflower oil, corn oil, soybean oil
- Vitamin K: kale, broccoli, parsley, Swiss chard, spinach

Consult with your physician before making any changes to your diet or supplemental regimen.

SIMVASTATIN (SIM-vuh-stat-in)

Brand Name: Zocor

About Simvastatin

Popularly known by its brand name Zocor, simvastatin is one of the widely prescribed statin drugs. The statins are used to reduce cholesterol and blood fats—and they work well in many people.

A report appearing in the medical journal *Lancet* described a study of 4,444 people suffering from coronary heart disease.[7] The participants took either simvastatin or a placebo for more than five years. Simvastatin reduced the total cholesterol by an average of 25 percent and the LDL "bad" cholesterol by an average of 35 percent, while raising the HDL "good" cholesterol by an average of 8 percent.

But as with all drugs, simvastatin has side effects—some of which may counterbalance its good effects. For example, simvastatin reduces the levels of coenzyme Q_{10} (CoQ_{10}) in the body. This can be deleterious to the heart, which relies on CoQ_{10} to keep its mitochondria (tiny cellular energy factories) in high gear. Some researchers fear that if taken for years on end, simvastatin could reduce CoQ_{10} levels to such an extent that patients could begin to suffer from congestive heart failure. And the drug must be taken for years on end, because simvastatin doesn't cure elevated cholesterol once and for all. Once you stop taking it, cholesterol levels rise again. Simvastatin may also reduce levels of beta-carotene and vitamin E, two antioxidants that help protect the cardiovascular system from the effects of oxidation.

Possible Side Effects

The drug's more common side effects include constipation, flatulence, stomach upset, and upper respiratory infections.

Which Nutrients Are Robbed

Taking this medicine may deplete your supply of, increase your need for, or interfere with the activity of:

- Beta-carotene
- Coenzyme Q_{10}
- Vitamin E

Additional Ways This Drug May Upset Your Nutritional Balance

Simvastatin can cause a feeling of bloating, heartburn, and nausea, all of which can upset your eating habits and possibly interfere with good nutrition.

This drug may cause blood levels of vitamin A to rise.

Restoring Your Nutritional Balance

To compensate for the nutrient loss caused by this drug, speak to your physician about taking 25,000 IU beta-carotene, 400 IU vitamin E, and 30–100 mg coenzyme Q_{10} per day.

You can also eat foods that contain the depleted nutrients:

- Beta-carotene: carrot, spinach, mango, cantaloupe, apricot nectar
- Vitamin E: wheat germ oil, almonds, safflower oil, corn oil, soybean oil
- Coenzyme Q_{10}: beef, chicken, trout, salmon, oranges, broccoli

Consult with your physician before making any changes to your diet or supplemental regimen.

SODIUM BICARBONATE (SOE-dee-um bye-KAR-bun-ate)

Brand Names: Citrocarbonate, Neut

About Sodium Bicarbonate

You probably know it as baking soda, a white powder that makes baked goods rise. Perhaps you even use it to brush your teeth. But as a medicine, sodium bicarbonate is most commonly used as an antacid. Inside the stomach, it releases bicarbonate, an alkaline substance that neutralizes stomach acid.

Sodium bicarbonate is also used to treat metabolic acidosis, a condition in which the blood has become too acidic. The problem can arise because of a metabolic problem, or from ingestion of something like wood alcohol or large doses of aspirin, which the body converts into acid. Poor kidney function and poorly controlled type 1 diabetes may also be to blame.

If your blood becomes too acidic, you will breathe deeper and faster, feel tired, and suffer from nausea and vomiting. If the problem grows worse, you'll feel drowsy, confused, and very weak. Your blood pressure may plummet, and you may even lapse into a coma and die.

Sodium bicarbonate may be used to rebalance the blood as part of the treatment of metabolic acidosis.

Possible Side Effects

The drug's side effects include metabolic alkalosis (the opposite of metabolic acidosis), distension of the stomach, and retention of excess water and sodium.

Which Nutrients Are Robbed

Taking this medicine may deplete your supply of, increase your need for, or interfere with the activity of:

- Calcium
- Potassium

Restoring Your Nutritional Balance

To compensate for the nutrient loss caused by this drug, speak to your physician about taking 1,200 mg calcium and 100–300 mg potassium per day.

You can also eat foods that contain the depleted nutrients:

- Calcium: milk, dried figs, Swiss cheese, yogurt, tofu
- Potassium: dried figs, California avocado, papaya, banana, dates

Consult with your physician before making any changes to your diet or supplemental regimen.

SODIUM CHLORIDE (SOE-dee-um KLOR-ide)

About Sodium Chloride

Thanks to French fries, pretzels, and other highly salted foods, most of us take in more salt (sodium chloride) that we should for good health. While too much sodium in the blood can contribute to major health problems, too little sodium in the blood (a condition called hyponatremia) can also be dangerous. This can result from drinking too much water or receiving a large quantity of intravenous liquid in the hospital that doesn't contain enough sodium. Chronic diarrhea, poor kidney function, heart failure, or cirrhosis of the liver can also be to blame. A sodium deficit could also be due to SIADH (syndrome of inappropriate secretion of antidiuretic hormone), or underactive adrenal glands that prompt the loss of too much sodium in the urine. Whatever the cause of a sodium deficiency, the results are potentially serious, including confusion, lethargy, seizures, muscle twitching, coma, and even death.

If the problem is mild, your doctor may simply recommend that you restrict your fluid intake for a while to let the water/sodium balance readjust. In more serious cases, a sodium chloride solution may be infused. Sodium chloride is also used in hemodialysis, blood transfusion, to clean wounds, and to moisturize the respiratory system.

Possible Side Effects

The drug's side effects include pulmonary edema, formation of blood clots (thrombosis), and vein inflammation (phlebitis).

Which Nutrients Are Robbed

Taking this medicine may deplete your supply of, increase your need for, or interfere with the activity of:

- Potassium

Restoring Your Nutritional Balance

To compensate for the nutrient loss caused by this drug, speak to your physician about taking 100–300 mg potassium per day.

You can also eat foods that contain the depleted nutrient:

- Potassium: dried figs, California avocado, papaya, banana, dates

Consult with your physician before making any changes to your diet or supplemental regimen.

SODIUM PHOSPHATE (SOE-dee-um FOSS-fate)

Brand Names: Fleet Enema, Fleet Phospho-Soda

About Sodium Phosphate

Constipation—the infrequent or incomplete passing of hard stool, or difficulty passing hard stools—can be caused by many things, chief of which are a lack of fiber in the diet and not drinking enough fluid. Poor bowel habits (such as waiting too long to have a bowel movement) may also be to blame. Many medications can contribute to constipation by slowing the movement of food through the intestines or drying out the stool, the most notorious of these being diuretics, calcium channel blockers, nonsteroidal anti-inflammatory drugs (NSAIDs), and narcotics. Other factors that can contribute to this uncomfortable condition include various endocrine, metabolic, and neurologic diseases; structural problems such as rectal prolapse and colonic stricture; eating disorders; and irritable bowel syndrome.

Constipation can bring on nausea and lack of appetite and cause straining during attempts to move the bowels. The straining, in turn, can cause hemorrhoids, damage to the large intestines, and diverticular disease, the formation of small "sacs" in the lining of the intestines that can become clogged with fecal matter and inflamed.

Sodium phosphate is a bowel cleanser used to relieve constipation, and clear the colon before surgery or procedures involving the bowel or rectum. It's an osmotic laxative, which means that it works by drawing water into the intestines and stimulating peristalsis (contraction of the muscles that push the intestinal contents through the bowel), which increases the urge to defecate.

Possible Side Effects

The drug's side effects include diarrhea, cramps, confusion, and weakness.

Which Nutrients Are Robbed

Taking this medicine may deplete your supply of, increase your need for, or interfere with the activity of:

- Calcium
- Potassium
- Magnesium
- Sodium

Additional Ways This Drug May Upset Your Nutritional Balance

Sodium phosphate can cause abdominal pain, nausea, and vomiting, all of which can upset your eating habits and possibly interfere with good nutrition. It can also cause diarrhea, which can hamper nutrient absorption.

Sodium phosphates can trigger hyperkalemia, or too much potassium, and hyperphosphatemia, or too much phosphate in the blood.

Restoring Your Nutritional Balance

To compensate for the nutrient loss caused by this drug, speak to your physician about taking 1,200 mg calcium and 500–1,000 mg magnesium per day. And ask your physician to consider the potential effects of sodium depletion and to monitor your potassium status.

You can also eat foods that contain the depleted nutrients:

- Calcium: milk, dried figs, Swiss cheese, yogurt, tofu
- Magnesium: Florida avocado, toasted wheat germ, almonds, shredded wheat cereal, pumpkin seeds

Consult with your physician before making any changes to your diet or supplemental regimen.

SODIUM POLYSTYRENE SULFONATE (SOE-dee-um pol-ee-STYE-reen SUL-fon-ate)

Brand Name: Kayexalate

About Sodium Polystyrene Sulfonate

You may have too much potassium in your blood (hyperkalemia) if you have Addison's disease, your kidneys aren't working properly, or you're taking drugs that interfere with the kidney's ability to excrete potassium. Or your bloodstream may be flooded with potassium after a severe burn or a crush injury that destroys a lot of muscle tissue, both of which can allow potassium to flow from damaged cells into the bloodstream.

Whatever the reason, hyperkalemia can cause nausea, vomiting, muscle fatigue, and irregular heartbeat. In severe cases, the heart may stop beating altogether.

Sodium polystyrene sulfonate is used to lower potassium levels that are mildly to moderately elevated. The drug works by "swapping" its sodium ions for potassium ions in the intestines, preventing the potassium ions from being absorbed.

Possible Side Effects

The drug's side effects include constipation, loss of appetite, and gastric irritation.

Which Nutrients Are Robbed

Taking this medicine may deplete your supply of, increase your need for, or interfere with the activity of:

- Calcium
- Magnesium
- Potassium

Additional Ways This Drug May Upset Your Nutritional Balance

Sodium polystyrene sulfonate can cause loss of appetite, nausea, and vomiting, all of which can upset your eating habits and possibly interfere with good nutrition.

Restoring Your Nutritional Balance

To compensate for the nutrient loss caused by this drug, speak to your physician about taking 1,200 mg calcium and 500–1,000 mg magnesium per day. And ask your physician to monitor your potassium status.

You can also eat foods that contain the depleted nutrients:

- Calcium: milk, dried figs, Swiss cheese, yogurt, tofu
- Magnesium: Florida avocado, toasted wheat germ, almonds, shredded wheat cereal, pumpkin seeds

Consult with your physician before making any changes to your diet or supplemental regimen.

SOTALOL (SOE-tuh-lole)

Brand Names: Betapace, Betapace AF, Sotacor

About Sotalol

Have you ever looked at an electrocardiogram (EKG), that long, thin strip of graph paper with a wiggly line on it? That line represents your heartbeat. Ideally, the line moves up and down in a very stable repeating pattern, with the same degree of highs and lows and the proper amount of space within each pattern and between each repetition.

The heartbeat itself is not a single action; it's a series of actions powered by an electrical current. Unfortunately, for various reasons, this sequence can be upset and the heartbeat can become irregular.

Sotalol is one of the medicines doctors use to treat deviations from the normal heartbeat pattern (arrhythmias), including certain times when the heart is beating too rapidly (a condition known as tachycardia). Sotalol is a beta-blocker that works by occupying certain receptors in the heart, thus interfering with the "beat fast" command and similar messages coming from the nervous system.

Possible Side Effects

The drug's more common side effects include stomach upset, trouble breathing, dizziness, fatigue, and a slow heartbeat.

Which Nutrients Are Robbed

Taking this medicine may deplete your supply of, increase your need for, or interfere with the activity of:

- Coenzyme Q_{10}
- Melatonin

Additional Ways This Drug May Upset Your Nutritional Balance

Sotalol can cause stomach discomfort, nausea, and vomiting, all of which can upset your eating habits and possibly interfere with good nutrition. It can also cause diarrhea, which can hamper nutrient absorption.

Restoring Your Nutritional Balance

To compensate for the nutrient loss caused by this drug, speak to your physician about taking 30–100 mg coenzyme Q_{10} and 1–3 mg melatonin per day.

You can also eat foods that contain the depleted nutrient:

- Coenzyme Q_{10}: beef, chicken, trout, salmon, oranges, broccoli

Consult with your physician before making any changes to your diet or supplemental regimen.

SPARFLOXACIN (spar-FLOKS-uh-sin)

Brand Name: Zagam

About Sparfloxacin

If you have to get pneumonia, you certainly don't want to get the hospital-acquired variety. In the well-scrubbed, antiseptic hospital environment, the germs that do survive are usually the hardiest—and often the hardest to kill. And just the fact that you're in the hospital (assuming you're a patient) suggests that your immune system may already have been weakened by an illness.

Community-acquired pneumonia, which strikes those living at home (as opposed to in a hospital or an institution), is usually fairly easy to cure if treatment is started soon enough and you're otherwise healthy. Several types of germs can cause community-acquired pneumonia, including *Streptococcus pneumoniae* and *Legionella pneumophilia* (the cause of Legionnaires' disease).

The typical victims of community-acquired pneumonia are children and senior citizens. Symptoms (which can vary depending on the bacteria that caused the pneumonia) may include fever, chills and shaking, a sputum-producing cough, fatigue, and muscle aches.

Fortunately, antibiotics such as sparfloxacin can cure community-acquired pneumonia caused by a variety of bacteria. Sparfloxacin, which works by preventing bacteria from reproducing itself, is also useful in treating bronchitis that has been made worse by invading bacteria.

Possible Side Effects

The drug's more common side effects include changes in the heart rhythm, agitation, anxiety, anemia, and stomach upset.

Which Nutrients Are Robbed

Taking this medicine may deplete your supply of, increase your need for, or interfere with the activity of:

- Biotin
- Inositol
- Thiamin
- Riboflavin
- Niacin
- Vitamin B$_6$

- Vitamin B$_{12}$
- Vitamin K
- Zinc
- *Bifidobacterium bifidum*
- *Lactobacillus acidophilus*

Additional Ways This Drug May Upset Your Nutritional Balance

Sparfloxacin can cause abdominal pain, changes in taste, nausea, and vomiting, all of which can upset your eating habits and possibly interfere with good nutrition. It can also cause diarrhea, which can hamper nutrient absorption.

Restoring Your Nutritional Balance

To compensate for the nutrient loss caused by this drug, speak to your physician about taking 500–1,000 mcg biotin, 250–1,000 mg inositol, 25–100 mg thiamin, 25–100 mg riboflavin, 50–100 mg niacin, 50–100 mg vitamin B$_6$, 500–1,000 mcg vitamin B$_{12}$, 60–80 mcg vitamin K, 50–200 mg zinc, 15 billion live *Bifidobacterium bifidum* organisms, and 15 billion live *Lactobacillus acidophilus* organisms per day.

You can also eat foods that contain the depleted nutrients:

- Biotin: beef liver, soybeans, rice bran, peanut butter, barley
- Inositol: cantaloupe, oranges, green beans, grapefruit juice, limes
- Thiamin: braised liver, turkey heart, roasted chicken, gefilte fish, sardines
- Riboflavin: dried sunflower seeds, orange juice, bulgur, spinach noodles, pine nuts
- Niacin: chicken breast, beef liver, mackerel, barley, bulgur
- Vitamin B$_6$: potato, banana, garbanzo beans, chicken breast, fortified oatmeal
- Vitamin B$_{12}$: beef liver, rainbow trout, sockeye salmon, beef, haddock
- Vitamin K: kale, broccoli, parsley, Swiss chard, spinach
- Zinc: oysters, beef shank, chicken, pork tenderloin, plain yogurt
- *Bifidobacterium bifidum*: Jerusalem artichokes, asparagus, garlic, and onions may stimulate the growth or activity of this probiotic

- *Lactobacillus acidophilus*: yogurt containing live lactobacillus cultures, kefir, acidophilus milk

Consult with your physician before making any changes to your diet or supplemental regimen.

SPIRONOLACTONE (speer-on-oh-LAK-tohn)

Brand Names: Aldactone, Novospiroton

About Spironolactone

About 5 million Americans suffer from heart failure. If you're less than 60 years old, your chances of developing it are less than 1 percent, but if you're over 80, the odds are 10 times that.

Heart failure doesn't mean that the heart is broken, just that it can't keep the blood zipping through the arteries and veins like it should. As a result, you feel tired, you may be short of breath, and fluid will accumulate in your legs, lungs, or elsewhere.

An important part of the treatment for heart failure is ridding the body of this excess fluid. To do so, your physician may prescribe diuretics such as spironolactone. Although not a rapid-acting diuretic, spironolactone does have an important property: It "spares" potassium. This means it prevents potassium from being washed away along with the excess fluid that's released from the body via the urine. This is important, because many diuretics prompt the excretion of large amounts of potassium and can cause a deficiency of this important mineral. A lack of potassium can trigger twitching muscles, paralysis, irregular heartbeat, and other problems.

Spironolactone is also used to treat the buildup of excess fluid in the body caused by ailments other than heart failure.

Possible Side Effects

The drug's more common side effects include stomach upset, breast development in men (gynecomastia), mental confusion, and drowsiness.

Which Nutrients Are Robbed

Taking this medicine may deplete your supply of, increase your need for, or interfere with the activity of:

- Magnesium
- Sodium
- Phosphorus

Additional Ways This Drug May Upset Your Nutritional Balance

Spironolactone can cause loss of appetite, nausea, and vomiting, all of which can upset your eating habits and possibly interfere with good nutrition. It can also cause diarrhea, which can hamper nutrient absorption.

This drug can also trigger hyperkalemia, or too much potassium, and hypermagnesemia, or too much magnesium in the blood.

Restoring Your Nutritional Balance

To compensate for the nutrient loss caused by this drug, speak to your physician about taking 700 mg phosphorus per day. And ask your physician to consider the potential effects of sodium depletion and to monitor your magnesium status.

A Note on Potassium: "Regular" diuretics lower potassium levels, while potassium-sparing diuretics do not—they may increase levels instead. It is not uncommon for doctors to prescribe two different diuretics. That's why you should speak to your physician about your potassium levels, and whether it is appropriate for you to take supplements or eat potassium-rich foods.

You can also eat foods that contain the depleted nutrient:

- Phosphorus: plain nonfat yogurt, lentils, salmon, milk, halibut

Consult with your physician before making any changes to your diet or supplemental regimen.

STANOZOLOL (stan-OH-zoe-lole)

Brand Name: Winstrol

About Stanozolol

One of the many important components of the immune system is the C1 inhibitor, part of the complement system that helps destroy foreign cells. If there isn't enough C1 inhibitor, or if it isn't working well and you're hit with a virus, injury, or stress, parts of your body will swell. This condition, called hereditary angioedema, is a genetic problem, *not* an allergic reaction.

The swelling may happen in the digestive tract, windpipe, throat, mouth, or under the skin, and can be accompanied by cramps, nausea, and vomiting. If the swelling occurs in the wrong place or is excessive, the unpleasant symptoms can give way to the deadly. For example, if your windpipe swells too much, you may not be able to breathe, a problem that could be fatal if you don't get emergency treatment.

Stanozolol, a steroid that encourages the body to produce more C1 inhibitor, is used as a long-term preventive treatment for hereditary angioedema.

Possible Side Effects

The drug's more common side effects include acne, enlargement of the breast in men (gynecomastia), bladder irritability, and an unusually prolonged penile erection.

Which Nutrients Are Robbed

Taking this medicine may deplete your supply of, increase your need for, or interfere with the activity of:

- Iron

Additional Ways This Drug May Upset Your Nutritional Balance

Stanozolol can cause nausea, which can upset your eating habits and possibly interfere with good nutrition. It can also cause diarrhea, which can hamper nutrient absorption.

This drug can also trigger hypercalcemia, or too much calcium in the blood.

Restoring Your Nutritional Balance

Ask you physician to consider the potential effects of iron depletion.

Consult with your physician before making any changes to your diet or supplemental regimen.

STAVUDINE (STAV-yoo-deen)

Brand Name: Zerit

About Stavudine

AIDS (acquired immunodeficiency syndrome) often begins quietly, with a fever, swollen lymph nodes, and other symptoms that resemble infectious mononucleosis. Some of these symptoms may disappear for a while, and years may pass before any new ones are noticed. Or relatively mild symptoms may appear and reappear several months after the initial infection.

At some point, however, the seriousness of the problem will become evident. As HIV (human immunodeficiency virus, the virus that causes AIDS) takes over and destroys more and more immune system cells, the body falls prey to infections that it could have handled easily if the immune defenses were intact. The yeast known as *Candida* may overgrow in the esophagus, making swallowing difficult. Pneumonia caused by the fungus *Pneumocystis carinii* may develop. Or perhaps some *Toxoplasma* bacteria that the body has been harboring since childhood may suddenly become active and move into the brain, causing headaches and seizures.

Whatever its symptoms, AIDS must be aggressively attacked with a combination of antiviral medicines. Stavudine is a reverse transcriptase inhibitor that inhibits the attempts of HIV to force the body's cells to manufacture clones of the virus.

Stavudine is combined with other antiviral drugs to promote the strongest effects with the fewest side effects and to slow the evolution of new, resistant strains of HIV.

Possible Side Effects

The drug's more common side effects include nerve damage, chills, fever, insomnia, nausea, vomiting, and diarrhea.

Which Nutrients Are Robbed

Taking this medicine may deplete your supply of, increase your need for, or interfere with the activity of:

- Vitamin B_{12}
- Zinc
- Copper
- Carnitine

Additional Ways This Drug May Upset Your Nutritional Balance

Stavudine can cause loss of appetite, abdominal pain, nausea, and vomiting, all of which can upset your eating habits and possibly interfere with good nutrition. It can also cause diarrhea, which can hamper nutrient absorption.

Restoring Your Nutritional Balance

To compensate for the nutrient loss caused by this drug, speak to your physician about taking 500–1,000 mcg vitamin B_{12}, 2 mcg copper, 50–200 mg zinc, and 250–1,000 mg carnitine per day.

You can also eat foods that contain the depleted nutrients:

- Vitamin B$_{12}$: beef liver, rainbow trout, sockeye salmon, beef, haddock
- Copper: beef liver, almonds, raw mushrooms, hazelnuts, lentils
- Zinc: oysters, beef shank, chicken, pork tenderloin, plain yogurt
- Carnitine: ground beef, pork, Canadian bacon, whole milk, cod

Consult with your physician before making any changes to your diet or supplemental regimen.

STREPTOMYCIN (strep-toe-MYE-sin)

About Streptomycin

Back in the 1800s, tuberculosis (TB) was a major problem in the western world, causing as many as 30 percent of all deaths. Indeed, up until the 1940s and 1950s, many hospitals had entire wards dedicated to the care of those who had the disease.

Although TB is much less of a problem in today's western world, it does exist, and it is still potentially fatal. The *Mycobacterium tuberculosis* bacteria that cause the disease are spread from person to person via airborne germs. As you inhale them, the battle for survival begins in your lungs, as your immune system tries to kill the bacteria or wall them off inside large immune system cells called macrophages. If your built-in defense systems are successful, you may never even know you were exposed to TB. If not, the next stage will depend on where the germs take up residence.

If the problem remains in your lungs, you will develop a cough, which may include yellow or green sputum and, eventually, streaks of blood. You may also suffer from night sweats, a loss of appetite, decreased energy, weight loss, and a general feeling of malaise.

If the bacteria settles in your bladder, there may be blood in the urine and pain upon urinating.

If your brain is the target, symptoms can include headache, drowsiness, nausea, and, eventually, coma.

If your joints are afflicted, you may suffer from symptoms resembling those of arthritis.

If the disease attacks the membrane surrounding your heart, you may develop fever, shortness of breath, and enlarged veins in the neck, as your heart struggles to pump blood.

For the past 50 or so years, physicians have used several drugs to attack TB, including streptomycin, which is always used in conjunction with other drugs, such as isoniazid and rifampin. Because it doesn't penetrate cell walls effectively, streptomycin zeroes in on the *Mycobacterium tuberculosis* it finds floating around outside the body's cells. Other drugs are used to carry on the fight inside the cells.

Possible Side Effects

The drug's side effects include low blood pressure, rash, joint pain, and difficulty breathing.

Which Nutrients Are Robbed

Taking this medicine may deplete your supply of, increase your need for, or interfere with the activity of:

- Calcium
- Magnesium
- Potassium
- *Bifidobacterium bifidum*
- *Lactobacillus acidophilus*

Additional Ways This Drug May Upset Your Nutritional Balance

Streptomycin can cause nausea and vomiting, which can upset your eating habits and possibly interfere with good nutrition.

Restoring Your Nutritional Balance

To compensate for the nutrient loss caused by this drug, speak to your physician about taking 1,200 mg calcium, 500–1,000 mg magnesium, 100–300 mg potassium, 15 billion live *Bifidobacterium bifidum* organisms, and 15 billion live *Lactobacillus acidophilus* organisms per day.

You can also eat foods that contain the depleted nutrients:

- Calcium: milk, dried figs, Swiss cheese, yogurt, tofu
- Magnesium: Florida avocado, toasted wheat germ, almonds, shredded wheat cereal, pumpkin seeds
- Potassium: dried figs, California avocado, papaya, banana, dates
- *Bifidobacterium bifidum*: Jerusalem artichokes, asparagus, garlic, and onions may stimulate the growth or activity of this probiotic
- *Lactobacillus acidophilus*: yogurt containing live lactobacillus cultures, kefir, acidophilus milk

Consult with your physician before making any changes to your diet or supplemental regimen.

SUCRALFATE (soo-KRAL-fate)

Brand Names: Carafate, Novo-Sucralate, Sulcrate, Sulcrate Suspension Plus

About Sucralfate

A duodenal ulcer is a raw, open wound that develops when the inner lining of the duodenum is eaten away. The duodenum, the first part of the small intestines, receives partially digested food laden with acid and digestive juices (such as pepsin) directly from the stomach, along with bile (a fluid necessary for the breakdown of fats) from the gallbladder. Like the stomach, the duodenum has a protective mucosal lining, but sometimes this lining fails. Perhaps it's because you secrete lots of acid, or the *Helicobacter pylori* bacteria in your digestive system have gotten out of control. Or maybe you smoke cigarettes or drink large amounts of alcohol, use certain medications (such as nonsteroidal anti-inflammatory drugs [NSAIDs]), or have some underlying disease. Whatever the reason, in serious cases, an ulcer may eat straight through the intestinal wall and allow the intestinal contents to leak into the abdominal cavity, causing infection, fever, and severe pain.

The classic symptom of a duodenal ulcer is a steadily burning, aching, or gnawing pain that generally strikes just below the breastbone. The pain can be mild to moderate, and is usually relieved for a couple of hours by eating, taking antacids, or drinking milk. There may also be bleeding in the intestinal lining, and the blood can make the stool bloody or dark and tarlike.

Sucralfate is believed to treat duodenal ulcers by shielding them from the corrosive action of acid, pepsin, and bile.

Possible Side Effects

The drug's side effects include constipation and rash.

Which Nutrients Are Robbed

Taking this medicine may deplete your supply of, increase your need for, or interfere with the activity of:

- Vitamin A
- Vitamin K
- Vitamin D
- Calcium
- Vitamin E
- Phosphorus

Restoring Your Nutritional Balance

To compensate for the nutrient loss caused by this drug, speak to your physician about taking 5,000 IU vitamin A, 400 IU vitamin D, 400 IU vitamin E, 60–80 mcg vitamin K, 1,200 mg calcium, and 700 mg phosphorus per day.

You can also eat foods that contain the depleted nutrients:

- Vitamin A: beef liver, chicken liver, cheese pizza, whole milk, cheddar cheese
- Vitamin D: salmon, mackerel, sardines, eel, fortified milk
- Vitamin E: wheat germ oil, almonds, safflower oil, corn oil, soybean oil
- Vitamin K: kale, broccoli, parsley, Swiss chard, spinach
- Calcium: milk, dried figs, Swiss cheese, yogurt, tofu
- Phosphorus: plain nonfat yogurt, lentils, salmon, milk, halibut

Consult with your physician before making any changes to your diet or supplemental regimen.

SULFADIAZINE (sul-fuh-DYE-uh-zeen)

Brand Names: Coptin, Microsulfon

About Sulfadiazine

In order to replicate, bacteria must manufacture DNA. But they don't simply push a biochemical button and watch new DNA pop out fully formed. Instead, they manufacture it step by step. Certain bacteria begin with PABA (para-aminobenzoic acid), which they use to make dihydrofolic acid, which is used to make the purines necessary to synthesize DNA.

This is a multistep manufacturing process, which means it can be stopped at several points. Sulfadiazine derails the process at step 1. The drug is structurally similar to PABA, so it "fools" the bacterial machinery into thinking that it's the original raw material. As a result, the DNA is not manufactured properly and the bacteria cannot replicate.

This deceptive behavior makes sulfadiazine helpful in halting bacterial infections of the urinary tract and combating toxoplasmosis, a parasitic infection that can cause general malaise, headache, sore throat, joint pain, and other problems. The disease can be even more dangerous if it's passed from mother to fetus, or if it strikes those with weakened immune systems.

Possible Side Effects

The drug's side effects include fever, thyroid problems, hepatitis, and jaundice.

Which Nutrients Are Robbed

Taking this medicine may deplete your supply of, increase your need for, or interfere with the activity of:

- Biotin
- Inositol
- Thiamin
- Riboflavin
- Niacin
- Vitamin B_6
- Vitamin B_{12}
- Vitamin K
- *Bifidobacterium bifidum*
- *Lactobacillus acidophilus*

Additional Ways This Drug May Upset Your Nutritional Balance

Sulfadiazine can cause loss of appetite, nausea, and vomiting, all of which can upset your eating habits and possibly interfere with good nutrition. It can also cause diarrhea, which can hamper nutrient absorption.

Restoring Your Nutritional Balance

To compensate for the nutrient loss caused by this drug, speak to your physician about taking 500–1,000 mcg biotin, 250–1,000 mg inositol, 25–100 mg thiamin, 25–100 mg riboflavin, 50–100 mg niacin, 50–100 mg vitamin B_6, 500–1,000 mcg vitamin B_{12}, 60–80 mcg vitamin K, 15 billion live *Bifidobacterium bifidum* organisms, and 15 billion live *Lactobacillus acidophilus* organisms per day.

You can also eat foods that contain the depleted nutrients:

- Biotin: beef liver, soybeans, rice bran, peanut butter, barley
- Inositol: cantaloupe, oranges, green beans, grapefruit juice, limes
- Thiamin: braised liver, turkey heart, roasted chicken, gefilte fish, sardines
- Riboflavin: dried sunflower seeds, orange juice, bulgur, spinach noodles, pine nuts
- Niacin: chicken breast, beef liver, mackerel, barley, bulgur
- Vitamin B_6: potato, banana, garbanzo beans, chicken breast, fortified oatmeal
- Vitamin B_{12}: beef liver, rainbow trout, sockeye salmon, beef, haddock
- Vitamin K: kale, broccoli, parsley, Swiss chard, spinach
- *Bifidobacterium bifidum*: Jerusalem artichokes, asparagus, garlic, and onions may stimulate the growth or activity of this probiotic
- *Lactobacillus acidophilus*: yogurt containing live lactobacillus cultures, kefir, acidophilus milk

Consult with your physician before making any changes to your diet or supplemental regimen.

SULFASALAZINE (sul-fuh-SAL-uh-zeen)

Brand Names: Apo-Sulfasalazine, Azulfidine, Azulfidine EN-Tabs, PMS-Sulfasalazine, Salazopyrin, Salazopyrin EN-Tabs, S.A.S.

About Sulfasalazine

Attacks, or flare-ups, of ulcerative colitis (chronic inflammation of the colon or large intestine) can be mild, causing moderate abdominal cramps and blood and mucus in the stool. Or they can be severe, causing abdominal pain, high fever, inflammation of the abdominal cavity, and serious diarrhea. In extreme cases, you may be rushing to the toilet a dozen or more times a day.

The inflammation and ulceration that are hallmarks of ulcerative colitis typically begin in or near the rectum and work their way backward, spreading along the length of the colon over time. We don't know exactly what causes the disease; an errant immune system and genetic predisposition are the chief supsects. Stress doesn't cause the disease, but it may make it worse.

Sulfasalazine helps to prevent future flare-ups by reducing inflammation in the colon, most likely by slowing the production of the prostaglandins, hormone-like substances that encourage inflammatory reactions.

Sulfasalazine may also be used to treat people with rheumatoid and juvenile rheumatoid arthritis who have not been helped by nonsteroidal anti-inflammatory drugs (NSAIDs) or other painkillers.

Possible Side Effects

The drug's more common side effects include headache, diarrhea, and low sperm count.

Which Nutrients Are Robbed

Taking this medicine may deplete your supply of, increase your need for, or interfere with the activity of:

- Folic acid
- Vitamin B_6
- Vitamin B_{12}

Additional Ways This Drug May Upset Your Nutritional Balance

Sulfasalazine can cause gastric distress, loss of appetite, nausea, and vomiting, all of which can upset your eating habits and possibly interfere with good nutrition. It can also cause diarrhea, which can hamper nutrient absorption.

Restoring Your Nutritional Balance

To compensate for the nutrient loss caused by this drug, speak to your physician about taking 400–800 mcg folic acid, 50–100 mg vitamin B_6, and 500–1,000 mcg vitamin B_{12} per day.

You can also eat foods that contain the depleted nutrients:

- Folic acid: beef liver, fortified breakfast cereals, spinach, great northern beans, asparagus
- Vitamin B_6: potato, banana, garbanzo beans, chicken breast, fortified oatmeal
- Vitamin B_{12}: beef liver, rainbow trout, sockeye salmon, beef, haddock

Consult with your physician before making any changes to your diet or supplemental regimen.

SULFISOXAZOLE (sul-fi-SOKS-uh-zole)

Brand Names: Apo-Sulfisoxazole, Gantrisin, Novo-Soxazole, Sulfizole

About Sulfisoxazole

We humans don't have the enzymes necessary to make the B vitamin folic acid on our own; we must get it from our food. Many bacteria, however, are able to make their own folic acid, a vital ingredient in the manufacture of their DNA. If DNA can be successfully replicated, new bacteria can be churned out. This means that preventing bacteria from making new DNA is a prime strategy for defeating them.

Sulfisoxazole interferes with the bacteria's ability to make folic acid. This makes sulfisoxazole a bacteriostatic drug, meaning that it prevents new bacteria from being made, as opposed to a bactericidal drug, which would kill the bacteria outright.

Because of its ability to stop the production of folic acid and therefore new bacteria cells, sulfisoxazole is used to treat certain bacterial infections of the urinary tract, ear, and other parts of the body.

Possible Side Effects

The drug's side effects include fever, thyroid dysfunction, and hepatitis.

Which Nutrients Are Robbed

Taking this medicine may deplete your supply of, increase your need for, or interfere with the activity of:

- Biotin
- Inositol
- Thiamin
- Riboflavin
- Niacin
- Vitamin B_6
- Vitamin B_{12}
- Vitamin K
- *Bifidobacterium bifidum*
- *Lactobacillus acidophilus*

Additional Ways This Drug May Upset Your Nutritional Balance

Sulfisoxazole can cause loss of appetite, nausea, and vomiting, all of which can upset your eating habits and possibly interfere with good nutrition. It can also cause diarrhea, which can hamper nutrient absorption.

Restoring Your Nutritional Balance

To compensate for the nutrient loss caused by this drug, speak to your physician about taking 500–1,000 mcg biotin, 250–1,000 mg inositol, 25–100 mg thiamin, 25–100 mg riboflavin, 50–100 mg niacin, 50–100 mg vitamin B_6, 500–1,000 mcg vitamin B_{12}, 60–80 mcg vitamin K, 15 billion live *Bifidobacterium bifidum* organisms, and 15 billion live *Lactobacillus acidophilus* organisms per day.

You can also eat foods that contain the depleted nutrients:

- Biotin: beef liver, soybeans, rice bran, peanut butter, barley
- Inositol: cantaloupe, oranges, green beans, grapefruit juice, limes
- Thiamin: braised liver, turkey heart, roasted chicken, gefilte fish, sardines
- Riboflavin: dried sunflower seeds, orange juice, bulgur, spinach noodles, pine nuts
- Niacin: chicken breast, beef liver, mackerel, barley, bulgur
- Vitamin B_6: potato, banana, garbanzo beans, chicken breast, fortified oatmeal
- Vitamin B_{12}: beef liver, rainbow trout, sockeye salmon, beef, haddock
- Vitamin K: kale, broccoli, parsley, Swiss chard, spinach
- *Bifidobacterium bifidum*: Jerusalem artichokes, asparagus, garlic, and onions may stimulate the growth or activity of this probiotic
- *Lactobacillus acidophilus*: yogurt containing live lactobacillus cultures, kefir, acidophilus milk

Consult with your physician before making any changes to your diet or supplemental regimen.

SULINDAC (sul-IN-dak)

Brand Names: Apo-Sulin, Clinoril, Novo-Sundac

About Sulindac

When you cut yourself, you may notice the skin in the area gets a little red. Redness is one of the signs of inflammation, a defensive and rebuilding process that goes on inside your body.

Here's how it works. When you cut or burn yourself, when body tissue is crushed, or when it's overrun by bacteria or other invaders, extra blood is rushed to the area, bringing with it nutrients, red blood cells, white blood cells, and more.

The white blood cells are immune system "soldiers" responsible for defense and cleanup. The macrophages are large cells that literally consume bacteria and other foreign particles. The basophils serve as the "buglers," calling neutrophils and eosinophils to the area. The neutrophils ingest foreign cells. Eosinophils do the same, and can also destroy parasites and certain cancer cells. There are also T-cells specifically programmed to kill only certain foreign or invading cells. At the height of the battle, the afflicted area may become red, swollen, sensitive to touch, and a little hot. The net result is something like you'd see at a major crime scene: The area is cordoned off, the bad guys are taken care of, and the cleanup crew is putting everything back to normal.

Unfortunately, when the inflammation response is too great, continues too long, or has no purpose, it can cause unnecessary pain and disability. That's where anti-inflammatory medicines like sulindac come in handy. Sulindac interferes with the inflammation process early on, before it gets well under way, reducing inflammatory reactions and pain. And if the inflammation happens to be in a joint, quelling it improves joint movement and mobility.

Thanks to its ability to reduce inflammation, sulindac is used to treat acute gouty arthritis, rheumatoid disorders, and other inflammatory conditions.

Possible Side Effects

The drug's more common side effects include water retention, dizziness, rash, and stomach upset.

Which Nutrients Are Robbed

Taking this medicine may deplete your supply of, increase your need for, or interfere with the activity of:

- Folic acid

Additional Ways This Drug May Upset Your Nutritional Balance

Sulindac can cause gastrointestinal pain, heartburn, loss of appetite, abdominal cramps, nausea, and vomiting, all of which can upset your eating habits and possibly interfere with good nutrition. It can also cause diarrhea, which can hamper nutrient absorption.

Restoring Your Nutritional Balance

To compensate for the nutrient loss caused by this drug, speak to your physician about taking 400–800 mcg folic acid per day.

You can also eat foods that contain the depleted nutrient:

- Folic acid: beef liver, fortified breakfast cereals, spinach, great northern beans, asparagus.

Consult with your physician before making any changes to your diet or supplemental regimen.

TACROLIMUS (tah-KROE-li-muss)

Brand Name: Prograf

About Tacrolimus

Lichen planus is an itchy skin disease that may be caused by an immune system reaction to certain infectious organisms, drugs, or chemicals, such as color film developing solution. The drugs that seem to trigger lichen planus (or lichen planus–like symptoms) include the nonsteroidal anti-inflammatory drugs (NSAIDs) used for pain and inflammation, the hydrochlorothiazide used for elevated blood pressure, and the antibiotics streptomycin and tetracycline.

Itching is a major symptom of the disease, as are red or purplish bumps that emerge and then grow into each other to form scaly patches on the skin. These patches often arise on the torso, but can also show up on the legs, wrists, mouth, vagina, and head of the penis. About half the people with lichen planus develop sores on the mouth.

Lichen planus may disappear on its own after a year or two, although it can last longer. The problems flares up and recedes, and you may or may not need treatment in between flares. In one form of the disease, ulcerations can develop on the soles of the feet and elsewhere.

Tacrolimus, an immunosuppressant that helps prevent the rejection of transplanted organs, may be used to treat lichen planus, especially the oral and vaginal varieties. Applied to the skin, tacrolimus relieves the symptoms but doesn't cure the underlying disease, so you may have to use it continually to prevent recurrences.

Possible Side Effects

The drug's more common side effects include tremor, high blood pressure, dizziness, rash, and urinary tract infection.

Which Nutrients Are Robbed

Taking this medicine may deplete your supply of, increase your need for, or interfere with the activity of:

- Calcium
- Phosphorus
- Magnesium
- Potassium

Additional Ways This Drug May Upset Your Nutritional Balance

Tacrolimus can cause abdominal pain, heartburn, nausea, and vomiting, all of which can upset your eating habits and possibly interfere with good nutrition. It can also cause diarrhea, which can hamper nutrient absorption.

This drug can also trigger hypercalcemia, or too much calcium, hyperphosphatemia, or too much phosphate, and hyperkalemia, or too much potassium in the blood.

Restoring Your Nutritional Balance

To compensate for the nutrient loss caused by this drug, speak to your physician about taking 500–1,000 mg magnesium per day. And ask your physician to monitor your calcium, phosphorus, and potassium status.

You can also eat foods that contain the depleted nutrient:

- Magnesium: Florida avocado, toasted wheat germ, almonds, shredded wheat cereal, pumpkin seeds

Consult with your physician before making any changes to your diet or supplemental regimen.

TETRACYCLINE (te-truh-SYE-kleen)

Brand Names: Achromycin Ophthalmic, Achromycin Topical, Apo-Tetra, Novo-Tetra, Nu-Tetra, Sumycin Oral, Topicycline Topical

About Tetracycline

Special kinds of bacteria called ehrlichioses can live only inside the cells of a human or an animal—specifically, inside the white blood cells found in the immune system.

You can become infected with these unusual invaders after being bitten by a tick or another "disease delivery" insect. Infection caused by ehrlichioses can cause depression of the white blood cell count, anemia, or problems with blood clotting. A week or two after being bitten, you may notice a severe headache, fever, aches, and general malaise, followed by diarrhea, vomiting, confusion, breathing difficulties, a cough and/or a rash. If the infection is serious enough, a coma or even death can result, although this doesn't happen very often, especially in those with strong immune systems who receive treatment right away.

Tetracycline is one of the standard treatments for infections caused by ehrlichioses. A broad-spectrum antibiotic that works against a variety of bacteria, tetracycline is also used to fight chlamydia, acne, the *Helicobacter pylori* bacteria associated with ulcers, as well as syphilis and gonorrhea in those who are allergic to penicillin.

Possible Side Effects

The drug's side effects include pericarditis (inflammation of the sac surrounding the heart), photosensitivity, and kidney damage.

Which Nutrients Are Robbed

Taking this medicine may deplete your supply of, increase your need for, or interfere with the activity of:

- Biotin
- Folic acid
- Inositol
- Thiamin
- Riboflavin
- Niacin
- Vitamin B_6
- Vitamin B_{12}
- Vitamin C
- Vitamin K
- Calcium
- Iron
- Magnesium
- Zinc
- *Bifidobacterium bifidum*
- *Lactobacillus acidophilus*

Additional Ways This Drug May Upset Your Nutritional Balance

Tetracycline can cause abdominal cramps, loss of appetite, nausea, and vomiting, all of which can upset your eating habits and possibly interfere with good nutrition. It can also cause diarrhea, which can hamper nutrient absorption.

Restoring Your Nutritional Balance

To compensate for the nutrient loss caused by this drug, speak to your physician about taking 500–1,000 mcg biotin, 400–800 mcg folic acid, 250–1,000 mg inositol, 25–100 mg thiamin, 25–100 mg riboflavin, 50–100 mg niacin, 50–100 mg vitamin B_6, 500–1,000 mcg vitamin B_{12}, 250–1,500 mg vitamin C, 60–80 mcg vitamin K, 1,200 mg calcium, 500–1,000 mg magnesium, 15 billion live *Bifidobacterium bifidum* organisms, and 15 billion live *Lactobacillus acidophilus* organisms per day. And ask your physician to consider the potential effects of iron depletion.

The citrate forms of calcium and magnesium may lower the levels of the tetracycline in your blood, so ask your physician which form of calcium and magnesium are best for you.

Zinc and tetracycline influence each other, so ask your physician how to handle a potential zinc deficiency.

You can also eat foods that contain the depleted nutrients:

- Biotin: beef liver, soybeans, rice bran, peanut butter, barley
- Folic acid: beef liver, fortified breakfast cereals, spinach, great northern beans, asparagus
- Inositol: cantaloupe, oranges, green beans, grapefruit juice, limes
- Thiamin: braised liver, turkey heart, roasted chicken, gefilte fish, sardines
- Riboflavin: dried sunflower seeds, orange juice, bulgur, spinach noodles, pine nuts
- Niacin: chicken breast, beef liver, mackerel, barley, bulgur
- Vitamin B_6: potato, banana, garbanzo beans, chicken breast, fortified oatmeal
- Vitamin B_{12}: beef liver, rainbow trout, sockeye salmon, beef, haddock
- Vitamin C: papaya, guava, red pepper, cantaloupe, black currants
- Vitamin K: kale, broccoli, parsley, Swiss chard, spinach
- Calcium: milk, dried figs, Swiss cheese, yogurt, tofu
- Magnesium: Florida avocado, toasted wheat germ, almonds, shredded wheat cereal, pumpkin seeds
- *Bifidobacterium bifidum*: Jerusalem artichokes, asparagus, garlic, and onions may stimulate the growth or activity of this probiotic

- *Lactobacillus acidophilus*: yogurt containing live lactobacillus cultures, kefir, acidophilus milk

Consult with your physician before making any changes to your diet or supplemental regimen.

THEOPHYLLINE (thee-OFF-i-lin)

Brand Names: Asmalix, Bronkodyl, Elixophyllin, Lanophyllin, Slo-bid, Theo-Dur, Uniphyl

About Theophylline

There's no describing the terror that can strike an asthmatic who wakes up in the middle of the night gasping for breath. Asthma has caused the muscles surrounding your airways to contract and restrict the flow of air. In a sense, it's like what happens when the muscles surrounding the blood vessels in the heart constrict and restrict the flow of blood to the heart. But instead of a heart attack, you suffer a "lung attack."

The squeezing of the airways is just the beginning of what happens during an asthma attack. The tissues that line the airways become inflamed and swollen, thick plugs of mucus form, and damaged cells are cast off. Just taking a breath can become a major effort.

Fortunately, for most people with asthma, the gasping for breath, wheezing, sweating, and terror is about as far as it goes. Asthma generally responds well to treatment, and rarely is an attack so severe that the victim can't get to his or her medicine or call someone before passing out.

Asthma strikes some 18 million Americans and is becoming more and more common. Theophylline is one of several drugs used to treat the disease. Although we don't know exactly how it works, theophylline may help prevent the contraction of the airway muscles, slow the release of asthma-causing chemicals, and/or inhibit inflammation.

Possible Side Effects

This drug's side effects include anxiety, rapid heartbeat, insomnia, chest pains, headache, nausea, and vomiting.

Which Nutrients Are Robbed

Taking this medicine may deplete your supply of, increase your need for, or interfere with the activity of:

- Thiamin
- Vitamin B_6
- Phosphorus

Additional Ways This Drug May Upset Your Nutritional Balance

Theophylline can cause nausea and vomiting, which can upset your eating habits and possibly interfere with good nutrition.

Restoring Your Nutritional Balance

To compensate for the nutrient loss caused by this drug, speak to your physician about taking 25–100 mg thiamin, 50–100 mg vitamin B_6, and 700 mg phosphorus per day.

You can also eat foods that contain the depleted nutrients:

- Thiamin: braised liver, turkey heart, roasted chicken, gefilte fish, sardines
- Vitamin B_6: potato, banana, garbanzo beans, chicken breast, fortified oatmeal
- Phosphorus: plain nonfat yogurt, lentils, salmon, milk, halibut

Consult with your physician before making any changes to your diet or supplemental regimen.

THIETHYLPERAZINE (thye-eth-il-PER-uh-zeen)

Brand Names: Norzine, Torecan

About Thiethylperazine

It certainly feels as if vomiting originates in the body. That is, you usually feel some unpleasant sensation in your stomach or the back of your throat that lets you know your stomach is about to forcibly discharge its contents. But the command to vomit actually originates in the brain.

Several areas in the brain can trigger the command to vomit. One of these, called the chemoreceptor trigger zone, can be set off by the actions of serotonin or dopamine. Thiethylperazine helps to reduce the urge to vomit by interfering with the actions of dopamine; in effect, keeping its biochemical finger off the "vomit button."

Possible Side Effects

The drug's more common side effects include blurred vision, drowsiness, dizziness, and dry nose.

Which Nutrients Are Robbed

Taking this medicine may deplete your supply of, increase your need for, or interfere with the activity of:

- Riboflavin
- Coenzyme Q_{10}

Restoring Your Nutritional Balance

To compensate for the nutrient loss caused by this drug, speak to your physician about taking 25–100 mg riboflavin and 30–100 mg coenzyme Q_{10} per day.

You can also eat foods that contain the depleted nutrients:

- Riboflavin: dried sunflower seeds, orange juice, bulgur, spinach noodles, pine nuts
- Coenzyme Q_{10}: beef, chicken, trout, salmon, oranges, broccoli

Consult with your physician before making any changes to your diet or supplemental regimen.

THIORIDAZINE (thye-oh-RID-uh-zeen)

Brand Names: Novo-Ridazine, Mellaril, Mellaril-S

About Thioridazine

We don't know for sure what causes schizophrenia, and we also don't know what cures it. But several theories attempt to explain it, and one of the most likely is the dopamine hypothesis.

Dopamine is a neurotrasmitter, one of the many chemicals that shuttle between brain cells carrying messages. Experts theorize that schizophrenia is related to excess dopamine activity. Researchers point to several links between dopamine and schizophrenia, such as:

- Amphetamines and other drugs that increase dopamine activity can make schizophrenia worse or trigger schizophrenic symptoms in people who don't have the disease.
- Brain scans have shown that dopamine receptors are denser in people with schizophrenia than they are in those who do not have the disease.
- Most drugs that help quell psychosis are very good at blocking dopamine receptors in the central nervous system.

The dopamine hypothesis is intriguing, but if excess dopamine activity were the cause, then drugs that decrease dopamine activity should solve the problem. However, they aren't a guaranteed cure. After you've had your first schizophrenia episode, medications that reduce dopamine activity can lower your risk of having a second one. The drugs can lower the odds substantially, from 70 to 80 percent to 23 to 30 percent, but they can't eliminate the risk entirely. So although it appears that we have several pieces connected, we haven't yet put the entire schizophrenia puzzle together. That's not unusual; the causes and cures of many diseases are not fully understood, nor are the reasons why many medicines work.

Thioridazine, like other antipsychotic medicines, interferes with the activity of dopamine in the central nervous system. Because newer drugs are believed to work better, thioridazine is generally reserved for people who have not been helped by other drugs.

Possible Side Effects

The drug's side effects include dizziness, drowsiness, urinary difficulties, and tremor.

Which Nutrients Are Robbed

Taking this medicine may deplete your supply of, increase your need for, or interfere with the activity of:

- Riboflavin
- Coenzyme Q_{10}

Additional Ways This Drug May Upset Your Nutritional Balance

Thioridazine can cause stomach pain, nausea, and vomiting, all of which can upset your eating habits and possibly interfere with good nutrition. It can also cause diarrhea, which can hamper nutrient absorption.

Restoring Your Nutritional Balance

To compensate for the nutrient loss caused by this drug, speak to your physician about taking 25–100 mg riboflavin and 30–100 mg coenzyme Q_{10} per day.

You can also eat foods that contain the depleted nutrients:

- Riboflavin: dried sunflower seeds, orange juice, bulgur, spinach noodles, pine nuts
- Coenzyme Q_{10}: beef, chicken, trout, salmon, oranges, broccoli

Consult with your physician before making any changes to your diet or supplemental regimen.

TICARCILLIN, TICARCILLIN PLUS CLAVULANATE POTASSIUM (tye-kar-SIL-in, klav-yoo-LAN-ate poe-TASS-ee-um)

Brand Names: Ticarcillin: Ticar
Ticarcillin and clavulanate potassium: Timentin

About Ticarcillin, Ticarcillin plus Clavulanate Potassium

Ticarcillin is a penicillin antibiotic that can be used to treat various infections of the skin and of the respiratory and urinary tracts, effectively controlling many strains of bacteria known as serratia, indole-positive proteus, and pseudomonas.

But ticarcillin isn't effective in treating staphylococcal infections, because these bacteria have developed a resistance to it. Staph bacteria make substances called beta-lactamase, which they squirt out when ticarcillin gets near. Beta-lactamase deactivates the medicine, and the bacteria can keep multiplying. This is a common problem; more and more bacteria are figuring out how to defeat our medicines.

One way to handle that problem is to keep coming up with new antibiotics that bacteria don't yet know how to destroy. Another is to protect existing medicines from beta-lactamase, which is why ticarcillin is sometimes combined with clavulanate potassium, a beta-lactamase inhibitor. Clavulanate potassium shields ticarcillin, allowing the medicine to do its job. The combination of these two medicines can fight the staph infections that ticarcillin alone cannot.

Possible Side Effects

The side effects with either ticarcillin or ticarcillin plus clavulanate potassium include confusion, convulsions, drowsiness, and rash.

Which Nutrients Are Robbed

Taking these medicines may deplete your supply of, increase your need for, or interfere with the activity of:

- Biotin
- Inositol
- Thiamin
- Riboflavin
- Niacin
- Vitamin B_6

- Vitamin B_{12}
- Vitamin K
- Potassium
- *Bifidobacterium bifidum*
- *Lactobacillus acidophilus*

Restoring Your Nutritional Balance

To compensate for the nutrient loss caused by these drugs, speak to your physician about taking 500–1,000 mcg biotin, 250–1,000 mg inositol, 25–100 mg thiamin, 25–100 mg riboflavin, 50–100 mg niacin, 50–100 mg vitamin B_6, 500–1,000 mcg vitamin B_{12}, 60–80 mcg vitamin K, 100–300 mg potassium, 15 billion live *Bifidobacterium bifidum* organisms, and 15 billion live *Lactobacillus acidophilus* organisms per day.

You can also eat foods that contain the depleted nutrients:

- Biotin: beef liver, soybeans, rice bran, peanut butter, barley
- Inositol: cantaloupe, oranges, green beans, grapefruit juice, limes
- Thiamin: braised liver, turkey heart, roasted chicken, gefilte fish, sardines
- Riboflavin: dried sunflower seeds, orange juice, bulgur, spinach noodles, pine nuts
- Niacin: chicken breast, beef liver, mackerel, barley, bulgur
- Vitamin B_6: potato, banana, garbanzo beans, chicken breast, fortified oatmeal
- Vitamin B_{12}: beef liver, rainbow trout, sockeye salmon, beef, haddock
- Vitamin K: kale, broccoli, parsley, Swiss chard, spinach
- Potassium: dried figs, California avocado, papaya, banana, dates
- *Bifidobacterium bifidum*: Jerusalem artichokes, asparagus, garlic, and onions may stimulate the growth or activity of this probiotic
- *Lactobacillus acidophilus*: yogurt containing live lactobacillus cultures, kefir, acidophilus milk

Consult with your physician before making any changes to your diet or supplemental regimen.

TILUDRONATE (tye-LOO-droe-nate)

Brand Name: Skelid

About Tiludronate

Most of us know that osteoporosis can cause the bones to become thin and more likely to fracture. But few of us know that there's an "opposite" disease that causes the bones to become overgrown.

Paget's disease causes an imbalance in the normal processes of remodeling bones—breaking them down and building them back up again. For unknown reasons, both the bone-building cells (osteoblasts) and the bone-breakdown cells (osteoclasts) become overactive, tearing down and rebuilding bone at a furious pace. The result is twofold: Not only is there too much bone being built in the affected area, but it's poor-quality, weakened bone tissue.

You may not have any symptoms, or you may feel a deep pain in your bones. The overgrown bones can cause additional pain by pressing on nearby nerves, or if they reside in or near a joint, they can throw the joint out of alignment, causing osteoarthritis.

Other symptoms of Paget's disease depend on the location of the overgrown, abnormal bone tissue. If it involves the bones in your skull, there can be pressure on the nerves, causing headaches or damage to the inner ear. If the nerves running from your ear to your brain are affected, you may suffer from dizziness and hearing problems. Paget's can also cause your skull to get larger, forcing you to buy a bigger hat. If your vertebrae become overgrown, your spine may weaken and collapse, leaving you with a "dowager's hump." The resulting pressure on the spinal nerves can cause anything from pain to paralysis of the legs.

Tiludronate, one of the medicines used to treat Paget's disease, works by slowing the action of the osteoclasts and thus the breakdown of bone tissue.

Possible Side Effects

The drug's more common side effects include chest pain, nausea, diarrhea, nasal and sinus inflammation, dizziness, and heartburn.

Which Nutrients Are Robbed

Taking this medicine may deplete your supply of, increase your need for, or interfere with the activity of:

- Calcium

Additional Ways This Drug May Upset Your Nutritional Balance

Tiludronate can cause heartburn, nausea, and vomiting, all of which can upset your eating habits and possibly interfere with good nutrition. It can also cause diarrhea, which can hamper nutrient absorption.

Restoring Your Nutritional Balance

To compensate for the nutrient loss caused by this drug, speak to your physician about taking 1,200 mg calcium per day.

You can also eat foods that contain the depleted nutrient:

- Calcium: milk, dried figs, Swiss cheese, yogurt, tofu

Consult with your physician before making any changes to your diet or supplemental regimen.

TIMOLOL (TYE-moe-lole)

Brand Names: Apo-Timol, Apo-Timop, Betimol Ophthalmic, Blocadren Oral, Gen-Timolol, Novo-Timol, Nu-Timolol, Timoptic Ophthalmic, Timoptic-XE Ophthalmic

About Timolol

Timolol is a beta-blocker used to treat glaucoma. Normally when we think of beta-blockers, we think of elevated blood pressure, angina, and other heart-related ailments. But doctors accidentally discovered that certain beta-blockers could also reduce the pressure inside the eyeball, which makes them useful for treating glaucoma.

A major cause of blindness, glaucoma is caused by the buildup of excessive fluid within the eyeball, which damages the optic nerve. One form of glaucoma begins with no obvious symptoms. But later on you may notice strange things, like blind spots, a loss of peripheral vision, and other problems. Another form of the disease hits hard and fast—if untreated it may rob you of your vision in just a few hours.

If the glaucoma has been triggered by an infection, a tumor, or an eye injury, the excessive pressure in the eyeball may fade away once the underlying problem has been handled. But sometimes there is no obvious trigger.

Medicines such as timolol can be used to reduce the pressure of glaucoma. When applied directly to the eye, timolol appears to work by lowering the production of fluid in the eye. Less fluid means less pressure. In addition to treating glaucoma, timolol taken in pill form is used to treat elevated blood pressure, migraine headaches, and other ailments.

Possible Side Effects

When used for glaucoma, the drug's side effects include pain in the eye and staining of the cornea. When used for other purposes, the drug can trigger insomnia, drowsiness, a slow heartbeat, and cold extremities.

Which Nutrients Are Robbed

Taking this medicine may deplete your supply of, increase your need for, or interfere with the activity of:

- Coenzyme Q_{10} • Melatonin

Additional Ways This Drug May Upset Your Nutritional Balance

Timolol can cause stomach discomfort, nausea, and vomiting, all of which can upset your eating habits and possibly interfere with good nutrition. It can also cause diarrhea, which can hamper nutrient absorption.

Restoring Your Nutritional Balance

To compensate for the nutrient loss caused by this drug, speak to your physician about taking 30–100 mg coenzyme Q_{10} and 1–3 mg melatonin per day.

You can also eat foods that contain the depleted nutrient:

- Coenzyme Q_{10}: beef, chicken, trout, salmon, oranges, broccoli

Consult with your physician before making any changes to your diet or supplemental regimen.

TOBRAMYCIN (toe-bruh-MYE-sin)

Brand Names: AKTob, Nebcin, Tobrex

About Tobramycin

We may think of a battle between the immune system and invading bacteria as a toe-to-toe slug 'em out, with each side using the biochemical equivalent of sledgehammers to bash the other into submission. But that's not how it works. True, there's some of that, with the giant macrophages attempting to engulf and devour the germs. But much of the battle is based on clever, constantly evolving tactics. It's safe to say that although many of the germs in your body today have the same names and characteristics as they did 30 years ago, they also have new weapons and survival strategies.

Fortunately, we have a variety of antibiotics that can attack bacteria in different ways. These include a group called the aminoglycosides, which worm their way through the bacteria's cellular membrane and take up residence inside the invader. Once inside, they interfere with the bacteria's protein manufacturing processes, causing it to misread its messenger RNA, so the wrong amino acids are put together. The resulting proteins just don't work, and the bacteria dies.

But many strains of bacteria have figured out how to keep the aminoglycosides at bay, primarily by secreting enzymes that deactivate them. They have also evolved in ways that keep these medicines from getting through their cell membranes.

Fortunately, a number of bacteria that cause severe infections still cannot resist aminoglycosides such as tobramycin. This means that tobramycin can be used to treat a variety of infections, including some affecting the eye.

Possible Side Effects

The drug's more common side effects include damage to hearing, nerves, and kidneys.

Which Nutrients Are Robbed

Taking this medicine may deplete your supply of, increase your need for, or interfere with the activity of:

- Biotin
- Inositol
- Thiamin
- Riboflavin
- Niacin
- Vitamin B_6
- Vitamin B_{12}
- Vitamin K
- Calcium
- Magnesium
- Potassium
- Sodium
- *Bifidobacterium bifidum*
- *Lactobacillus acidophilus*

Restoring Your Nutritional Balance

To compensate for the nutrient loss caused by this drug, speak to your physician about taking 500–1,000 mcg biotin, 250–1,000 mg inositol, 25–100 mg thiamin, 25–100 mg riboflavin, 50–100 mg niacin, 50–100 mg vitamin B_6,

500–1,000 mcg vitamin B$_{12}$, 60–80 mcg vitamin K, 1,200 mg calcium, 500–1,000 mg magnesium, 100–300 mg potassium, 15 billion live *Bifidobacterium bifidum* organisms, and 15 billion live *Lactobacillus acidophilus* organisms per day. And ask your physician to consider the potential effects of sodium depletion.

You can also eat foods that contain the depleted nutrients:

- Biotin: beef liver, soybeans, rice bran, peanut butter, barley
- Inositol: cantaloupe, oranges, green beans, grapefruit juice, limes
- Thiamin: braised liver, turkey heart, roasted chicken, gefilte fish, sardines
- Riboflavin: dried sunflower seeds, orange juice, bulgur, spinach noodles, pine nuts
- Niacin: chicken breast, beef liver, mackerel, barley, bulgur
- Vitamin B$_6$: potato, banana, garbanzo beans, chicken breast, fortified oatmeal
- Vitamin B$_{12}$: beef liver, rainbow trout, sockeye salmon, beef, haddock
- Vitamin K: kale, broccoli, parsley, Swiss chard, spinach
- Calcium: milk, dried figs, Swiss cheese, yogurt, tofu
- Magnesium: Florida avocado, toasted wheat germ, almonds, shredded wheat cereal, pumpkin seeds
- Potassium: dried figs, California avocado, papaya, banana, dates
- *Bifidobacterium bifidum*: Jerusalem artichokes, asparagus, garlic, and onions may stimulate the growth or activity of this probiotic
- *Lactobacillus acidophilus*: yogurt containing live lactobacillus cultures, kefir, acidophilus milk

Consult with your physician before making any changes to your diet or supplemental regimen.

TOLAZAMIDE (tole-AZ-uh-mide)

Brand Name: Tolinase

About Tolazamide

Tolazamide is a member of the sulfonylurea group of medicines, which have long been used to treat type 2 diabetes.

Diabetes is a disease of access and excess. Certain cells in the body are unable to access (or accept) the glucose in the blood, even though they desperately need it. So the excess glucose in the bloodstream builds up to higher and higher levels that can eventually cause damage to the blood vessels, nerves, kidneys, and eyes, among other body tissues and organs.

How does this happen? After a meal, carbohydrates from your food or drink are converted into glucose, which flows through the bloodstream destined for hungry cells. But when it reaches certain cells that need it, it can't just float in by itself. It needs the help of a hormone called insulin.

You can think of insulin as a tugboat nudging a ship into place at a dock. The insulin tugs and pushes blood glucose into docking sites on cell membranes, where it can be taken up by the cells. After delivering the glucose, the insulin is reabsorbed by the body.

But sometimes, the insulin can't deliver its cargo. The undelivered blood sugar backs up in the bloodstream, rising to unhealthy levels and causing diabetes. With type 1 diabetes, the body doesn't make enough insulin to do the job. With type 2 diabetes, the body may make adequate amounts of insulin, but the cells don't respond to it the way they should. It's as if the cellular docks are at least partially shut down, and the normal amount of tugboats can't nudge the glucose into place.

Tolazamide and the other sulfonylureas work by encouraging the pancreas to produce more insulin. In a sense, the body produces many more tugboats than ordinarily necessary to get the insulin into place, forcing the docks to open and receive the goods.

Tolazamide is used to treat mild to moderately severe type 2 diabetes.

Possible Side Effects

The drug's side effects include rash, yellowing of the skin or whites of the eyes, and low blood sugar.

Which Nutrients Are Robbed

Taking this medicine may deplete your supply of, increase your need for, or interfere with the activity of:

- Coenzyme Q_{10}

Additional Ways This Drug May Upset Your Nutritional Balance

Tolazamide can cause loss of appetite, stomach upset, nausea, and vomiting, all of which can upset your eating habits and possibly interfere with good nutrition.

Restoring Your Nutritional Balance

To compensate for the nutrient loss caused by this drug, speak to your physician about taking 30–100 mg coenzyme Q_{10} per day.

You can also eat foods that contain the depleted nutrient:

- Coenzyme Q_{10}: beef, chicken, trout, salmon, oranges, broccoli

Consult with your physician before making any changes to your diet or supplemental regimen.

TOLBUTAMIDE (tole-BYOO-tuh-mide)

Brand Names: Apo-Tolbutamide, Novo-Butamide, Orinase

About Tolbutamide

Tolbutamide is used to treat mild to moderately severe type 2 diabetes. It works by encouraging the pancreas to produce more insulin, which helps to shepherd excess blood glucose into select body cells, where it can be used for fuel or stored for future use.

Tolbutamide has a short half-life of four to five hours, which means that half of a dose of the medicine is metabolized, or used up, within a relatively short period of time. This is important because diabetes medications can go overboard and produce the opposite effect: That is, they can push the blood sugar down too far, causing low blood sugar (hypoglycemia). Since tolbutamide is used up quickly, it's safer for the elderly, who can't tolerate low blood sugar for long.

Possible Side Effects

The drug's side effects include headache, and high or low blood sugar.

Which Nutrients Are Robbed

Taking this medicine may deplete your supply of, increase your need for, or interfere with the activity of:

- Coenzyme Q_{10}

Additional Ways This Drug May Upset Your Nutritional Balance

Tolbutamide can cause loss of appetite, stomach upset, nausea, and vomiting, all of which can upset your eating habits and possibly interfere with good nutrition.

Restoring Your Nutritional Balance

To compensate for the nutrient loss caused by this drug, speak to your physician about taking 30–100 mg coenzyme Q_{10} per day.

You can also eat foods that contain the depleted nutrient:

- Coenzyme Q_{10}: beef, chicken, trout, salmon, oranges, broccoli

Consult with your physician before making any changes to your diet or supplemental regimen.

TOLMETIN (TOLE-met-in)

Brand Names: Novo-Tolmetin, Tolectin, Tolectin DS

About Tolmetin

The words "rheumatoid arthritis" usually call to mind the gnarled hands of a senior citizen, but this disease can also strike youngsters. In fact, close to 300,000 American children under the age of seventeen suffer from symptoms of this disease. When it strikes children, it's called juvenile rheumatoid arthritis, or JRA.

The junior version is very much like the adult form, causing inflammation of the joints and/or connective tissues. Symptoms include pain, swelling and stiffness of the joints, and possibly fever, eye inflammation, swollen lymph nodes, inflammation of the lining of the heart, and other problems.

Doctors give youngsters with JRA a variety of drugs, including tolmetin, which helps relieve pain and inflammation. The drug's painkilling properties kick into action an hour or two after it's taken, but it takes a few days or weeks for tolmetin to begin to reduce the swelling.

Possible Side Effects

The drug's more common side effects include high blood pressure, depression, weight gain or loss, and stomach upset.

Which Nutrients Are Robbed

Taking this medicine may deplete your supply of, increase your need for, or interfere with the activity of:

- Folic acid

Additional Ways This Drug May Upset Your Nutritional Balance

Tolmetin can cause abdominal pain, gastritis, heartburn, nausea, and vomiting, all of which can upset your eating habits and possibly interfere with good nutrition. It can also cause diarrhea, which can hamper nutrient absorption.

Restoring Your Nutritional Balance

To compensate for the nutrient loss caused by this drug, speak to your physician about taking 400–800 mcg folic acid per day.

You can also eat foods that contain the depleted nutrient:

- Folic acid: beef liver, fortified breakfast cereals, spinach, great northern beans, asparagus

Consult with your physician before making any changes to your diet or supplemental regimen.

TORSEMIDE (TOR-se-mide)

Brand Name: Demadex

About Torsemide

Doctors use diuretics to flush out the excess fluid seen in congestive heart failure, kidney disease, and other ailments. There are different kinds of diuretics, including the loop diuretics.

Inside the kidneys, blood flows into tiny funnel-shaped areas called nephrons, where fluid and various substances are filtered out. What's left—what will become the urine—flows into a very squiggly tube. At one point the tube drops straight down, does a U-turn, and heads back up. This is called the loop of Henle. Loop diuretics get their name from the fact that they perform their medicinal chores in Henle's loop.

Torsemide, a loop diuretic, works by preventing the reabsorption of

sodium and chloride and sending them off for excretion. Because the combination of sodium and chloride (table salt) draws water, these minerals
"pull" water out of the body as they are excreted. This makes torsemide useful for treating elevated blood pressure, congestive heart failure, or other
conditions in which fluid builds up within the body.

Possible Side Effects

The drug's more common side effects include headache, excessive urination, dizziness, and diarrhea.

Which Nutrients Are Robbed

Taking this medicine may deplete your supply of, increase your need for,
or interfere with the activity of:

- Thiamin
- Vitamin B_6
- Vitamin C
- Calcium
- Chloride
- Magnesium
- Potassium
- Sodium
- Zinc

Additional Ways This Drug May Upset Your Nutritional Balance

Torsemide can cause a feeling of bloating, heartburn, and nausea, all of
which can upset your eating habits and possibly interfere with good nutrition.
It can also cause diarrhea, which can hamper nutrient absorption.

Restoring Your Nutritional Balance

To compensate for the nutrient loss caused by this drug, speak to your
physician about taking 25–100 mg thiamin, 50–100 mg vitamin B_6, 250–1,500
mg vitamin C, 1,200 mg calcium, 500–1,000 mg magnesium, and 50–200 mg
zinc per day. And ask your physician to consider the potential effects of
sodium and chloride depletion.

A Note on Potassium: "Regular" diuretics lower potassium levels, while
potassium-sparing diuretics do not—they may increase levels instead. It is
not uncommon for doctors to prescribe two different diuretics. That's why
you should speak to your physician about your potassium levels, and whether
it is appropriate for you to take supplements or eat potassium-rich foods.

You can also eat foods that contain the depleted nutrients:

- Thiamin: braised liver, turkey heart, roasted chicken, gefilte fish, sardines
- Vitamin B_6: potato, banana, garbanzo beans, chicken breast, fortified
  oatmeal

- Vitamin C: papaya, guava, red pepper, cantaloupe, black currants
- Calcium: milk, dried figs, Swiss cheese, yogurt, tofu
- Magnesium: Florida avocado, toasted wheat germ, almonds, shredded wheat cereal, pumpkin seeds
- Zinc: oysters, beef shank, chicken, pork tenderloin, plain yogurt

Consult with your physician before making any changes to your diet or supplemental regimen.

TRANDOLAPRIL, TRANDOLAPRIL PLUS VERAPAMIL
(tran-DOE-luh-pril, ver-AP-uh-mil)

Brand Names: Trandolapril: Mavik
Trandolapril plus verapamil: Tarka

About Trandolapril, Trandolapril plus Verapamil

The body has several ways to raise the blood pressure, and you definitely want to be able to raise it, and fast, at the right time. It's only when blood pressure goes up inappropriately that you have a problem. Unfortunately, some 50 million Americans have chronically elevated blood pressure, or hypertension. Some 15 million of those who have hypertension don't even know they have the problem, so they aren't doing anything to treat it. And of the 35 million who do know, almost two-thirds are either getting inadequate treatment or no treatment at all.

Trandolapril is an ACE inhibitor, which means that it inhibits, or derails, ACE. ACE stands for angiotensin converting enzyme, a substance that converts the relatively inactive angiotensin I into the active angiotensin II, a blood pressure–raising powerhouse. By inhibiting this conversion, trandolapril helps to stifle the internal biochemical "urge" to raise blood pressure, thus keeping the pressure down to safer levels.

Trandolapril may be used alone or combined with verapamil. A calcium channel blocker, verapamil combats elevated blood pressure by slowing the movement of calcium into the muscles surrounding the small arteries. These muscles need calcium to work, so depriving them of this mineral makes it harder for them to contract and narrow the blood's passageway. (Narrowed arteries can raise the pressure.) By keeping the blood vessels open and wide, verapamil helps the blood pressure fall to more normal levels.

Trandolapril is used to treat elevated blood pressure and problems with the heart's left ventricle after a heart attack. Trandolapril plus verapamil is often prescribed for hypertension when either drug by itself isn't producing the desired result.

Possible Side Effects

Trandolapril's side effects include a lack of energy and strength, fainting, a slow heartbeat, and intermittent limping. Verapamil's side effects include constipation, slow heartbeat, and fatigue.

Which Nutrients Are Robbed

Taking these medicines may deplete your supply of, increase your need for, or interfere with the activity of:

- Calcium
- Zinc

Additional Ways This Drug May Upset Your Nutritional Balance

Trandolapril can cause heartburn and nausea, while verapamil can cause nausea. These side effects can upset your eating habits and possibly interfere with good nutrition.

Trandolapril can also trigger hyperkalemia, or too much potassium in the blood.

Restoring Your Nutritional Balance

To compensate for the nutrient loss caused by this drug, speak to your physician about taking 1,200 mg calcium and 50–200 mg zinc per day.

You can also eat foods that contain the depleted nutrients:

- Calcium: milk, dried figs, Swiss cheese, yogurt, tofu
- Zinc: oysters, beef shank, chicken, pork tenderloin, plain yogurt

Consult with your physician before making any changes to your diet or supplemental regimen.

TRIAMCINOLONE (trye-am-SIN-oh-lohn)

Brand Names: Amcort, Aristocort ("regular," A, Forte, Intralesional), Aristospan (Intra-Articular, Intralesional), Atolone, Azmacort, Delta-Tritex, Flutex, Kenacort, Kenaject-40, Kenalog ("regular," -10, -40, H, in

Orabase), Kenonel, Nasacort ("regular," AQ), Tac (-3, -40), Triacet, Triam (-A, Forte), Triderm, Tri-Kort, Trilog, Trilone, Tri-Nasal Spray, Tristoject

About Triamcinolone

Systemic lupus erythematosus (often referred to as lupus, or SLE) is a puzzling disease that prefers women to men, striking females eight times more often than males. Women are particularly at risk during their childbearing years. Yet experts are still uncertain about what causes lupus, why it strikes women much more often than men, and how to cure it. We have many theories, but no definitive answers.

Lupus is an autoimmune disease, which means that the immune system's antibodies, designed to destroy invaders, turn against healthy body tissue. We don't know why this happens, although stress, certain infections, and pregnancy seem to be predisposing factors.

Depending on which part of the body is attacked, symptoms may include fever, weight loss, fatigue, nausea, diarrhea, rashes, and joint pain. Women may have menstrual difficulties, there may be problems with the heart and lungs, and exposure to sunlight may cause skin eruptions.

Triamcinolone is used to ease lupus-related skin eruptions, as well as to treat allergic rhinitis, bronchial asthma, adrenocortical insufficiency, rheumatic disorders, allergies, and other diseases in which inflammation or an errant immune system is a problem.

Possible Side Effects

The drug's side effects include stomach upset, elevated blood pressure, fever, and vertigo.

Which Nutrients Are Robbed

Taking this medicine may deplete your supply of, increase your need for, or interfere with the activity of:

- Vitamin A
- Vitamin B_6
- Folic acid
- Vitamin C
- Vitamin D
- Vitamin K
- Calcium
- Magnesium
- Potassium
- Selenium
- Zinc

Additional Ways This Drug May Upset Your Nutritional Balance

Triamcinolone can cause abdominal distension, heartburn, and nausea, all of which can upset your eating habits and possibly interfere with good nutrition. It can also cause diarrhea, which can hamper nutrient absorption.

Restoring Your Nutritional Balance

To compensate for the nutrient loss caused by this drug, speak to your physician about taking 5,000 IU vitamin A, 50–100 mg vitamin B$_6$, 400–800 mcg folic acid, 250–1,500 mg vitamin C, 400 IU vitamin D, 60–80 mcg vitamin K, 1,200 mg calcium, 500–1,000 mg magnesium, 100–300 mg potassium, 20–100 mcg selenium, and 50–200 mg zinc per day.

You can also eat foods that contain the depleted nutrients:

- Vitamin A: beef liver, chicken liver, cheese pizza, whole milk, cheddar cheese
- Vitamin B$_6$: potato, banana, garbanzo beans, chicken breast, fortified oatmeal
- Folic acid: beef liver, fortified breakfast cereals, spinach, great northern beans, asparagus
- Vitamin C: papaya, guava, red pepper, cantaloupe, black currants
- Vitamin D: salmon, mackerel, sardines, eel, fortified milk
- Vitamin K: kale, broccoli, parsley, Swiss chard, spinach
- Calcium: milk, dried figs, Swiss cheese, yogurt, tofu
- Magnesium: Florida avocado, toasted wheat germ, almonds, shredded wheat cereal, pumpkin seeds
- Potassium: dried figs, California avocado, papaya, banana, dates
- Selenium: Brazil nuts, tuna, beef liver, turkey breast, spaghetti with meat sauce
- Zinc: oysters, beef shank, chicken, pork tenderloin, plain yogurt

Consult with your physician before making any changes to your diet or supplemental regimen.

TRIAMTERENE (trye-AM-ter-een)

Brand Name: Dyrenium

About Triamterene

Triamterene is a diuretic designed to draw fluid out of the body. Your doctor may want to use it if you have elevated blood pressure. Having less fluid in the blood means the heart doesn't have to work quite as hard to pump it through the circulatory system, so the blood pressure will drop. Your doctor may also prescribe triamterene if you have an accumulation of fluid in your abdominal cavity (a condition called ascites) or congestive heart failure, which can cause a buildup of fluid in your feet, ankles, lungs, or elsewhere.

Although triamterene is not as powerful as some other diuretics, it is often used because it "spares" potassium. Some diuretics flush potassium and other substances out of the body along with the excess fluid, which may cause muscle spasms, paralysis, and other problems. But triamterene helps the kidneys hold on to potassium, so the excess water goes out, but potassium stays.

Triamterene taken alone is not effective for everyone who has a problem with fluid buildup, so it's often combined with other diuretics. But whether alone or in combination, triamterene does spare potassium and is used to treat hypertension, congestive heart failure, ascites, and other conditions involving excess fluid.

Possible Side Effects

The drug's side effects include cramps, excessively high potassium levels, and kidney stones.

Which Nutrients Are Robbed

Taking this medicine may deplete your supply of, increase your need for, or interfere with the activity of:

- Folic acid
- Calcium
- Magnesium
- Zinc

Additional Ways This Drug May Upset Your Nutritional Balance

Triamterene can trigger hyperkalemia, or too much potassium in the blood.

Restoring Your Nutritional Balance

To compensate for the nutrient loss caused by this drug, speak to your physician about taking 400–800 mcg folic acid, 1,200 mg calcium, and 50–200 mg zinc per day.

There is some concern that potassium-sparing diuretics such as triamterene may cause the body to retain magnesium, so ask your physician to monitor your magnesium level.

A Note on Potassium: "Regular" diuretics lower potassium levels, while potassium-sparing diuretics do not—they may increase levels instead. It is not uncommon for doctors to prescribe two different diuretics. That's why you should speak to your physician about your potassium levels, and whether it is appropriate for you to take supplements or eat potassium-rich foods.

You can also eat foods that contain the depleted nutrients:

- Folic acid: beef liver, fortified breakfast cereals, spinach, great northern beans, asparagus
- Calcium: milk, dried figs, Swiss cheese, yogurt, tofu
- Zinc: oysters, beef shank, chicken, pork tenderloin, plain yogurt

Consult with your physician before making any changes to your diet or supplemental regimen.

TRIFLUOPERAZINE (trye-floo-oh-PER-uh-zeen)

Brand Names: Stelazine, Novo-Trifluzine

About Trifluoperazine

There's no obvious sign—like a fever or red spots on the skin—to announce that schizophrenia has set in. Instead, doctors look for a pattern of behaviors that may include:

- Seeing or hearing people or things that aren't there
- Losing contact with reality
- Feeling like someone is watching you, or perhaps some device is monitoring you
- Behaving inappropriately
- Radically changing your appearance for no apparent reason
- Losing interest in important events at work, school, or home
- Becoming inappropriately angry or fearful
- Having trouble concentrating
- Moving your arms and legs without purpose
- Withdrawing from social situations

If these behaviors are not caused by a tumor, Huntington's disease, thyroid disease, or another ailment, schizophrenia may be suspected.

We don't fully understand what causes the disease, or why certain drugs can help control the symptoms. One of the more likely hypotheses is that schizophrenia is linked to excess activity of the neurotransmitter dopamine in the brain.

Trifluoperazine is sometimes prescribed for schizophrenia. Although it doesn't cure the underlying problem, it does reduce both dopamine activity in the brain and the symptoms of schizophrenia.

Possible Side Effects

The drug's side effects include stomach upset, heart attack, skin discoloration, nasal congestion, and liver damage.

Which Nutrients Are Robbed

Taking this medicine may deplete your supply of, increase your need for, or interfere with the activity of:

- Riboflavin
- Coenzyme Q_{10}

Additional Ways This Drug May Upset Your Nutritional Balance

Trifluoperazine can cause low blood sugar (hypoglycemia), stomach pain, nausea, and vomiting, all of which can upset your eating habits and possibly interfere with good nutrition.

Restoring Your Nutritional Balance

To compensate for the nutrient loss caused by this drug, speak to your physician about taking 25–100 mg riboflavin and 30–100 mg coenzyme Q_{10} per day.

You can also eat foods that contain the depleted nutrients:

- Riboflavin: dried sunflower seeds, orange juice, bulgur, spinach noodles, pine nuts
- Coenzyme Q_{10}: beef, chicken, trout, salmon, oranges, broccoli

Consult with your physician before making any changes to your diet or supplemental regimen.

TRIMETHOPRIM (trye-METH-oh-prim)

Brand Names: Primsol, Proloprim, Trimpex

About Trimethoprim

Trimethoprim is an antibiotic that works by interfering with the conversion of dihydrofolic acid into DNA inside the bacterial cell. Unable to manufacture new DNA, the bacterium cannot replicate itself and the invading bacterial army cannot grow. Trimethoprim may be used for infections of the urinary tract, or combined with sulfamethoxazole to treat respiratory tract infections, *Pneumocystis carinii* pneumonia, shigellosis, and salmonella infections.

Salmonella typhi is the bacteria that causes typhoid fever, a disease that turned an unknown Wild West cook named Mary Mallon into the infamous Typhoid Mary. This bacteria is found in the urine and stools of infected people. We don't know how Mary got typhoid, but sanitary conditions being what they were—or were not—back then, she probably transferred the germs to her hands after visiting the outhouse. Then she passed them to the food she prepared and served to unsuspecting customers. (Her symptoms must have been mild enough that she could continue cooking and serving food.)

Mary's customers became infected when the bacteria entered their digestive systems and passed into their bloodstreams. Their first symptoms, which probably appeared a week or two later, may have included fever, headache, sore throat, constipation, loss of appetite, abdominal and joint pain, and a nonproductive cough. As the high fever continued, they became delirious and exhausted. Some of them developed pink spots on the chest and abdomen or gastrointestinal bleeding. Within a couple weeks, perhaps 25 percent of Typhoid Mary's victims died.

Today, antibiotic treatments for typhoid can cure almost everyone. One of the antibiotics used is trimethoprim, which is given in combination with sulfamethoxazole to treat typhoid.

Possible Side Effects

Trimethoprim's side effects include stomach upset, fever, rash, and changes in the white blood cells.

Which Nutrients Are Robbed

Taking this medicine may deplete your supply of, increase your need for, or interfere with the activity of:

- Biotin
- Folic acid
- Inositol
- Thiamin
- Riboflavin
- Niacin

- Vitamin B_6
- Vitamin B_{12}
- Vitamin K
- Sodium
- *Bifidobacterium bifidum*
- *Lactobacillus acidophilus*

Additional Ways This Drug May Upset Your Nutritional Balance

Trimethoprim can cause nausea and vomiting, which can upset your eating habits and possibly interfere with good nutrition.

This drug can also trigger hyperkalemia, or too much potassium in the blood.

Restoring Your Nutritional Balance

To compensate for the nutrient loss caused by this drug, speak to your physician about taking 500–1,000 mcg biotin, 400–800 mcg folic acid, 250–1,000 mg inositol, 25–100 mg thiamin, 25–100 mg riboflavin, 50–100 mg niacin, 50–100 mg vitamin B_6, 500–1,000 mcg vitamin B_{12}, 60–80 mcg vitamin K, 15 billion live *Bifidobacterium bifidum* organisms, and 15 billion live *Lactobacillus acidophilus* organisms per day. And ask your physician to consider the potential effects of sodium depletion.

You can also eat foods that contain the depleted nutrients:

- Biotin: beef liver, soybeans, rice bran, peanut butter, barley
- Folic acid: beef liver, fortified breakfast cereals, spinach, great northern beans, asparagus
- Inositol: cantaloupe, oranges, green beans, grapefruit juice, limes
- Thiamin: braised liver, turkey heart, roasted chicken, gefilte fish, sardines
- Riboflavin: dried sunflower seeds, orange juice, bulgur, spinach noodles, pine nuts
- Niacin: chicken breast, beef liver, mackerel, barley, bulgur
- Vitamin B_6: potato, banana, garbanzo beans, chicken breast, fortified oatmeal
- Vitamin B_{12}: beef liver, rainbow trout, sockeye salmon, beef, haddock
- Vitamin K: kale, broccoli, parsley, Swiss chard, spinach
- *Bifidobacterium bifidum*: Jerusalem artichokes, asparagus, garlic, and onions may stimulate the growth or activity of this probiotic
- *Lactobacillus acidophilus*: yogurt containing live lactobacillus cultures, kefir, acidophilus milk

Consult with your physician before making any changes to your diet or supplemental regimen.

TRIMIPRAMINE (trye-MI-prah-meen)

Brand Names: Apo-Trimip, Novo-Tripramine, Nu-Trimipramine,
Rhotrimine, Surmontil

About Trimipramine

It's not at all rare for a drug that was developed for one purpose to be used for another. In fact, that happened with an entire group of drugs known as the tricyclic antidepressants. At first, researchers thought that these drugs would be used as antihistamines that had a sedative effect. Then it appeared that the tricyclics were good for combating psychoses. Finally, it was accidentally discovered that they were effective as antidepressants.

The tricyclics, so-named for their three-ringed chemical structure, go to work right on the nerve endings, where chemical messengers called neurotransmitters shuttle messages from one nerve cell to another. Some of these neurotransmitters, such as serotonin and norepinephrine, help to lift the mood. Thus, it's good to have a full supply of these two, ready to speed a "we're happy!" message through the nervous system.

Of course, you wouldn't want your brain to be overflowing with "we're happy" messages all the time. That would rob you of your incentive to work and take care of yourself, perhaps even to feed yourself. That's why the body has reuptake pumps to pull away the excess. Trimipramine and the other tricyclics work by blocking these reuptake pumps and allowing serotonin and norepinephrine to remain in action longer and build up to higher levels.

Possible Side Effects

The drug's side effects include low blood pressure, heart palpitations, headache, and insomnia.

Which Nutrients Are Robbed

Taking this medicine may deplete your supply of, increase your need for, or interfere with the activity of:

- Riboflavin
- Coenzyme Q_{10}
- Sodium

Additional Ways This Drug May Upset Your Nutritional Balance

Trimipramine can cause changes in taste, heartburn, loss of appetite, nausea, and vomiting, all of which can upset your eating habits and possibly interfere with good nutrition. It can also cause diarrhea, which can hamper nutrient absorption.

Restoring Your Nutritional Balance

To compensate for the nutrient loss caused by this drug, speak to your physician about taking 25–100 mg riboflavin and 30–100 mg coenzyme Q_{10} per day. And ask your physician to consider the potential effects of sodium depletion.

You can also eat foods that contain the depleted nutrients:

- Riboflavin: dried sunflower seeds, orange juice, bulgur, spinach noodles, pine nuts
- Coenzyme Q_{10}: beef, chicken, trout, salmon, oranges, broccoli

Consult with your physician before making any changes to your diet or supplemental regimen.

TROVAFLOXACIN (TROE-vuh-floks-uh-sin)

Brand Name: Trovan

About Trovafloxacin

Everybody suffers from occasional bacterial infections, such as respiratory infections, conjunctivitis, a mild infection that settles in a cut or scrape, and so on. Most come and go without much problem, while other, more serious infections (perhaps a bladder or prostate infection) are usually taken care of with a short course of antibiotics. But there are a few, such as bacterial pneumonia, that demand stronger treatments.

Most bacterial infections are kept to limited areas within the body. But if the bacteria escape from the site of the infection and invade the bloodstream (a condition known as sepsis), you may develop chills, shaking, weakness, and fever. In severe cases, the body may go into septic shock, a condition in which the bacteria in the bloodstream trigger a crash in blood pressure and malfunction of the organs, which can be fatal.

But even if the bacteria stay out of the bloodstream, if they continue to grow at the site of the infection, they can devour nearby healthy tissues. In the most serious cases, an infected limb may have to be amputated.

Before taking such drastic measures, doctors may prescribe an antibiotic such as trovafloxacin. Used for hospital-acquired and community-acquired infections, as well as gynecological, pelvic, and skin infections that have reached crisis proportions, trovafloxacin can cause potentially fatal liver reactions. For this reason, it is administered only in hospitals or other in-patient facilities.

Possible Side Effects

The drug's more common side effects include severe liver damage, dizziness, nausea, and headache.

Which Nutrients Are Robbed

Taking this medicine may deplete your supply of, increase your need for, or interfere with the activity of:

- Biotin
- Inositol
- Thiamin
- Riboflavin
- Niacin
- Vitamin B_6
- Vitamin B_{12}
- Vitamin K
- Zinc
- *Bifidobacterium bifidum*
- *Lactobacillus acidophilus*

Additional Ways This Drug May Upset Your Nutritional Balance

Trovafloxacin can cause abdominal pain, nausea, and vomiting, all of which can upset your eating habits and possibly interfere with good nutrition.

Restoring Your Nutritional Balance

To compensate for the nutrient loss caused by this drug, speak to your physician about taking 500–1,000 mcg biotin, 250–1,000 mg inositol, 25–100 mg thiamin, 25–100 mg riboflavin, 50–100 mg niacin, 50–100 mg vitamin B_6, 500–1,000 mcg vitamin B_{12}, 60–80 mcg vitamin K, 50–200 mg zinc, 15 billion live *Bifidobacterium bifidum* organisms, and 15 billion live *Lactobacillus acidophilus* organisms per day.

You can also eat foods that contain the depleted nutrients:

- Biotin: beef liver, soybeans, rice bran, peanut butter, barley
- Inositol: cantaloupe, oranges, green beans, grapefruit juice, limes

- Thiamin: braised liver, turkey heart, roasted chicken, gefilte fish, sardines
- Riboflavin: dried sunflower seeds, orange juice, bulgur, spinach noodles, pine nuts
- Niacin: chicken breast, beef liver, mackerel, barley, bulgur
- Vitamin B_6: potato, banana, garbanzo beans, chicken breast, fortified oatmeal
- Vitamin B_{12}: beef liver, rainbow trout, sockeye salmon, beef, haddock
- Vitamin K: kale, broccoli, parsley, Swiss chard, spinach
- Zinc: oysters, beef shank, chicken, pork tenderloin, plain yogurt
- *Bifidobacterium bifidum:* Jerusalem artichokes, asparagus, garlic, and onions may stimulate the growth or activity of this probiotic
- *Lactobacillus acidophilus:* yogurt containing live lactobacillus cultures, kefir, acidophilus milk

Consult with your physician before making any changes to your diet or supplemental regimen.

VALPROIC ACID (val-PROE-ik ASS-id)

Brand Names: Alti-Valproic, Depakene, Depakote, Deproic, Dom-Valproic, Med-Valproic, Novo-Valproic, PMS-Volproic Acid

About Valproic Acid

Valproic acid is used to treat different types of seizures and the mania seen in bipolar disorder. It's also used to prevent migraine headaches.

Valproic acid increases the levels of a substance called GABA in the brain, although exactly how it does this and whether it's the increase in GABA that actually quells seizures is not clear. There's also evidence suggesting that valproic acid changes the way potassium is handled in the brain. Although no one is sure whether either of these mechanisms affect seizures, valproic acid *does* seem to be effective in treating certain types of seizures.

Valproic acid is also used to help prevent migraine headaches (although once again, exactly how it works hasn't been established) and to calm mania. It's believed to be as good as lithium in the early stages of treatment for bipolar disorder and may be an effective substitute for those who don't respond to lithium.

Possible Side Effects

The drug's more common side effects include excessive sleepiness, dizziness, nausea, diarrhea, and hair loss.

Which Nutrients Are Robbed

Taking this medicine may deplete your supply of, increase your need for, or interfere with the activity of:

- Folic acid
- Vitamin B_{12}
- Vitamin D
- Selenium
- Sodium
- Carnitine
- Melatonin

Additional Ways This Drug May Upset Your Nutritional Balance

Valproic acid can cause abdominal pain, loss of appetite, nausea, and vomiting, all of which can upset your eating habits and possibly interfere with good nutrition. It can also cause diarrhea, which can hamper nutrient absorption.

Restoring Your Nutritional Balance

To compensate for the nutrient loss caused by this drug, speak to your physician about taking 500–1,000 mcg vitamin B_{12}, 400 IU vitamin D, 20–100 mcg selenium, 250–1,000 mg carnitine, and 1–3 mg melatonin per day. And ask your physician to consider the potential effects of sodium depletion. Taking folic acid can increase the risk of seizures in some people, so speak to your physician about the use of this nutrient.

You can also eat foods that contain the depleted nutrients:

- Vitamin B_{12}: beef liver, rainbow trout, sockeye salmon, beef, haddock
- Vitamin D: salmon, mackerel, sardines, eel, fortified milk
- Selenium: Brazil nuts, tuna, beef liver, turkey breast, spaghetti with meat sauce
- Carnitine: ground beef, pork, Canadian bacon, whole milk, cod

Consult with your physician before making any changes to your diet or supplemental regimen.

ZALCITABINE (zal-SITE-uh-been)

Brand Name: Hivid

About Zalcitabine

A virus is a tiny parasite that can't live or reproduce on its own. In fact, it's relatively helpless and harmless until it finds its way into a host body—like yours. Once inside, it eases into a body cell where it releases its own DNA or RNA, which takes control of the cell, forcing it to make thousands of copies of the virus. Besides becoming a reluctant "womb" for the virus, the infected cell may lose control over its own functions, become cancerous, or even die.

Antiviral drugs work in several ways, preventing viruses from getting into host cells, hijacking the cell's "machinery," or releasing the newly made viruses. Zalcitabine, which is used to treat HIV infections, is an antiretroviral, which means that it works against viruses that store their genetic information in the form of RNA, rather than DNA. Specifically, the drug is a nucleoside reverse transcriptase inhibitor that prevents HIV from replicating itself inside the human body.

Possible Side Effects

The drug's more common side effects include nerve damage, fever, and malaise.

Which Nutrients Are Robbed

Taking this medicine may deplete your supply of, increase your need for, or interfere with the activity of:

- Carnitine
- Vitamin B_{12}
- Calcium
- Copper
- Magnesium
- Sodium
- Zinc

Additional Ways This Drug May Upset Your Nutritional Balance

Zalcitabine can cause loss of appetite, abdominal pain, low blood sugar (hypoglycemia), nausea, and vomiting, all of which can upset your eating habits and possibly interfere with good nutrition. It can also cause diarrhea, which can hamper nutrient absorption.

Restoring Your Nutritional Balance

To compensate for the nutrient loss caused by this drug, speak to your physician about taking 250–1,000 mg carnitine, 500–1,000 mcg vitamin B_{12}, 1,200 mg calcium, 2 mcg copper, 500–1,000 mg magnesium, and 50–200 mg zinc per day. And ask your physician to consider the potential effects of sodium depletion.

You can also eat foods that contain the depleted nutrients:

- Carnitine: ground beef, pork, Canadian bacon, whole milk, cod
- Vitamin B_{12}: beef liver, rainbow trout, sockeye salmon, beef, haddock
- Calcium: milk, dried figs, Swiss cheese, yogurt, tofu
- Copper: beef liver, almonds, raw mushrooms, hazelnuts, lentils
- Magnesium: Florida avocado, toasted wheat germ, almonds, shredded wheat cereal, pumpkin seeds
- Zinc: oysters, beef shank, chicken, pork tenderloin, plain yogurt

Consult with your physician before making any changes to your diet or supplemental regimen.

ZIDOVUDINE, ZIDOVUDINE PLUS LAMIVUDINE, ZIDOVUDINE PLUS LAMIVUDINE PLUS ABACAVIR

(zye-DOE-vyoo-deen, la-MI-vyoo-deen, uh-BAK-uh-veer)

Brand Names: Zidovudine: Apo-Zidovudine, Novo-AZT, Retrovir
Zidovudine plus lamivudine: AZT + 3TC
Zidovudine plus lamivudine plus abacavir: Trizivir

About Zidovudine, Zidovudine plus Lamivudine, and Zidovudine plus Lamivudine plus Abacavir

Acquired immunodeficiency syndrome (AIDS) is an inexorable, deadly disease that slowly destroys the immune system, leaving the body defenseless against a number of opportunistic infections it would likely shrug off were its natural defenses intact.

AIDS is caused by the human immunodeficiency virus (HIV), which invades the body's cells and turns them into factories that manufacture copies of the virus. But HIV doesn't simply keep the cells busy making virus clones; it ultimately destroys those cells. Because it attacks cells belonging to the immune system, HIV eventually weakens the body's ability to respond to certain infections and cancers.

Zidovudine isn't a cure for AIDS, but it does slow the progression of the disease and increase survival time. This drug is a reverse transcriptase inhibitor, which means that it acts on the virus while it's inside the body's cells. A virus must safely penetrate a cell, uncoat its own nucleic acid, and get the cell to manufacture the DNA and RNA that the virus needs to replicate itself. Then the virus clones are released from the cell to go off and hijack other cells. Zidovudine works by inhibiting the manufacture of new nucleic acids that would be used to make virus clones.

Zidovudine is used in conjunction with other antiviral medications to treat HIV. Drugs are often combined to attack the virus in different ways at the same time and to slow the development of resistant strains. Zidovudine may be combined with lamivudine or with lamivudine plus abacavir. Both lamivudine and abacavir interfere with viral replication.

Possible Side Effects

Zidovudine's more common side effects include severe headache, nausea, vomiting, and pain. Lamivudine's more common side effects include headache, fatigue, and musculoskeletal pain, and abacavir's more common side effects include nausea, vomiting, elevated blood fats, fever, and diarrhea.

Which Nutrients Are Robbed

Taking these medicines may deplete your supply of, increase your need for, or interfere with the activity of:

- Vitamin B$_{12}$
- Copper
- Zinc
- Carnitine

Additional Ways These Drugs May Upset Your Nutritional Balance

The drugs making up this combination treatment can cause loss of appetite, nausea, and vomiting, all of which can upset your eating habits and possibly interfere with good nutrition. In addition, lamivudine can cause abdominal pain, and heartburn. These side effects can upset your eating habits and possibly interfere with good nutrition.

All three drugs can cause diarrhea, which can hamper nutrient absorption.

Restoring Your Nutritional Balance

To compensate for the nutrient loss caused by this drug, speak to your physician about taking 500–1,000 mcg vitamin B$_{12}$, 2 mcg copper, 50–200 mg zinc, and 250–1,000 mg carnitine per day.

You can also eat foods that contain the depleted nutrients:

- Vitamin B$_{12}$: beef liver, rainbow trout, sockeye salmon, beef, haddock
- Copper: beef liver, almonds, raw mushrooms, hazelnuts, lentils
- Zinc: oysters, beef shank, chicken, pork tenderloin, plain yogurt
- Carnitine: ground beef, pork, Canadian bacon, whole milk, cod

Consult with your physician before making any changes to your diet or supplemental regimen.

ZOLEDRONIC ACID (ZOE-le-dron-nik ASS-id)

Brand Name: Zometa

About Zoledronic Acid

Cancer brings to mind a lot of images, none of them pleasant, but there's one we probably wouldn't think about: excessive amounts of calcium in the bloodstream, or hypercalcemia.

Cancers of the lungs, ovaries, and kidneys can cause the secretion of large amounts of a protein that increases blood levels of calcium. Cancers that destroy bone tissue, which is where the body's calcium is banked, can release a flood of this mineral into the body tissues and blood. Still other cancers can raise calcium levels in different ways, although we don't know exactly how they do so.

Having too much calcium in the blood can actually be as dangerous as having too little, causing muscle weakness, abnormal heart rhythms, nausea and vomiting, and other problems; it can even lead to coma and death.

Unfortunately, cancer-driven hypercalcemia is very difficult to treat. One of the drugs used is zoledronic acid, which works by helping the bones resist breakdown and thus hold on to their calcium stores.

Possible Side Effects

The drug's more common side effects include fever, anemia, muscle pain, and breathing difficulty.

Which Nutrients Are Robbed

Taking this medicine may deplete your supply of, increase your need for, or interfere with the activity of:

- Calcium
- Phosphorus
- Magnesium
- Potassium

Additional Ways This Drug May Upset Your Nutritional Balance

Zoledronic acid can cause abdominal pain and loss of appetite, which can upset your eating habits and possibly interfere with good nutrition. It can also cause diarrhea, which can hamper nutrient absorption.

This drug can also trigger hypermagnesemia, or too much magnesium in the blood.

Restoring Your Nutritional Balance

To compensate for the nutrient loss caused by this drug, speak to your physician about taking 700 mg phosphorus and 100–300 mg potassium per day. And ask your physician to monitor your calcium and magnesium status.

You can also eat foods that contain the depleted nutrients:

- Phosphorus: plain nonfat yogurt, lentils, salmon, milk, halibut
- Potassium: dried figs, California avocado, papaya, banana, dates

Consult with your physician before making any changes to your diet or supplemental regimen.

ZONISAMIDE (zoe-NISS-uh-mide)

Brand Name: Zonegran

About Zonisamide

During a seizure, neurons in the brain lose control. Instead of passing on a message like "contract a muscle" at the proper time and with the proper amount of emphasis, they begin screaming the message over and over again.

Normally, when you walk, certain neurons will pass the message "contract left calf muscle" from the brain to the calf at the appropriate time. But imagine what would happen if they suddenly began screaming, over and over and as rapidly as possible, "CONTRACT LEFT CALF MUSCLE NOW! CONTRACT LEFT CALF MUSCLE NOW! CONTRACT LEFT CALF MUSCLE NOW!" Your left leg would begin to flail. Now imagine what would happen if this occurred in a part of the brain that controlled several muscles.

With what's known as a simple partial seizure, this rapid and incessant screaming of orders happens on just one side of the brain, and in a limited area. This means that only the parts of the body controlled by that part of the brain will respond. Fortunately, simple partial seizures are limited in scope and duration, with the victim completely conscious and watching, perhaps, his left arm shaking and wondering why.

Zonisamide is one of the drugs used to treat partial seizures. As with other antiseizure drugs, we don't know exactly how it works, although we can say that it appears to affect the way sodium and calcium are handled by the brain.

Possible Side Effects

The drug's more common side effects include excessive sleepiness, dizziness, and loss of appetite.

Which Nutrients Are Robbed

Taking this medicine may deplete your supply of, increase your need for, or interfere with the activity of:

- Biotin
- Folic acid
- Inositol
- Thiamin
- Calcium

Additional Ways This Drug May Upset Your Nutritional Balance

Zonisamide can cause loss of appetite, abdominal pain, changes in taste, nausea, and vomiting, all of which can upset your eating habits and possibly interfere with good nutrition. It can also cause diarrhea, which can hamper nutrient absorption.

Restoring Your Nutritional Balance

To compensate for the nutrient loss caused by this drug, speak to your physician about taking 500–1,000 mcg biotin, 250–1,000 mg inositol, 25–100 mg thiamin, and 1,200 mg calcium per day. Taking folic acid can increase the risk of seizures in some people, so speak to your physician about the use of this nutrient.

You can also eat foods that contain the depleted nutrients:

- Biotin: beef liver, soybeans, rice bran, peanut butter, barley
- Inositol: cantaloupe, oranges, green beans, grapefruit juice, limes
- Thiamin: braised liver, turkey heart, roasted chicken, gefilte fish, sardines
- Calcium: milk, dried figs, Swiss cheese, yogurt, tofu

Consult with your physician before making any changes to your diet or supplemental regimen.

Chapter One: Nutrient Robbery

1. Folkers, K., et al., "Lovastatin Decreases Coenzyme Q Levels in Humans," Proceedings of the National Academy of Sciences of the United States of America, 1990; 87(22): 8931–34.

2. Langsjoen, P., "Introduction to Coenzyme Q_{10}." Accessible at http://tishcon. com/coenzyme10.html. Viewed September 9, 2003.

Chapter Two: The Nutrients and Other Substances at Risk

1. Bucher, H. C., R. J. Cook, G. H. Guyatt, et al., "Effects of Dietary Calcium Supplementation on Blood Pressure: A Meta-analysis of Randomized Controlled Trials," Journal of the American Medical Association, 1996, 275(13): 1016–1022.

2. Atallah, A. N., G. J. Hofmeyr, and L. Duley, "Calcium Supplementation During Pregnancy for Preventing Hypertensive Disorders and Related Problems," Cochrane Database Syst Rev 2000;(3):CD001059. See also Villar J., and J. M. Belizan, "Same Nutrients, Different Hypotheses: Disparities in Trials of Calcium Supplementation During Pregnancy," American Journal of Clinical Nutrition,2000;71(Suppl):1375S–1379S.

3. Sano, M., K. Bell, and L. Cote, "Doubleblind Parallel Design Pilot Study of Acetyl Levocarnitine in Patients with Alzheimer's Disease," Archives of Neurology, 1992; 49:1137–41.

4. Spagnoli, A., U. Lucca, G. Menasce, et al., "Long-term Acetyl-L-Carnitine Treatment in Alzheimer's Disease," Neurology, 1991; 41:1726–32.

5. Anderson, R.A., N. Cheng, N.A. Bryden, et al., "Elevated Intakes of Supplemental Chromium Improve Glucose and Insulin Variable in Individuals with Type II Diabetes," Diabetes, 1997;46:1786–1791.

6. Roeback, J. R., K. M. Hla, L. E. Chambles, et al., "Effects of Chromium Supplementation on Serum High-density Lipoprotein Cholesterol Levels in Men Taking ß-blockers: A Randomized, Controlled Trial," Annals of Internal Medicine, 1991;115:917–924.

7. Jameson, S., "Statistical Data Support Prediction of Death Within 6 Months on Low Levels of Coenzyme Q_{10} and Other Entities," *The Clinical Investigator*, 1993; 71:S137–S139.

8. Singh, R. B., G. S. Wander, A. Rastogi, et al., "Randomized, Double-blind, Placebo-controlled Trial of Coenzyme Q_{10} in Patients with Acute Myocardial Infarction," *Cardiovascular Drugs and Therapy*, 1998;12:347–353.

9. Soja, A. M., and S. A. Mortensen, "Treatment of Congestive Heart Failure with Coenzyme Q_{10} Illuminated by Meta-analysis of Clinical Trials," *Molecular Aspects of Medicine*, 1997;18:S159–S168.

10. Morisco, C., B. Trimarco, and M. Condorelli, "Effect of Coenzyme Q_{10} Therapy in Patients with Congestive Heart Failure: A Long-term Multicenter Randomized Study," *The Clinical Investigator*, 1993;71:S134–S136.

11. Ascherio, A., E. B. Rimm, E. L. Giovannucci, et al., "A Prospective Study of Nutritional Factors and Hypertension among U.S. Men," *Circulation*, 1992;86:1475–1484.

12. Lissoni, P., G. Tancini, S. Barni, et al., "Treatment of Cancer Chemotherapy-induced Toxicity with the Pineal Hormone Melatonin," *Supportive Care in Cancer*, 1997; 5:126–129.

13. Lissoni, P., S. Barni, M. Mandala, et al., "Decreased Toxicity and Increased Efficacy of Cancer Chemotherapy Using the Pineal Hormone Melatonin in Metastatic Solid Tumor Patients with Poor Clinical Status," *European Journal of Cancer*, 1999; 35: 1688–1692.

14. Schoenen, J., J. Jacquy, and M. Lenaerts, "Effectiveness of High-dose Riboflavin in Migraine Prophylaxis: A Randomized, Controlled Trial," *Neurology*, 1998;50:466–470.

15. Arthritis Foundation 2002 Supplement Guide. Accessible at http://www.arthritis.org/conditions/supplement guide/herbs_h_s.asp. Viewed April 4, 2004.

16. Suadicani, P., H. O. Hein, and F. Gyntelberg, "Serum Selenium Concentration and Risk of Ischemic Heart Disease in a Prospective Cohort of 3,000 Males," *Arterioscleros*, 1992;96:33–42.

17. Rimm, E. B., W. C. Willett, F. B. Hu, et al., "Folate and Vitamin B_6 from Diet and Supplements in Relation to Risk of Coronary Heart Disease Among Women," *Journal of the American Medical Association*, 1998;279:359–364.

18. Folsom, A. R., F. J. Nieto, P. G. McGovern, et al., "Prospective Study of Coronary Heart Disease Incidence in Relation to Fasting Total Homocysteine, Related Genetic Polymorphisms, and B Vitamins: The Atherosclerosis Risk in Communities (ARIC) Study," *Circulation*, 1998;98:204–210.

19. Vitamin B_{12}. Facts about Dietary Supplements. Clinical Nutrition Service, Warren Grant Magnuson Clinical Center, Office of Dietary Supplements, National Institutes of Health, January 2001.

20. Hunt, C., N. K. Chakravorty, G. Annan, et al., "The Clinical Effects of Vitamin C Supplementation in Elderly Hospitalized Patients with Acute Respiratory Infections," *International Journal of Vitamin and Nutrition Research*, 1994;64:212–219.

21. Nyyssonen, K., M. T. Parviainen, R. Salonen, et al., "Vitamin C Deficiency and Risk of Myocardial Infarction: Prospective Study of Men from Eastern Finland," *British Medical Journal*, 1997;314:634–638.

22. Hankinson, S. E., M. J. Stampfer, J. M. Seddon, et al., "Nutrient Intake and Cataract Extraction in Women: A Prospective Study," *British Medical Journal*. 1992;305:335–339.

23. Sano, M., C. Ernesto, R. G. Thomas, et al., "A Controlled Trial of Selegiline, Alphatocopherol, or Both as Treatment for Alzheimer's Disease: The Alzheimer's Disease Cooperative Study," *New England Journal of Medicine*, 1997;336:1216–1222.

24. Prasad, A. S., J. T. Fitzgerald, B. Bao, et al., "Duration of Symptoms and Plasma Cytokine Levels in Patients with the Common Cold Treated with Zinc Acetate: A Randomized, Double-blind, Placebo-controlled Trial," *Annals of Internal Medicine*, 2000;133:245–252.

25. Mossad, S. B., M. L. Macknin, S. V. Medendorp, et al., "Zinc Gluconate Lozenges for Treating the Common Cold: A Randomized, Double-blind, Placebo-controlled Study," *Annals of Internal Medicine*, 1996;125:81–88.

26. Age-Related Eye Disease Study Research Group, "A Randomized, Placebo-controlled, Clinical Trial of High-dose Supplementation with Vitamins C and E, Beta-carotene, and Zinc for Age-related Macular Degeneration and Vision Loss," AREDS report no. 8, *Archives of Ophthalmology*, 2001;119:1417–1436.

Chapter Three: Drugs That Rob You of Nutrients, A to Z

1.. American Heart Association Journal Report, "Lifetime Risk for Heart Failure: One in Five." Accessible at http://www.americanheart.org/presenter.jhjtml?identifies=3006313. Viewed February 11, 2004.

2. Lowder, J. L., D. P. Shackelford, D. Holbert, et al., "A Randomized, Controlled Trial to Compare Ketorolac Tromethamine Versus Placebo After Cesarean Section to Reduce Pain and Narcotic Usage," *American Journal of Obstetrics and Gynecology*, 2003; 189(6):1559–62. Abstract.

3. Diblasio, C. J., M. E. Snyder, M. W. Kattan, et al., "Ketorolac: Safe and Effective Analgesia for the Management of Renal Cortical Tumors with Partial Nephrectomy," *Journal of Urology*, 2004;171(3):1062–1065. Abstract.

4. "Progress Toward Disease Resolution: Have We Improved the Treatment of GERD and Other Acid-related Disorders?" Transcript of presentations by the faculty of Digestive Disease Week, Atlanta, Georgia, May 20, 2001. Accessible at http://www.medscape.com/viewprogram/136_pnt.Viewed February 19, 2004.

5. "Fast Facts About Pain." American Pain Foundation, http://www.painfoundation.org/medres/medresfacts.tmpl, viewed March 23, 2001; "Pain Legislation S. 941/H.R. 2188 and H.R. 2260/S. 1272," Office of Legislative Policy and Analysis, National Institutes of Health, http://search.nic.nih.gov/search97cgi/s97_cgi, viewed September 4, 2000.

6. American Heart Association Journal Report, February 25, 2003. "ACE inhibitor drug reduces heart failure in high-risk patient." Accessible at http://www.americanheart.org/presenter.jhjtml?identifier=3009056. Viewed February 11, 2004.

7. [No authors listed] "Randomised Trial of Cholesterol Lowering in 4,444 Patients with Coronary Heart Disease: The Scandinavian Simvastatin Survival Study," *Lancet*, 1994;344(8934):1383–1389.

INDEX OF DRUGS AND NUTRIENTS

ABOUT THE AUTHORS

Frederic Vagnini, M.D., is medical director of The Cardiovascular Wellness Centers of New York and was assistant clinical professor of surgery at Cornell University for twenty-five years. He hosts *The Heart Show*, a call-in radio program on WOR 710 AM in New York. He is the coauthor of *The Carbohydrate Addict's Healthy Heart Program*.

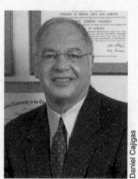

Daniel Cajigas

Barry Fox, Ph.D., is the coauthor of many medical books, including the number-one bestseller *The Arthritis Cure*. He is chair of the Consumer Advisory Council of the American Nutraceutical Association.

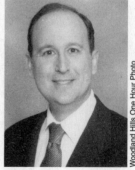

Woodland Hills One Hour Photo